'Imagine watching a country and people you love being ravaged by a disease that seems unstoppable. Imagine shaping emergency operations one minute and pleading with distant leaders the next, all the while not knowing whether what you are doing will ever be enough. *Getting to Zero* takes us behind the scenes to the harrowing frontlines of the Ebola epidemic – highlighting a set of lessons that an inter-connected world would ignore at our peril. A compelling read.'
Samantha Power, former US Ambassador to the UN

'A brave, bold, yet humble account of the Ebola outbreak in Sierra Leone. This is vital reading to help us all do better next time.'
David Miliband, President and CEO of the International Rescue Committee

'Walsh and Johnson represent the best of international intervention. This book reveals the complexities and level of cooperation that made "getting to zero" possible. Offers excellent insight into those trying times.'
O.B. Sisay, Director of the Situation Room at the National Ebola Response Centre, Sierra Leone

'A detailed, up-close-and-personal perspective on the Ebola epidemic in Sierra Leone, important for all who want to understand what it is to confront a terrible health threat.'
Tom Frieden, former Director of the Centers for Disease Control and Prevention

'A frank, beautifully written, and essential guide to the lessons learned from the heart of the outbreak. Their first-hand experiences in battling this terrible disease will take your breath away. A must read.'
Tulip Mazumdar, Global Health Correspondent for BBC News

About the authors

DR SINEAD WALSH has worked for Ireland's Department of Foreign Affairs and Trade since 2009. She was a Senior Fellow at the Harvard Humanitarian Initiative in 2016/17. Prior to this, she served as the Ambassador of Ireland to Sierra Leone and Liberia and the Head of Irish Aid in the two countries, based in Freetown from 2011 to 2016. Her first role with the Department was as a Development Specialist in the Civil Society Section.

Before joining the government, Sinead spent ten years in the NGO sector, predominantly with Concern Worldwide, working in India, Pakistan, Rwanda and South Sudan, as well as in a global advocacy role. She has a BA in English from Harvard University, an MSc in development studies from University College Dublin and a PhD in social policy from the London School of Economics.

DR OLIVER JOHNSON is a visiting lecturer in global health at King's College London. He was based in Freetown from 2013 to 2015 working as the Director of the King's Sierra Leone Partnership.

Oliver has previously worked as Director of Strategy and teaching fellow at the King's Centre for Global Health and as Policy Director for the All-Party Parliamentary Group on Global Health. He studied medicine at King's College London and international health at University College London.

Oliver was awarded an OBE in the 2015 Queen's Birthday Honours in recognition of his leadership role in the British response to the Ebola outbreak.

Sinead is donating her proceeds from the book to St Joseph's School in Makeni, Northern Sierra Leone. St Joseph's educates and supports children with hearing impairments and other disabilities, including Ebola survivors. www.friendsofstjosephskids.org

Oliver is donating his proceeds from the book towards projects to support training opportunities for health workers in Sierra Leone.

GETTING TO ZERO

A Doctor and a Diplomat on the Ebola Frontline

SINEAD WALSH AND OLIVER JOHNSON

ZED

Getting to Zero: A Doctor and a Diplomat on the Ebola Frontline was first published in 2018 by Zed Books Ltd, The Foundry, 17 Oval Way, London SE11 5RR, UK.

www.zedbooks.net

Typeset in Bulmer by Swales and Willis Ltd, Exeter, Devon
Index by Rohan Bolton
Cover design by Emma J. Hardy
Cover photo © Espen Rasmussen/Panos

A catalogue record for this book is available from the British Library.

ISBN 978-1-78699-247-5 hb
ISBN 978-1-78699-248-2 pb
ISBN 978-1-78699-249-9 pdf
ISBN 978-1-78699-250-5 epub
ISBN 978-1-78699-251-2 mobi

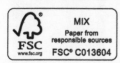

Printed and bound by CPI Group (UK) Ltd, Croydon, CR0 4YY

Contents

Acknowledgements

Sinead would like to warmly thank the staff team of the Embassy of Ireland during Ebola, without whom none of the work in this book would have been possible: Paula Molloy, Emma Mulhern, Teta Lincoln, Lorna Stafford, Davida Macauley, Abubakar Kargbo, Gibril Kargbo, Allie Kamara, Desmond Tucker, Fatmata Mansaray and Ramatu Mansaray. More broadly, she would also like to thank her colleagues at the Department of Foreign Affairs and Trade of Ireland for their support during the crisis and on this book, particularly Niall Burgess and Michael Gaffey.

She is grateful to colleagues and friends in Freetown and internationally who provided great support during the crisis: Peter West, Sister Mary Sweeney, Sonia Walia, Esmee de-Jong, Roeland Monasch, Kathleen Fitzgibbon, John Hoover, Daniel Kertesz, Kate Airey, Ato Brown, Yvonne Aki-Sawyerr, OB Sisay, Yoti Zabulon, David Nabarro, Peter Graaff, Bintou Keita, Peter Rees-Gildea, Ed Davis, Memuna Forna, Hussien Ibrahim, Jatin Hiranandani, Philippe Maughan, Fiona McLysaght, Saffea Senessie, Amanda McClelland, Amanda Tiffany, Ibrahim Dakhlala, Eric Eccles-James and the late, great Joy Samake. These and other colleagues were generous with their time on the book, particularly Paul Richards, Chukwu-Emeka Chikezie, Kande-Bure O'Bai Kamara, Chris Lane, Claire Bader, Ian Norton, Martin Cormican, David Harris, John Raine and Luisa Enria.

Sinead would also like to thank the Harvard Humanitarian Initiative within the Harvard T. Chan School of Public Health for their warm hospitality during her year in residence to write the book, especially Susan Tannehill and Theresa Lund. She is also extremely grateful to Harvard Medical School's Department of Global Health and Social Medicine for their support, including financial support to conduct some of the later interviews. Special thanks to Paul Farmer, Ishaan Desai, Katherine Kralievits and Jennifer Puccetti.

For wonderful moral support during Ebola and beyond, Sinead would like to thank her parents, Gay and Joe Walsh, and family members Brian, Joseph, James, Deirdre and Paddy Walsh; Louise Collins; Helen Thornton; Steve Landon; Martina, Brian, Emily, Oscar and Fionnuala Rowe. She would also like to thank Neal McCarthy, Bhakti Mirchandani, Aine Bhreathnach, Caroline Johnston, Jane Kelly Rogers, Alison O'Connor, Fionnuala Gilsenan, Kate Golden and Jennie Timoney.

Oliver would particularly like to thank his colleagues; although his story was written as an individual memoir, everything he did was as part of a team. Many also helped with the writing process. It was impossible to recognise everyone's contribution in the retelling of events, but he would specifically like to acknowledge Marta Lado, Suzanne Thomas, Dan Youkee, Colin Brown, Amardeep Kamboz, Andy Hall, Ibrahim Kabia, Terry Gibson, Max Manning-Lowe, Jo Dunlop, Ahmed Seedat, Paul Arkell, Sakib Rokadiya, Will Pooley, Katy Lowe, Peter Baker, Stacey Mearns, Karine Mussaud, Leanne Brady, Kate Clay and Chris Curry.

In addition, he is grateful to the Sierra Leonean colleagues who stood shoulder-to-shoulder with him throughout, at Connaught Hospital and beyond: TB Kamara, Eva Hanciles, Cecilia Kamara, Alie Wurie, Susan Mohammed, Lovetta Jawara, Mohamed

Sillah, Tamba Senessie, Foday Sahr and Mohamed Boie Jalloh, amongst others.

He would also like to thank his colleagues at King's in London for their support: Andy Leather, Rachel Parr, Jill Lockett, John Rees, Martin Prince and Robert Lechler. And from the wider international community: Susan Elden, Kate Airey, Katherine Owen, Laura Miller, Michael Duff, Donal Brown, Peter West, Christopher Whitty, Daniel Kertesz, Andy Garrow, Ali Readhead, Kate Dooley, Victoria Parkinson, Ian Crozier, Oliver Morgan and Les Roberts.

We would both like to thank David Harris and Les Roberts for extremely helpful external reviews of the manuscript.

On a personal level, Oliver would not have been able to stay strong during the response or to write this book without his parents, Jane and Michael, and his siblings Jeremy, Alix and Ben. His close friends were a huge support, as were his Freetown family, particularly Kallie Kallon and Thaimu Bangura.

We would both like to thank our intern Madeleine Joung for her high levels of commitment, diligence and skill. We would also like to thank Ekemini Ekpo for excellent proofreading. We are grateful to individuals who advised us on the book writing process including David Lewis, Michaela Wrong and Nigel Crisp.

We would like to warmly thank all of our interviewees for their time and insights.

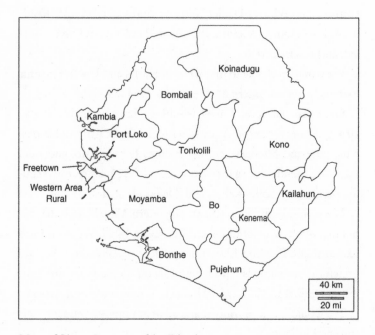

Map of Sierra Leone and its Districts

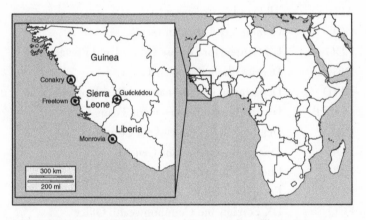

Map of Africa and the Subregion Surrounding Sierra Leone

Abbreviations

AGI	Africa Governance Initiative
AFRO	WHO Regional Office for Africa
APC	All People's Congress
CCC	Community Care Centre
CDC	US Centers for Disease Control and Prevention
DERC	District Ebola Response Centre
DFID	Department for International Development
DHMT	District Health Management Team
DRC	Democratic Republic of the Congo
EOC	Emergency Operations Centre
ETU	Ebola Treatment Unit
EU	European Union
FCO	UK Foreign and Commonwealth Office
GOARN	Global Outbreak Alert and Response Network
IMC	International Medical Corps
IRC	International Rescue Committee
ISAT	International Security Advisory Team
JIATF	Joint Inter-Agency Taskforce
Med-evac	Medical Evacuation
MSF	Médecins sans Frontières
NERC	National Ebola Response Centre
NGO	non-governmental organisation
OCHA	United Nations Office for the Coordination of Humanitarian Affairs

PIH	Partners in Health
PPE	personal protective equipment
RAF	Royal Air Force
RUF	Revolutionary United Front
SLPP	Sierra Leone People's Party
SMAC	Social Mobilisation Action Consortium
UK	United Kingdom
UN	United Nations
UNESCO	United Nations Educational, Scientific and Cultural Organization
UNFPA	United Nations Population Fund
UNICEF	United Nations Children's Fund
UNMEER	United Nations Mission for Ebola Emergency Response
US	United States
WHO	World Health Organization

Preface

The 25th known outbreak of Ebola virus infection is unlike any of the previous epidemics. It has already killed over 2,800 people – more than all previous epidemics combined; it's affecting virtually the entire territory of three countries, involving rural areas, major urban centers, and capital cities; it has been going on for almost a year; and it is occurring in West Africa, where no Ebola outbreak had previously occurred. Above all, the epidemic seems out of control and has evolved into a major humanitarian crisis that has finally mobilized the world, with responses ranging from an emergency health mission launched by the United Nations Security Council to proposed military-style interventions and the global provision of emergency aid.[1]

These were the opening words from an editorial published on 23 September 2014 in a leading medical journal. The editorial was co-authored by Professor Peter Piot, who had helped to discover the Ebola virus nearly forty years before. That same day, the US Centers for Disease Control and Prevention in Atlanta released the results of new mathematical modelling on the outbreak that stunned health officials across the globe: the number of new Ebola cases was doubling every two to four weeks and, in the worst-case scenario, the virus could infect 1.4 million people in Sierra Leone and Liberia by 20 January 2015.[2,3]

This dramatic warning went far beyond anything anyone had imagined possible. What had started as a local outbreak had evolved into a regional epidemic and was now becoming both a global crisis and a major humanitarian emergency. "Indeed," Professor Piot and his colleague wrote, "there is a very real danger of a complete breakdown in civic society, as desperate communities understandably lose faith in the established systems."[4]

In the words of one Norwegian epidemiologist at the time, "It seems very hard to stop this now, but I think we all just have to believe that it is possible."[5]

* * * * *

By September 2014, Freetown, the capital of Sierra Leone, had become the eye of this unprecedented storm, one into which the two authors of this book – Oliver Johnson and Sinead Walsh – had been thrust.

Oliver: I was a twenty-eight-year-old British doctor leading a small medical team embedded in the country's main hospital, having found myself running its Ebola isolation unit after the Sierra Leonean doctor in charge had been killed by the virus. My colleagues and I were completely overwhelmed, taking turns enduring long stints wearing stifling protective suits, able to do little more than provide the most basic care to patients and remove dead bodies. Together, we were trying against all odds to keep the hospital open. The Ebola unit was full, as it had been for weeks, and a queue of sick and dying patients continued to grow outside the hospital gates. Between shifts, I was shuttling between emergency planning meetings and live TV interviews, trying to raise awareness of what was going on and pleading with the international community for reinforcements.

Sinead: I was working just a few miles down the road as Ireland's Ambassador, trying to amplify voices like Oliver's at national and international levels. I was then thirty-six years old and had been in Sierra Leone for three years. As one of the international diplomats with the most experience in Sierra Leone, I had thrown myself into efforts to raise the alarm and rapidly scale up the response. Through media interviews and urgent briefings over the phone to Dublin, Brussels, Geneva and New York, I had been working to alert the world to the growing catastrophe that had, at last, gotten the attention of the White House, Downing Street and the UN Security Council. Meanwhile, on the ground in Freetown, I was helping bring together UN agencies and international donors to properly resource and support the response. In addition, I was meeting frequently with the country's president and senior ministers, who had ultimately imposed a last-resort State of Emergency, quarantining households and whole districts of the country to try to halt the further spread of the disease.

We had both found ourselves unexpectedly playing central roles in the response. We had not gone looking for Ebola; rather it had come to our doorstep. And we had each found our own ways to fight back.

* * * * *

Although we interacted with each other several times during the response, we did not get to know each other well until many months later, when the epidemic was in its final stages. It was at a weekend yoga retreat at a beach near Freetown, of all places, that we first started chatting about our shared experiences and frustrations with the response, and about how some of the initial accounts of the outbreak that we were reading did not reflect what we had lived through. That's when the idea for this book began. In it, we aim to tell the story of what happened before, during and after the Ebola epidemic in Sierra Leone, and to draw out key lessons and recommendations so that the next time such a crisis happens, the same mistakes won't be repeated.

Why is learning from this Ebola epidemic important? Because a whole set of twenty-first-century trends like increasing high-speed international travel, drug resistance and shifting disease patterns due to climate change mean that we are likely to see more severe disease outbreaks with global ramifications in the coming years. Bill Gates believes that there is a "reasonable probability" that the world will experience an outbreak in the next ten to fifteen years that could kill more than thirty million people.[6]

We can't avoid disease outbreaks, some of which, like Ebola, are unpredictable. However, there *are* ways we can ensure that the next major outbreak does not needlessly destroy as many lives as Ebola did and we aim to highlight these. This book also contains insights on responding to humanitarian emergencies in general, as well as better navigating long-term development programming to address the root causes of these crises.

So we believe that learning from the Ebola crisis is vital. But we initially had our hesitations about writing a book. This was partly because we felt Sierra Leonean voices ought to be at the centre of the literature for this subject. We are also acutely aware of the huge number of people, living and dead, who made enormous sacrifices and contributions during the crisis, many of which remain unknown and untold. We struggled with the notion of doing justice to this topic, given the enormity of all that happened.

Nonetheless, we believed that our roles in the response made our experiences relevant, so we decided to write about them. To present a more complete picture, we supplemented our experiences with the perspectives of others who were better placed than us to talk about certain events. This also meant challenging our own perceptions with different points of view. In particular, Sinead took a year off work when the Ebola crisis was over and spent it doing in-depth interviews with eighty-five people who were involved in the response in Sierra Leone. These ranged from Ebola survivors and frontline health workers to the President of Sierra Leone and the Secretary General of the UN. She also read several hundred documents on the topic which helped us to deepen our understanding on the issues involved.

We hope the resulting book will serve as an engaging account, in our own voices, of an extraordinary moment in world history that will be accessible to the general reader, whilst also providing valuable insight to students and professionals.

This book is critical of others, but also critical of ourselves and the mistakes we made. We recognise that, like us, the majority of people engaged in the Ebola response did the best they could at the time, in often-chaotic environments. We are also aware that we are writing with the benefit of hindsight. We hope that our commentary will be understood as being motivated by the desire to contribute to a more informed debate about the crisis and to prevent the same mistakes from happening again.

While we made significant efforts to cross-check all information used, any mistakes in this book are entirely our own responsibility. The views in this book are our own personal ones and do not represent those of the Government of Ireland or of King's College London.

ONE | New beginnings: Sierra Leone before the outbreak of Ebola

SINEAD

A first taste of Sierra Leone

In September 2011, I arrived in Freetown to head up the Irish government's presence in Sierra Leone, with responsibility also for neighbouring Liberia. But this was not my first time in the country. I had visited Sierra Leone six years earlier: a visit which, in hindsight, gave me great insights into the country and its history.

In 2005, three years after the end of the civil war in Sierra Leone, I was working in South Sudan. One of my best friends was based in Liberia at the time, and another in Sierra Leone, so it seemed like a trip to West Africa was in order. The three of us agreed to meet up in Freetown. My friend there sold us on the beaches of the long Sierra Leonean coastline, which she said were the most stunning she had ever seen.

It was a long trip from East Africa and I was exhausted by the time I got to Freetown, but even so I loved it immediately. As I drove to the guesthouse, the city centre was full of activity, accompanied by music blaring from omnipresent radios. Around me were thousands of people hustling to make a living, from street vendors cooking sweetcorn on the pavement to women in bright colours selling peanuts and bananas to motorists sitting in traffic. Compared with my hut in rural South Sudan, even post-war Sierra Leone seemed luxurious. Our YMCA guesthouse in the city centre had running water, and I was able to go to a restaurant to order a cold drink from a fridge powered by a noisy generator outside. I was truly on holiday.

But while the Sierra Leoneans I met during my visit welcomed me warmly, they were puzzled as to why I was there. I hadn't thought about it beforehand, but I was probably one of the first tourists to come to Sierra Leone since the end of the eleven-year war.

All week I fielded questions from confused Sierra Leoneans: "So you're doing a consultancy project for the UN or an NGO then?"

"Nope, just taking a holiday, having a look around."

"Having a look around after finishing your consultancy, you mean?"

And so it went. I tried to convince people that there was no reason why anyone wouldn't want to visit Sierra Leone, now that it was peaceful. They weren't convinced though, and I'm pretty sure they had me down as some kind of Irish CIA agent! It was clear, though, that to gain an insight into the country I would need to understand the conflict and its causes.

A cow grazes where it is tethered

The civil war was as brutal as it was long. By its end in 2002, 50,000 Sierra Leoneans had died, many thousands more had been maimed, and two million people, approximately half of the country's population at the time, had been displaced. A lot of the country's educated elite went abroad, some never to return. International media coverage of mass amputations by rebel forces often portrayed the conflict as barbaric and senseless. However, the conflict had very real causes. Many historical accounts of the war have traced its roots back to Sierra Leone's post-independence period.

Initially, there were high hopes for a bright future when Sierra Leone, a country about the same size as Ireland, became independent from Britain in 1961. The country had abundant natural and mineral resources, including iron ore, diamonds, gold, bauxite and rutile.[1] It was the site of Fourah Bay College, founded in 1827 and the oldest university in West Africa. The college attracted students from all over the continent, earning Freetown the title 'the Athens of Africa'.[2] Sierra Leone was also one of the first countries in sub-Saharan Africa to transition power from an incumbent party, the Sierra Leone People's Party (SLPP), to an opposition party, the All People's Congress (APC), in an election in 1967.

However, it did not take long for political problems to emerge. The initial peaceful transfer of power was very quickly followed by a coup and two counter-coups that exposed the first cracks in the new democratic process. These cracks widened when the winner of that 1967 election, Siaka Stevens of the APC, was disinclined to give up power once it was restored to him in the second counter-coup. He retained the presidency until his retirement in 1985.

The Siaka Stevens era has often been cited as the period when Sierra Leone entered into deep economic decline.[3] From the late 1970s, large-scale iron and diamond mining plummeted, as many of the best deposits were exhausted. This made the country more dependent on international aid.[4]

Perhaps more fundamentally, the period was defined by declining accountability as the state became principally a source of personal accumulation for individuals, rather than a provider of basic services to the broader population. The Krio phrase *usay den tay kaw na de i go it* (a cow grazes where it is tethered) is associated with this period.[5] What this meant was that civil servants were expected to find ways to supplement their incomes, and those of their extended families and supporters, within their line of work. This applied whether they were cabinet ministers or traffic police-men on the streets and, clearly, they could only 'eat' by making dodgy business deals and seeking bribes from the population.

Siaka Stevens did not invent corruption in Sierra Leone, but, in liaison with his cronies, he took it to a new level, with the infor-malisation of the country's diamond sector as its centrepiece. This capture of the state by the elite and the distrust of govern-ment that it created are seen by many as root causes of the war.

The immediate trigger of the civil war was the 1991 invasion of Kailahun, a district in the southeast of the country, by a group calling itself the Revolutionary United Front (RUF). This group of Sierra Leonean rebels was aided by the forces of Charles Tay-lor, the warlord from Liberia who had started the civil war there two years earlier. They began a campaign which, over the course of the long war, included killings, mass rape, amputations, kid-nappings and looting. Often fuelled by drugs and alcohol, the rebels abducted local people and forced them to become soldiers, exploited some women as sex slaves ('bush wives'), all the while looting enough from local villages to sustain themselves.

In 1992, they reached the diamond fields of Kono district and, with the help of sponsors in Freetown and abroad, used Sierra Leone's diamond wealth to buy more weapons, drugs, and food to keep the war going.[6] Diamonds had been fuel for corruption since their discovery in the 1930s, as they were small enough to smuggle easily out of the country without paying any tax. Anyone who has seen the movie *Blood Diamond* will remember the scene when Leonardo DiCaprio tries to smuggle goats out of Sierra Leone with diamonds sewn into their backs.

One of the most extraordinary things about the war is that the country was brought to its knees for eleven years by a rebel force that initially numbered only about a hundred, with some support from Taylor but without any strong political, religious or ethnic base.[7]

This only makes sense when you understand two things. Firstly, from its history of slavery to colonialism to the post-independence era, the Sierra Leonean population had been left largely impoverished and had suffered much injustice. Although the country's patronage system had often extended beyond corrupt government officials to members of their extended families, their ethnic groups and others, there were still many people marginalised and without access to basic services. Resentment festered. Anger against this injustice proved a powerful rallying cry for many of the rebels.

Secondly, it is important to understand how crippled Sierra Leone's army was at that time. The army had been turned into a ceremonial force by Siaka Stevens, who maintained a separate security force for himself, the SSD (officially the 'State Security Department', although their brutality earned them the nickname 'Siaka Stevens' Dogs').[8] Many of the soldiers who went out to fight the rebels ended up engaging in looting themselves. This led to Sierra Leoneans speaking of a hybrid type of fighter: a 'sobel', soldier by day, rebel by night.[9]

The war finally ended in 2002, a result of internal splits within the RUF and international military assistance to the government, most notably from the Guinean army. Other important assistance came from Nigeria and the UN, including the latter's imposition of an arms embargo and sanctions against Charles Taylor in Liberia.[10] A UK military intervention in Freetown in mid-2000 was particularly visible and is well-remembered by the populace.

Simmering after-effects
A lot had changed in the three years after the war. As my friends and I explored the bustling streets of central Freetown and hiked

in the rolling hills of its outskirts in 2005, it seemed like any
other African city, and we found it hard to believe that the war
had ended so recently. But one evening, a few days into our trip,
we got a glimpse of some of the dynamics lingering beneath the
surface.

We had gone to a restaurant on the local beach for dinner,
and afterwards took a taxi back to the YMCA through dimly lit
streets. We were completely absorbed in our conversation and
didn't realise during the journey that the red-eyed driver was
drunk. After he parked at the guesthouse, we paid him the usual
fare, including a bit of a tip, but he rejected it angrily, throwing
the money on the ground and demanding ten times that amount.
I started to feel uneasy. We were new to the country and we were
out of our depth.

It had been quiet on the street when we had parked, but it
was the middle of the city centre and a small crowd of curious
onlookers quickly emerged from the darkness. Since most people in Freetown didn't have electricity in their houses, which
were sometimes therefore stiflingly hot, people commonly hung
around outside in the evenings, chatting with neighbours or just
enjoying the breeze until it was time to go to sleep.

Two middle-aged men approached us, having quickly sized
up the situation, and, in a mixture of Krio and English, they
offered to take over the negotiations with the increasingly hysterical driver. We accepted with gratitude and some relief. The
men took the driver to one side and tried to calm him down, but
to no avail.

Eventually, the two men came back to where we were standing and advised us to put the money through the window of
the taxi and go inside the guesthouse. As they walked us to the
gate, one of the men said that the driver was probably a former
rebel, as many of them had been given support in disarmament

programmes after the war to set up as taxi drivers, but some still had drink or drug problems. We thanked the men and went to our rooms, but were soon roused by more shouting when the taxi driver tried – unsuccessfully – to climb over the guesthouse fence to find us. At this point, the guesthouse staff called the police, who quickly came and sorted things out. After a few pleasant and peaceful days, it was a reminder that the after-effects of the war were very real, even if they were not easily visible.

The scars of colonialism

My visit also gave me fascinating insights into pre-war Sierra Leone. My friends and I went to a beach called River Number Two, which still had the iconic lopsided palm tree that had featured in the Bounty chocolate bar 'Taste of Paradise' advertisement of the 1980s. We then waded across the shallow river to the neighbouring Tokeh beach, with its miles and miles of white sand. It was completely deserted and, as we walked along it, we came across abandoned rowing boats with faded multi-coloured paint that had the label 'Club Med'. It turned out that an international tour company had been in the process of setting up an operation there when the civil war broke out in 1991. The tourist industry had completely collapsed with the war, and with the media coverage and the *Blood Diamond* reputation, things didn't look great for post-war tourism either.

Another day we hired a boat to go upriver to Bunce Island. Once on the island, we walked around the remnants of one of about forty slave castles that Europeans had built on the West African coast during the Atlantic slave trade. During the second half of the eighteenth century, British and European traders had shipped thousands of captives via Bunce Island to places like South Carolina and Georgia, where their experience in growing rice was highly sought after for the booming rice industry in early

America. Slavery had enormously negative impacts on the African societies affected, and often created a deep sense of distrust of foreigners.

While the slave trade was still going on, a group of British abolitionists chose this stretch of coastline as a place to resettle freed slaves, including those who had fought alongside the British in the American Revolutionary War.[11] Different waves of freed slaves from London, Nova Scotia and Jamaica arrived on the coast between 1787 and 1800.[12] They ultimately formed a new ethnic group, the Krio people, and the settlement 'Freetown' was born.

Freetown became a British colony soon thereafter in 1808, but the rest of Sierra Leone was governed much more loosely by Britain after 1896 as a 'protectorate', with different rules and laws applied. It was not until 1947 that all of Sierra Leone became a British colony.[13] Historians have discussed this dual system of governing as representative of the 'divide and rule' strategy of the coloniser which "sowed seeds of distrust, competition and intransigence" between different groups in society.[14]

This division between the Freetown peninsula and the rest of the country became evident during the civil war. The war didn't affect Freetown for its first six years, until 1997. Many residents of Freetown, notably the elite and including many government officials, were largely oblivious of the war until it came to their doorstep.[15] We were to see this division rear its head again during the Ebola crisis.

Other dynamics that hark back to the impact of colonialism on Sierra Leone also came to the fore during the Ebola crisis. Two of these are the related issues of corruption and low capacity of the formal state. One historian talks about the "intimate connections between current formal government incapacity and the colonial past" when he describes how colonial officials often did side deals with powerful individuals at the local level to make profits from resources like diamonds and to keep the peace. This system helped to create a parallel political authority, promoting the decay of the formal state.[16]

Major players that, for better and for worse, were central to this parallel political authority during the Ebola crisis were the country's chiefs. Rather than replacing pre-existing local authorities, the British colonisers left them in place and, in some cases, strengthened their authority. The post-independence state therefore inherited a reliance on local power bases such as chiefs.[17]

Sierra Leone has 149 chiefdoms, each headed by a Paramount Chief. Generally, these chiefs are male, from a ruling clan, and they rule for life. There are also lower levels of chief, all the way down to the village level. Officially chiefs have a limited set of responsibilities vis-à-vis the formal government, such as running local courts to implement by-laws. But in practice, particularly in the rural areas, the chieftaincy system is the main authority that many Sierra Leoneans know and interact with in their daily lives.

Everybody agrees that chiefs are hugely significant, particularly in rural Sierra Leone. There is, however, a major debate as to whether this is a good or a bad thing. On the one hand, there have been issues over the years about the accountability of chiefs, abuses of power by some, and grievances of youth and women who feel marginalised by the system. On the other hand, chiefs have also been central to attempts at democratisation and decentralisation.[18] Many Sierra Leoneans trust their chiefs more than the formal state, despite efforts by the government over the years to bring government 'closer to the people' by decentralising various central-level ministries and agencies. So alongside chiefs and the 'traditional' authority system, there are parliamentarians and local government structures across all fourteen districts of the country.[19]

Getting things done in Sierra Leone requires local leaders, whether or not formal government structures are also involved. My first experience of this came when, after the trip to Bunce Island, my friends and I headed back to Freetown. As our boat docked at the port, a few young men came unsolicited to 'help' us disembark, and afterwards I discovered one of them had stolen my Nokia phone, which I had astutely stored in a phone-shaped external pocket of my handbag. My friends, both lawyers, were keen that we pursue justice as a matter of principle, so we took ourselves to the ramshackle police station nearby.

There wasn't much space inside so I went in alone and made a complaint to the policeman on duty. He nodded sympathetically, opened a case file and wrote down the details, while not really giving me any hope that I would see my phone again. As I was doing this, my friends got chatting outside to a few community leaders who had shown up to see what the problem was. Having listened to my friends explaining the situation, the community leaders were not happy that the only tourists in many months were going to leave with a sour taste in their mouths. They came in to the station and spoke in Krio over my head to the policeman, "*Leh wi go fen de tifman bo, ya?*" (We're going to find the thief, ok brother?). The policeman gladly assented and two hours later we left the station with the phone. This would have been impressive in any busy city and I had a bit of a spring in my step knowing that this kind of community action was possible in post-war Sierra Leone.

OLIVER

First sight
I first set foot on Freetown's rich red soil in July 2009, clambering down from the speedboat that had carried me from the country's small international airport at Lungi across the bay to the capital.

This journey, often through choppy waters, was a rite of passage shared by everyone who visited the country. The steep hills that ringed the capital had made it difficult to build an airport closer to the city itself, and the main alternative to the hair-raising thirty-minute sea journey was a circuitous and potentially dangerous road trip that would take several hours.

I was starting my final year of medical school at King's College London and had arrived with a fellow medic to spend a month studying at the Ola During Children's Hospital on the east side of Freetown. The subsequent four weeks proved to be gruelling and intense. Because we were on a tight budget, we were staying in a dilapidated guesthouse that was sandwiched between a cemetery and a burning rubbish dump that gave off plumes of plastic smoke, filling our shared room with acrid soot.

The guesthouse was run by a group of young guys. Their leader was a man in his twenties with disfiguring facial burns and only one arm, who was determined not to live with the many amputees in the neighbouring 'amputees village' run by an international NGO. At first, these guys seemed intimidating, until we discovered how diligent they were about housekeeping. One would burst into our room each morning carrying a bucket of water on his head, since the plumbing didn't work, and proceed to dig out a pair of my boxers from a drawer to use as a duster while I was still asleep in bed!

They took us under their wing and would sit with us in the evenings, telling stories about how they had hidden and protected each other as children during the war. On the weekends, they would take us out to their favourite bars and were fiercely protective of us wherever we went. Like most young Sierra Leoneans, they were very sharp dressers, piecing together colour-coordinated outfits from the second-hand market in town and generally looking at our drab British clothing with scorn.

The traffic between our guesthouse and the hospital was terrible, so each morning we would set out on an hour-long trek across the city on foot. We often arrived soaked from the monsoon rains and fatigued from navigating the potholed roads that were dangerously congested with pedestrians, motorbikes and impatient trucks

The country's main paediatrics hospital had just one specialist, who was supported by a handful of other doctors, most of whom had graduated only recently. We spent as much time as we could with one of the doctors, Dr Ayeshatu Mustapha, a brilliant and dedicated young woman who took us under her wing. She would sit behind an enormous wooden desk for long shifts each day as dozens of parents and grandparents crowded into her office. The most common illness was malaria, which was endemic in the country. The parasite was not only a constant problem for adults, forcing them to take days off work to recover, but was also a significant cause of death amongst children.

We had read that Sierra Leone had the highest child mortality rate in the world, with nearly one in every five children dying before the age of five, and it was easy for us to believe this statistic.[20] When we were near the entrance of the hospital, we would often be approached by desperate families carrying the limp body of a dying child, and we would hurriedly direct them to Dr Mustapha. Despite her heroic efforts, more often than not the child would be either dead already or too unwell to resuscitate with the paltry drugs and equipment at her disposal. The calm of the hospital would then be punctuated by the screams and wails of the grieving family. It was a sound we heard all too regularly.

The situation outside of Freetown was similar. The French anthropologist Mariane Ferme, who spent decades doing ethnographic research in rural Sierra Leone, writes about the patient experience:

For most rural Sierra Leoneans, getting to hospital involves long, uncomfortable, and expensive journeys, navigating Kafka-esque bureaucracies. Repeated payments are required and long waits are interspersed with inconclusive interactions with medical personnel. After all this, one often returns home as one had left or dies from the journey's hardships and lack of care.[21]

One Saturday morning in the intensive care unit, which was really just a smaller ward with a couple of oxygen concentrators, a teenage girl was carried in by her father, with her mother and grandmother in tow. She was in the middle of a seizure and was clearly very sick. Instead of treating the girl, however, the nurses angrily berated the family in Krio.

I asked one of them what was going on. "We know this girl, she was here in this unit until yesterday, but her family took her away," she explained. "They said they couldn't afford the fees, but we know they took her to a traditional healer instead, because the grandmother believes in those things and because it's cheaper."

Of course, the girl had just become sicker. The sister-in-charge was furious, telling the family that she would leave their daughter to die so they would learn their lesson when it came to their other children.

Horrified, I rushed to find the doctor on call, who came to see for himself but was reluctant to intervene. I suspect that he, like the nurses, was thoroughly exhausted by the failing health system and was numbed by the constant death. Even in my short time at the hospital, my sense of disillusionment and helplessness had been growing by the day, and as a result my compassion had started to ebb away. After the family sobbingly begged the staff to help, they eventually set to work trying to save the girl. She passed away a few minutes later.

Despite the high mortality rate, and the shortage of practically everything at the hospital, colleagues on the ground told me things were improving. A small international NGO called Welbodi Partnership had been established to help support the hospital, and their work was already having an impact. Electricity and running water had largely been restored and morale was actually better than it had been. I heard that plans were underway at the national level for a flagship programme to provide free health care for under-fives, pregnant women and new mothers to try to tackle the extremely high maternal and child mortality rates. This would include an increase in staff salaries and the provision of additional medical supplies.

I returned to the UK with a sense of cautious optimism. Although it had been a tough few weeks, I had been inspired by colleagues like Dr Mustapha and reminded that overcoming these sorts of challenges was why I had chosen to study medicine in the first place. I left knowing that I wanted to be part of Sierra Leone's renewal in the coming years.

SINEAD

Back to Sierra Leone

In September 2011, I went back to Freetown, this time to live. I had joined the Irish government after ten years in the NGO sector, mostly focused in Africa. My heart was still very much in the continent and I had jumped when the opportunity came up to be posted to Sierra Leone. In my five years there, I was to fall in love with this vibrant, fascinating, troubled country.

In the intervening years since my first visit, Sierra Leone had stabilised further and I found a peaceful country with remarkably little crime. The country had moved so definitively away from conflict that the UN peacekeeping mission for Sierra Leone had closed in 2007. After their intervention during the war, the UK had provided enormous support to radically reform the military.

The army had improved so much that Sierra Leone was starting to send its soldiers to assist with peacekeeping efforts in other countries, such as Somalia and Sudan.[22]

One of the first things I noticed as I started to travel around the country was the ubiquitous mini-vans (locally known as 'poda podas') with colourful signs on their back windows. Initially, I was puzzled by a sign that read 'God loves Allah', but my driver explained that in Sierra Leone, where the population was mostly Muslim but with a significant Christian minority, it was not uncommon to be 'ChrisMus', a term which I'm fairly certain was coined in Sierra Leone and meant to consider yourself both Christian and Muslim.

Every time I went to a formal meeting, there would be both Muslim and Christian prayers at the beginning. Many people would put their hands together for "Our Father, who art in Heaven . . . " and then, two minutes later, hold them out flat and recite "*Bismillahir Rahmanir Raheem . . .*". Indeed, I soon found myself with a Sierra Leonean friend who was Christian, but fasted for Ramadan. Cultural and spiritual institutions, like the male and female 'secret societies' which are influential in local and national politics, also cut across religious lines.[23] This went beyond the religious tolerance we strive for in other countries; this was a close embrace.

In my first few months I would cycle somewhere different in the city every weekend. I had always been an inveterate cyclist and over the years in different countries I had found it a very useful way to get my bearings, particularly since I have an appalling sense of direction. I should say my cycling did raise a few eyebrows in Freetown, where steep hills and unpredictable traffic deterred most prospective riders, Sierra Leonean and international alike.

What struck me on those early rides was the number of children everywhere. The population was booming, fast climbing towards seven million. But neither the education system nor the economy were keeping up. Despite the improvements that had taken place since the end of the war, Sierra Leone in 2011 remained the eighth poorest country in the world.[24] Less than half of the adults in the population could read and, while most children started primary school, poverty meant that only one in five males in the population had ended up with some secondary school education, with the number dropping to one in ten for females.[25,26] There was a long way to go.

My two hats

I often get asked: what do ambassadors do? Lots of people have preconceptions about the role that involve cocktail parties and the consumption of Ferrero Rocher chocolates.

In reality, the answer varies significantly depending on which country you are representing and which country you are in. In the Embassy of Ireland in Freetown, just as in every other Irish embassy, we supported our citizens with services such as passport renewals, helped Irish companies navigate the local business environment and issued visas for Sierra Leoneans to visit Ireland. However, since the volume of tourism and trade between Ireland and Sierra Leone was modest, these activities took up the minority of my time.

Most of my time was spent on two other areas. The first is something that all ambassadors do: political and diplomatic engagement with the host government. The second was unusual for an ambassador to do: management of the aid programme. I had this second hat because, unlike many other countries, Ireland combines its diplomatic and aid functions under one department, the Department of Foreign Affairs and Trade. So, during my time in Freetown, I had a dual role. It was perfect for me. My background was in aid work, but I had always had a special interest in politics, governance and human rights, areas that diplomats regularly engage with.

To give an example of what my job looked like in practice, a lot of my work in my first year was on preparations for the 2012 elections. On any given day leading up to the elections, I might spend the morning in a meeting alongside other diplomats, such as the British High Commissioner and the US Ambassador, having a discussion with political parties about the safeguards that existed against vote rigging.[27] In the afternoon, I might meet with aid donors – such as the UK Department for International Development (DFID) or the US Agency for International Development (USAID) – and Sierra Leonean government representatives about the details of organising the elections and how each aspect would be funded. In the evening, there might be a working dinner in a local hotel with a visiting election monitoring team from the European Union or the African Union, during which we would try to help them to understand the local context.

Because Sierra Leone was such a poor country, aid from other countries made up a significant portion of the national income – 19% on my arrival in 2011.[28] The funders that provided this aid might be from individual governments such as Ireland (Irish Aid) or the UK (DFID), or from donors representing multiple governments grouped together, such as the World Bank or the EU.[29] Donors might give money directly to the government, or we might fund the UN or NGOs to work alongside them.

Ireland led the international community on nutrition in Sierra Leone. We funded UNICEF and various NGOs to support government clinics around the country to provide better nutrition for pregnant women and children. This was the domain of my deputy, Paula Molloy. Paula, a thirty-year-old diplomat, was from Dublin like me and she was a highly competent and yet relaxed presence. She somehow managed to keep everything going on a hundred different fronts at the Embassy while I was dashing around. The other Irish staffer was our programme advisor, Emma Mulhern from Donegal, a petite dynamo who led our work on women's and girls' rights.

This was the sum total of our programme staff, although we were lucky enough to have six phenomenal Sierra Leonean colleagues working on areas such as administration, finance and the issuing of visas. With no postal system, very poor supplies of water and power, and huge difficulties getting spare parts and skilled people to help if anything broke, 'administration' in Sierra Leone was an absolutely critical skill-set in any office. Somehow, our Sierra Leonean staff managed to ensure that the Embassy presented an efficient, calm and well-functioning exterior, when the reality was more like the proverbial duck paddling furiously underwater, as our lives were plagued with generator nightmares and printers that could never be fixed.

The Embassy itself was, like many offices in Freetown, a large house that we had converted for our purposes. I loved the way the building, painted in lemon yellow, felt comfortable rather than industrial. I especially liked the fact that all our external interactions took place downstairs, in the reception room with the Irish and EU flags, or around the gleaming mahogany table in the conference room. Upstairs was 'staff only' and I enjoyed being able to sit at my desk wearing flip flops, a cardigan and one of my many brightly coloured hairbands. Since most of my formal meetings were outside of the office, I kept a black jacket and a pair of dress shoes in the car, and our driver, Allie Kamara, was tasked with making sure that, in between making phone calls in the car and dashing to the next meeting, I remembered to put the jacket and shoes on and take the hairband off before I met anyone important.

Since most of our operations were in Sierra Leone, I spent most of my time there. I also spent a few days each month visiting

Liberia, where we had a small sub-office. Our health advisor, an extraordinarily energetic Liberian woman named Teta Lincoln, managed our Liberian health programme day-to-day, working closely with the Ministry there on the building blocks for the health system, such as salaries for staff and medical supplies for the hospitals and clinics around the country.

Dissatisfied: Sierra Leone pre-Ebola

President Ernest Bai Koroma of the APC party first came to power in 2007 and ran for a second term in 2012. Ernest, as he was fondly known by his supporters, was a tall, white-haired and deliberative man, then in his late fifties.

The evening the 2012 election results were being declared, I remember sitting in the packed and stiflingly hot National Election Commission conference room waiting for the announcement. There were parliamentary and local government elections on the same day, but the big question was who would win the presidential race, because this was where most of the power lay in the government. There was a wide consensus that President Koroma would be the top candidate; the question was whether he would get the 55% necessary to win in the first round of voting.

The Election Commission was on top of a hill in the centre of Freetown, and tens of thousands of people all over the capital below were tuning their radio sets to the Commissioner's speech. When she announced that President Koroma had won "fifty . . . eight– ", the rest of her sentence was drowned out by the roar of euphoric APC supporters on the twilit streets of the city, a roar which seemed to shake the building in which we sat.

My diplomatic colleagues and I drove a few hundred metres down the road to the State House for an impromptu celebration. The gleaming white painted building, with a tower in its centre that overlooked the town below, had been the seat of government in Sierra Leone since colonial times. It would actually have been easier to walk there, but it would have seemed disrespectful to the Presidential Guard manning the majestic gates, who saluted us on the way in. We drove through the gateposts adorned with the national crest.

I got a text message from one of the President's advisors to say proceedings were about to start, so I jumped out of the car, dashed past the flags and through the main entrance, where a large wooden placard kept record of the Presidents of the Republic of Sierra Leone. The gathering was on the second floor in a large red-carpeted meeting hall and the President and his closest colleagues were mingling when we arrived. The room was already quite full, so the huge ornate wooden doors were soon locked as the President approached the podium to give his speech.

Soon, though, a bunch more APC supporters arrived and wanted to hear the speech too, so much so that they banged on the door for the entire speech, meaning that many at the back of the room couldn't hear the President's words. It was the kind of moment that I came to see as representing a uniquely democratic and non-hierarchical aspect of Sierra Leone. No one took the banging on the door badly. No presidential security guards rushed out to tell the supporters to behave. Everybody simply smiled good-naturedly and shook their heads at the enthusiasm of the supporters.

The President spoke about what he wanted to achieve in his second term. His 'Agenda for Prosperity' included building more roads and infrastructure for water and electricity; creating jobs for the many unemployed youth; continuing the Free Health Care Initiative for pregnant women and children under five; and providing increased support to agriculture.

I think many of us in the room that evening thought that at least some of these lofty objectives were achievable. It was an optimistic time. The economy had been growing fast, some 15% in 2012.[30] This was mostly because the iron ore industry had begun to boom in the north of the country and global iron ore prices were high.

Growing discontent

Fast-forward fifteen months to February 2014. We were in the same room at State House, but the scene looked very different. This time, we sat around a big wooden conference table, with President Koroma at the head, looking tired and frustrated. The much-hyped Agenda for Prosperity had gotten off to a very slow start. Iron ore prices were down. The earlier economic growth had not trickled down to the majority of the population, and they knew it. There was growing discontent in Freetown. Residents were exasperated by poor and irregular water and power supplies. Unemployment or underemployment of youth was estimated at 70%.[31] That day, we had a discussion about what the government should do, specifically about how they should put food on the table of the average Sierra Leonean.

I, along with other international donors, expressed the view that there were fundamental issues underlying the visible problems. One issue was quality of education. While attendance numbers had been growing in schools, there were big questions about how much kids were actually learning. How prepared would they be for the jobs market? Another related issue was capacity within government. The World Bank estimated in 2012 that Sierra Leone only had a quarter of the professional and technical staff it needed to run the government.[32]

And finally, corruption was rampant. In July 2013, Sierra Leone earned the dubious accolade of having the highest bribery rate in the world – a survey by Transparency International found that 84% of Sierra Leoneans had paid a bribe in the past year.

These issues were deep, and there were no quick fixes. This, though, was where we stood in the spring of 2014.

OLIVER

Setting up

After graduating from medical school, I made the unusual decision not to do my internship as a junior doctor, much to the consternation of my supervisors in the hospital. The month I had spent in Sierra Leone in 2009 had reinforced my interest in improving the design and management of health systems in developing countries. So instead of working as a clinician, I joined the faculty of a new Centre for Global Health at King's College London that focused on teaching global health and strengthening health systems in Africa. King's was joining forces with its three major South London teaching hospitals and was eager to grow its global health programme. The director of the centre was Andy Leather, a humble yet charismatic surgeon in his early fifties who had set up a partnership between King's and Somaliland about a decade before. He was a wonderful mentor and gave me lots of space to set up new projects.

I was keen for Sierra Leone to be considered as one of the countries for our expansion. Andy was very supportive and travelled out with me in 2011 to meet prospective partners there. The government-run medical school in Freetown asked us to collaborate, and we won a small grant from DFID for us to help develop a new curriculum and improve the teaching facilities. I was leading the project and was eager to live in Africa, so requested to relocate to Freetown. Luckily the Vice-Principal at King's was fully behind our vision and gave me the green light to move there in January 2013. Three other doctors, who also had an interest in global health and happened to be friends from medical school, volunteered to join me for the first six months and we all squeezed into the house I rented there.

Soon after I arrived, I was summoned by the Minister of Health and Sanitation to discuss the partnership.[33] The Ministry was spread over two floors of a huge government office block called the Youyi Building, which had been built, along with the adjacent national stadium, in the 1970s by the Chinese government.

The building had seen better days. The lifts had long since stopped working. There was no internet apart from mobile phone dongles, which downloaded emails at a glacial pace, when they worked at all, onto computers often plagued by viruses.

Each section within the Ministry, such as the Directorate of Primary Health Care, normally consisted of just a director, a secretary and maybe one or two programme officers. It was starkly different from UN agencies such as UNICEF, or the international health NGOs such as Save the Children, where you would find teams of technical staff that had access to generators, Wi-Fi, a fleet of vehicles and a professional support team of accountants, grants managers and administrators.

The Minister, Miatta Kargbo, was welcoming but also intimidating. A dynamic woman in her late 30s, she had been made a minister a few months previously, having studied in the US and worked in the corporate sector there. "Forget about the medical school, that's not my priority," she told us. "Connaught is this country's main hospital and I want your help in overhauling it to make it a flagship hospital for this country." After a discussion with my colleagues in London, we agreed to take this on as well, not that she'd given us much say in the matter . . .

Connaught Hospital
Sierra Leone's main hospital had been constructed in 1913 and sat squeezed between the downtown business district and a shelf of

steep cliffs. These cliffs would once have led directly down to the sea, but they now loomed over a large shanty town called Kroo Bay, which had crept out onto a landfill that had emerged from the build-up of trash during the civil war. A whitewashed colonial Emergency Department formed the front of the hospital building, at the centre of which was a large gated arch. This entrance led through to a grassy central courtyard that was criss-crossed by covered walkways that connected the various wards and clinics within.

Connaught had survived the civil war largely unscathed but had fared less well with the subsequent efforts by international donors to refurbish it. Some of its doorways were randomly bricked up, and a previously reliable plumbing system was replaced with another that was crippled by leaks and water shortages. This was typical of so much of the reconstruction that had taken place in the health sector since the war, from the Freetown hospitals to rural clinics.

Looking at the national picture, a director at the Ministry described how donors had funded the government to double the number of primary health clinics since 2002.[34] The new clinics, however, were often hastily constructed. Some that he visited had "cracked walls, leaky roofs, and so few cupboards that supplies like syringes and medical registers had to be stacked on the floor". He attributed this to "a piecemeal and hurried approach to investment in health-care infrastructure". The health budget was simply not enough, with the government spending only $13 per person on health each year (a minimum of $86 is recommended to provide a minimum package of care).[35,36]

As a result, the Ministry was "unable to equip all of these new facilities and cover staff and operational costs, as its budget [had] not risen to match the system's expansion".[37] A national policy document noted that only half of these clinics had more than two staff members and that 7% had no staff at all.[38] This meant that, in reality, there was little in the way of community health services, something that the Ministry director described as "an empty promise in physical form".

Back at Connaught, older Sierra Leoneans, particularly those from the Krio elite whose ancestors had settled in Freetown, would reminisce about a very different hospital from their child-hood memories of the 1950s and 1960s: immaculate wards kept tidy by disciplined nurses in their pristine uniforms, large depart-ments of specialist doctors that were the envy of West Africa, and in the private wing, liveried waiters bringing afternoon tea on sil-ver plates to the balconies of patients' rooms.

Those halcyon days were long gone and the Connaught Hos-pital I knew had suffered thirty years of unforgiving decline. The civil war may have spared the hospital building but it had gutted its staff. Most senior doctors, nurses and other professionals had packed their bags and left during the conflict, largely to Britain and the United States. They had seen few opportunities and great risk to themselves and their families if they stayed. Of the few who remained, many had reached retirement. Others, by choosing to remain in the country, had sacrificed their opportunity for further training, preventing their careers and expertise from developing.

In total, the country had only a little over a hundred doctors working clinically in the public sector, and even if you included doctors working in the private sector, this was approximately just one doctor per 45,000 people.[39] This compared to about one per 350 people in the UK.[40]

With so few senior staff at the hospital, the new generation of medical and nursing graduates lacked teachers and role models. Coupled with the toxic effects of political interference, wherein the governing elite would routinely intervene to prevent health workers in their extended family from being disciplined or sent on unpopular postings, you had a recipe for an unruly, often-absent and poorly performing workforce. Control of Connaught had also become tightly centralised, and the hospital leadership would need written permission from the Ministry for even minor actions such as reprimanding staff or changing the use of a ward.

Despite this unenviable training climate, a few dedicated professionals and strong leaders were starting to emerge. Amongst these was Dr Martin Salia, a doctor in his early forties who had completed his surgical training abroad. This made him one of the first of the new generation to become a specialist. His dedication and restless energy saw him shuttle between the Methodist NGO Hospital he ran and Connaught, where he performed surgery and was in charge of the Emergency Department. He was an inspiration to his juniors and the kind of leader that I believed could drive the reform of the health sector at large.

Let them fall by their own weight

Reformers faced a strong headwind, however, in the form of entrenched interests and resistance to change. At the root of this was the fact that staff were poorly paid, with junior doctors earning just a few hundred dollars a month, after having completed eight years of medical school. They therefore relied on other sources of funding to supplement their meagre income from the government and make ends meet.

For some, this would involve leaving work early to run a private clinic, or even seeing private patients at government facilities. Although having multiple jobs was officially forbidden, some other health workers would look to the overseas aid sector for extra income. One international NGO discovered through a routine audit that over thirty of their staff were also on the Ministry payroll.

Some health workers were not paid a salary by government at all; many nurses worked as volunteers and turned up for shifts at the hospital each day in the hope that they would eventually be put onto the government payroll.

The only way for many health workers at Connaught to make a reasonable living was to rely on the sprawling black market that underpinned every transaction within the hospital. Patient names would rarely appear in the registration log as the finance clerks would simply pocket the admission fee. Drugs and medical equipment such as gloves or syringes often had to be bought for an inflated price from the handbag of a ward nurse, with patients discouraged from buying them at the hospital pharmacy. Medical interventions, such as putting in a drip or inserting a catheter, might require a further cash transaction, whilst relatives would be expected to perform basic nursing tasks like bathing and feeding the patients themselves.

An extreme example, which was documented in a Ministry report, was of "porters and other non-clinical staff pretending to be doctors in the [Emergency] Department and accepting fees directly from patients".[41] One particular porter was well known for this, and in one case, I was told that a patient had to have their arm amputated to correct one of his botched jobs. I remember a meeting when the Minister had asked whether anyone knew about the actions of this dangerous porter, to which a senior doctor replied, "This man, we all know him, he has been 'treating' patients since back when I was a junior doctor." But, of course, nothing had been done.

This lack of accountability would become a recurring theme. Few people were willing to take action against allegations of misconduct for fear of reprisal. You never knew how someone might be politically connected through their family, their ethnic group, their church or their secret society. Colleagues would shake their heads, recognising my naïveté, and tell me it was useless to try to interfere. They would repeat a common expression that I came to hate: "We should let them fall by their own weight."

All this might make the hospital seem like a depressing place to work, and at times it was. It is not hard to imagine why so many doctors and nurses had had their spirits broken and given up their seemingly futile efforts to make improvements, choosing instead to leave or simply stop resisting.

Redeeming qualities

There was, however, still the odd oasis within the hospital where pockets of good care and motivated staff could be found. Dr Matthew Vandy was a wonderful lead for the ophthalmology department, which was supported by Sightsavers International. They provided free eye care, performing thousands of cataract surgeries per year, and had a neatly painted waiting room and cheerful staff. In the main operating theatre building, there was a 7 a.m. surgical team meeting each day, where the surgeons would meet with their junior doctors to give advice on difficult patients and grill them on best practice. There was also the ear, nose and throat clinic, a shabby warren of rooms presided over by a visiting Cuban specialist who, despite his limited English and famous temper, provided excellent care to countless patients and mentored the department's nurses to be highly skilled professionals.

Overall, however, there was not much international support for the staff at the hospital, and the little there was tended to be narrowly focused around particular diseases or groups of patients. These are described in the trade as 'vertical programmes' since they tend to ignore the wider health system issues. A group of authors from the World Health Organization noted that, although there had been a substantial increase in international funding for health in Sierra Leone over the past decade, "most of this aid has been allocated to combat human immunodeficiency virus [HIV] infection, malaria and tuberculosis, with much of the residual going to maternal and child health services. Therefore, relatively little external aid was left to support overall development of health systems."[42]

For example, the HIV service at Connaught, supported by the Global Fund, was run out of a virtually autonomous clinic, with its own pharmacy and medical records system. This approach contributed to the fragmentation of the systems of the hospital. Furthermore, some staff in the HIV programme received additional financial incentives or a separate salary. Health workers would therefore flock towards these donor-funded programmes, leaving critical posts on the general wards unfilled. So while vertical programmes could be an effective way of delivering a targeted health programme, many had an unhelpful distorting effect.

We were trying to take a different approach with the King's partnership, supporting the improvement of the health system more widely over the long term. Rather than coming with our own agenda, we tried to be led by our local colleagues' priorities and to focus on strengthening the hospital as a whole, rather than just cherry picking a particular aspect such as the children's ward, the pharmacy or the finance department. After all, the different functions of the hospital were interconnected – there was no point teaching a nurse to wash their hands properly if there was no running water in the taps, soap in the storeroom or a budget to pay for it all.

Although some of the King's volunteers did clinical shifts a few times a week, our main focus wasn't on treating patients but on addressing the root causes of the hospital's challenges. It was fascinating and exhilarating work and we were all on a steep learning curve, gaining new skills and experience that we quickly realised would be invaluable when we returned back to work in the UK health service.

Our team on the ground was small, but we were able to call on the help of senior doctors and academics back at King's in London, which made it possible for us to handle some of the varied requests we received from Connaught, from the idea of introducing an electronic patient records system to advising on hospital design or researching the cause of surgical wound infections.

Whilst we had lots of technical expertise and volunteer energy, we had very little in the way of funding. We operated off a tiny budget made up of our DFID grant, some funding from King's for my salary, and whatever donations we could scrounge from friends and family. This made our lives quite different from many of our international colleagues. For example, until I learnt to drive at the Freetown driving school and bought a car, the team would have to queue for an age outside the hospital each afternoon before eventually squeezing into the back of a shared local taxi to get home. And our evenings would be spent in the dark, relying on our head torches to cook, as we didn't have a generator.

We were incredibly fortunate to recruit a committed and qualified team of volunteers. The term 'volunteer' can mean different things, but for us at King's it meant that we didn't pay a salary. At first, the doctors who came out had to pay their own living costs, as we were only able to afford the cost of their flights. As time went on, we were able to pay most of them a stipend of a few hundred pounds each month and provide accommodation. This was still tough for people, especially those with loans or mortgages to cover back home but, in a way, it was a filter which meant that everyone on the team was highly motivated.

Inch by inch
A few months after I arrived, the Minister established a taskforce to turn things around and detoxify Connaught's reputation as 'the place where you go to die'. This became a flagship project

for President Koroma for his second term in office and progress had to be reported to State House. An alliance formed between the new Minister and a fearless anaesthetist called Dr Eva Han-ciles, who had recently returned to Sierra Leone after decades of work in Ireland and the UK. A lively woman in her fifties, she had short cropped hair and was always colourfully dressed. Caring passionately about the hospital, she could often be heard reprimanding junior staff for some infringement or checking that patients had the right receipts and hadn't had to pay a bribe. She was an exception to the norm and wasn't afraid to challenge her colleagues, which often got her into hot water.

She and the Minister drew together a coalition of the willing from within the institution and outside of it, to try to make radical changes to its systems and culture. The King's team was asked to work alongside them to provide support and technical advice.

Meaningful changes started to be made, albeit in the teeth of an old guard who often frustrated and resisted change. Two committed young accountants were posted to the hospital to take over the finance department. Revenue collection was centralised and a receipt system was established, resulting in a doubling of the hospital's income. We worked with a delightful nurse called Sister Hajara Serry, who herself had only recently qualified, to introduce a triage system at the gate. This meant that the sickest patients could be prioritised and directed to a new resuscitation room. Some of the accountability problems, such as the porters pretending to be doctors, were finally dealt with. The hospital drew up a detailed plan for starting to train specialist doctors locally.

It fell to Dr TB Kamara, the head of the hospital, to adjudi-cate between the different factions within the hospital. Widely respected as the country's most senior surgeon, Dr Kamara was a slender man nearing retirement with a cautious demeanour, behind which lay considerable empathy and resolve. Years later, he would recount at a conference in London the comments he had made to the hospital management committee after our first meeting: "This partnership with King's seems promising, but can they be serious when their leader is so young?" We quickly developed a close working relationship, though, and I would spend hours each day sitting on the sofas in his office clutching a sheaf of papers for him to sign, waiting for my turn to get his attention as he dealt with the various officials and staff that would turn up unannounced to meet him. He supported improvements where possible whilst keeping the peace and ensuring the hospital continued running on a day-to-day basis.

The hospital was starting its long and arduous transition to a more functional state, but with its shortage of trained staff, weak governance and creaking infrastructure, it was completely unprepared for the tsunami of Ebola cases that would soon arrive at its gates.

TWO | A dubious start: Ebola in Guinea

OLIVER

Something strange and sinister in a remote forest
The first news I heard about unexplained deaths in West Africa came from an update on the BBC website on 18 March 2014. The report suggested that something strange and sinister was brewing in a remote forest area in Guinea. The King's team, eight of us by this stage, were sitting in our cramped office in the hospital management building, huddled with our laptops around a couple of shared desks. Next to me was Dr Marta Lado, a vivacious Spanish infectious diseases specialist who had arrived a week before as a new long-term volunteer. Her compassion and energy had immediately established her as a dominant force within the team.

Tropical diseases are probably the most exciting and mysterious corner of the medical world, at least for global health types like us. They are still largely uncharted territory, with very little known about many of them. Chief amongst tropical diseases are viral haemorrhagic fevers, which only a tiny fraction of doctors on the planet can expect to encounter during the course of their careers. They are so rare, contagious and deadly that they inspire both fear and fascination in equal measure within the medical community.

This news from Guinea therefore kicked off an excited discussion amongst the team about what the cause of these mysterious deaths might be. At this stage, it seemed extremely unlikely that this small outbreak in a neighbouring country would affect us in Freetown. Marta joked that she should dust off her copy of *Principles of Medicine in Africa*, the tropical medicine textbook tucked away on a shelf above our heads, so she could study up on these obscure conditions just in case.

A few days later, on 21 March 2014, the cause of the outbreak was confirmed as Ebola Haemorrhagic Fever.

Ebola is not the kind of thing that is regularly taught at a London medical school, so what I knew about the virus at this stage came mostly from the 1995 Hollywood disaster movie *Outbreak*. In that film, characters played by Dustin Hoffman, Rene Russo and Morgan Freeman battle a deadly Ebola-like outbreak in small-town America. Fortunately, most of my team had studied tropical medicine and they quickly got me up to speed about the disease.

In popular culture, Ebola is usually depicted as causing massive bleeding, typically from the eyes and nose. However, bleeding is actually quite an unusual and late symptom. In reality, a person infected with Ebola can take between two and twenty-one days before they start to show any symptoms at all. This is known as the incubation period. At first, the illness might seem quite mild, with just a fever, a sore throat, a headache and maybe some general muscle ache. At this early stage, Ebola therefore looks and feels just like other common diseases in West Africa, such as the flu or malaria, which makes it difficult to diagnose based on symptoms alone. A blood sample needs to be lab-tested to determine whether it is Ebola.

As the illness progresses, patients may start to get quite severe vomiting and diarrhoea. This can cause them to lose up to ten litres of fluid per day, resulting in dehydration that can quickly prove fatal. Patients start to feel weak and become increasingly confused until they become unresponsive. As the kidneys fail, the patient may experience hiccupping and, towards the end, occasionally suffer bleeding, which can be very difficult to stop. The disease can progress very quickly: an otherwise healthy person could progress from their first symptom to death in under a week. On average, fewer than half of Ebola patients survive their illness.

There is no specific treatment for the Ebola virus, but supportive care can improve a patient's chances of survival. This includes making sure they receive lots of fluids to prevent dehydration and giving them antibiotics to prevent a secondary bacterial infection from occurring whilst their bodies are in a weakened state.

What makes Ebola so dangerous is not just its deadliness, but its contagiousness. When a person is first infected, the amount of virus in their body is very low, and it is mostly contained within their blood and organs. At this stage, they are unlikely to infect anybody except health workers who come into contact with their blood. As the disease progresses, however, the amount of virus in the body increases exponentially such that there can be more than ten million individual virus particles in one millilitre of blood.[1] The virus also starts to get into the patient's other body fluids such as their vomit, faeces, urine, sweat, teardrops, and even breast milk or semen.

As they get sicker, patients can therefore become highly contagious, particularly to the people caring for them. Anything from getting splattered with sprayed vomit to touching a dirty sheet can bring you into contact with infected body fluids. If you then introduce the virus into your body through an open cut, or by rubbing your eyes or eating without washing your hands properly, you too can become infected. When people die of Ebola, their corpse can remain infectious for more than a week and those who touch that corpse to prepare the body for burial can be exposed.

Despite all this, unless you are caring for an Ebola patient or involved in conducting burials, the risk of contracting Ebola is extremely low, since Ebola is not airborne. Professor Peter Piot made this point in a media interview: "I wouldn't be worried to sit next to someone with Ebola virus on the Tube as long as they don't vomit on you or something. This is an infection that requires very close contact."[2] However, this point was massively misunderstood, both in Sierra Leone and internationally, leading to fear, panic and hysteria. This had lots of implications for the response, as we will see.

SINEAD

A mysterious disease

Though it was very concerning to read about what was going on across the border in Guinea, for my colleagues and me it was all quite abstract. Despite Guinea's capital, Conakry, being only a five-hour drive from Freetown, we had no engagement with the country.

Over time, the full story of how the outbreak had started was gradually pieced together. On 28 December 2013 in a small village called Meliandou in southern Guinea, a one-year-old boy, Emile Ouamouno, died after a brief intense fever.[3] Tragically, the death of an infant in rural West Africa was hardly unusual. But when Emile's sister, his pregnant mother and his grandmother died soon afterwards, it was evident something more dangerous was happening.

Before her death, Emile's grandmother Koumba had gone to the nearby city of Guéckédou for hospital treatment, and unknowingly passed the infection on to health workers, who in turn carried it to other villages.[4] It took Guinean authorities and international organisations until March to diagnose the mysterious illness as Ebola, which they could only do after sending lab samples to France for testing. By that time, there were forty-nine suspected cases and twenty-nine deaths.[5]

It seems likely that Emile contracted Ebola by playing in a tree near his home where there were bat droppings, as bats are one of the wild animals thought to spread Ebola. Nobody really knows though – forty years after the discovery of the Ebola virus, we are still not sure exactly how it passes from animals to humans.

The first recorded outbreaks of Ebola happened in 1976 in areas that are now in South Sudan and the Democratic Republic of the Congo (DRC). The virus was named after the Ebola River that flowed near the affected village of Yambuku in the DRC, as scientists wanted to avoid stigmatising the village itself. Until 2014, that 1976 outbreak, which killed 280 people – 88% of those infected – was the deadliest Ebola outbreak in history.[6] Out of the thirty-four outbreaks that had taken place up to 2014, six outbreaks had each killed more than 100 people, although seventeen other outbreaks had killed fewer than ten people or none at all.[7]

In other words, previous Ebola outbreaks had ranged widely in size and severity. But one common feature of these previous outbreaks was that they did not have a very large geographic spread, usually affecting only a small number of villages or towns before being contained.

Indeed, my own vague impression of Ebola from my years in East Africa was of a disease that only hit remote forested areas. I had heard rumours about the disease now and again when it emerged somewhat near where I was. While I had worked in Rwanda in 2001, there had been an outbreak across the border in Uganda, and when I had worked in South Sudan in 2005, I had heard stories about an outbreak that had happened the year before in the south-west of the country. The accounts were always horrifying, but also other-worldly and distant. It never occurred to me that this might be a disease that could reach where I was.

The Twitter duel

When Ebola was finally confirmed in Guinea on 21 March, there were only three international organisations with significant experience of the disease: the UN's World Health Organization (WHO); the US Centers for Disease Control and Prevention (CDC); and the NGO Médecins Sans Frontières (MSF). But WHO and MSF could not even come close to agreeing on the seriousness of the crisis in Guinea. This was a pattern that we would see for several months to come, in Guinea, Sierra Leone and beyond. After MSF called the outbreak in Guinea "unprecedented" on 31 March, having spent two weeks witnessing the situation in Guéckédou, a three-day Twitter battle followed during which the official WHO spokesperson in Geneva warned MSF not to "overblow" or "exaggerate" the situation.[8]

Both WHO and MSF had experienced many of the previous outbreaks in East and Central Africa. So why were they describing the Guinea outbreak so differently? In hindsight, I think there are probably two answers to that question.

Firstly, some people in WHO were too caught up in the fact that previous epidemics had been geographically limited and assumed this would be the same. On 23 March, the organisation's spokesperson tweeted: "Ebola has always remained a very localised event." In contrast, MSF were looking at the facts on the ground and saw what was different this time around.[9] As a senior MSF epidemiologist noted: "the sick and their caregivers were moving on a scale we'd never seen before. Even the dead were being transported [for funerals] from one village to another."[10] It later emerged that some people in WHO were also very worried, but internal political dynamics meant their voices were not being heard.

The second reason why the descriptions by the two organisations were so at odds related to their differing agendas. MSF's priorities were humanitarian; they wanted to stop Ebola and save lives. The WHO offices in the region, while they no doubt wanted the same thing, were also trying to maintain good relations with their host governments. This was certainly my own impression from the encounters I had had with WHO and MSF before Ebola. In fact, I had never actually thought of them as being comparable before. Any of my interactions with MSF had been with passionate chain-smoking French-speaking humanitarians, often railing against governments but very committed to serving local populations, whereas I had only ever come across WHO in capital cities, within their offices or in Ministry meeting rooms. I had experienced them as pleasant, knowledgeable about technical aspects of health, and very much focused on supporting host governments.

This additional political priority of WHO was hardly surprising, since countries like Guinea and Sierra Leone are members of WHO's global governance structure. Its 194 member states make up the World Health Assembly, which is the primary decision-making body for WHO. As members, ministers of health from each region nominate the regional representative of WHO, who in turn nominates the representatives that will lead the WHO offices in each country.[11]

This close relationship between host countries and the respective WHO offices was usually a good thing, since collaboration was vital for WHO to fulfil its mandate of helping to strengthen health systems.[12] The tension arose with Ebola in the spring of 2014 when the public health reality diverged from the political and economic priorities of the affected countries.

This happened when the government of Guinea decided that Ebola was bad for business. Anxious not to scare away airlines or mining companies, they promoted "positive communication" about the outbreak and downplayed its seriousness.[13] There were widespread reports of health officials having "massaged" the numbers.[14] From a public health standpoint, this was deeply problematic as transparency is key in an outbreak response: you can't stop a disease from spreading if you are not open about who is already infected and where they are. Nevertheless, this 'positive communication' was the priority of the host government and seems to have played into what has been termed WHO's "decidedly anti-alarmist approach" at the time.[15]

There were other problems that also prevented WHO from being a strong leader on Ebola at this juncture in Guinea.[16] WHO's constitution states that regional issues should largely be handled by regional offices, rather than by the headquarters in Geneva.[17] The responsibility for the Ebola crisis in West Africa therefore fell to the WHO's regional office in Congo-Brazzaville, known as 'AFRO'. But AFRO and its country offices were ill-equipped to handle Ebola.[18]

One reason was shortages of money and people. Most of WHO's budget, nearly 80%, is made up of voluntary donations by member states which can fluctuate from year to year.[19] WHO's budget was slashed by nearly a billion dollars in 2011, in part as a consequence of the financial crisis in donor countries. Consequently its global emergency response budget was halved and its emergency unit lost nearly two-thirds of its staff.[20,21,22] Specifically, AFRO lost nine of its twelve emergency response specialists and its overall budget went from $26m in 2011 to $11m in 2014.[23,24]

Another issue was the quality of WHO staff at the country level. A *New York Times* article noted that the WHO representatives in Guinea, Sierra Leone and Liberia were viewed as "earnest but overmatched".[25] The article also cited the United States Representative on the Executive Board of WHO under President

Obama as saying the WHO Africa office had long been seen as "a place where politics often trumps substance" and where key appointees "often are not the cream of the crop".

All this left us with a weak and politicised WHO Regional Office to support a poorly equipped WHO country office in dealing with this unprecedented outbreak.

Ebola crosses the border

MSF were particularly worried about cross-border spread, as the hotspot in Guéckédou was near the borders with Sierra Leone and Liberia. In fact, for many residents of the area, borders were irrelevant. The Kissi people had lived in and travelled throughout this region for centuries before it was subdivided into Sierra Leone, Liberia and Guinea by administrative borders during colonial times, and they continued to do so in March 2014.

As a case in point, on 17 March a thirty-year-old Liberian woman, Tewa Joseph, went to the Guinea side of the border to pick up her ailing sister and bring her to a hospital in Lofa county, northern Liberia.[26] Her sister died a few days later and Tewa started having symptoms of Ebola. She went back to the hospital on 26 March but, suspecting it was Ebola after hearing the announcement from Guinea, the staff initially refused her entry as they didn't have any protective clothing. A few days later, Tewa took a twelve-hour taxi ride, passing through the capital Monrovia, to her husband's workplace at the Firestone Plantation on the other side of the capital.[27,28] She was seeking treatment for the virus which she had just seen kill her sister, but she died soon after her arrival in Firestone.[29]

I happened to be in Monrovia at the time and was due to go to monitor one of our projects on violence against women in a part of town called Chicken Soup Factory with my Liberian colleague. However, just as we were driving there, Teta got a call from our partner International Rescue Committee (IRC). "Chicken Soup Factory has been closed", Teta relayed back to me from the front seat of the car. "Closed?" I said, "You mean the centre where we were supposed to meet the women?" Teta listened some more. "No, that whole area is closed," she said. It turned out that Tewa Joseph had stopped off there on her trip from Lofa and health officials had cordoned off the area for something called 'contact tracing'.

This was my introduction to the three actions that have to be undertaken simultaneously in an Ebola response (or, as I learnt, in any outbreak response).

The first task is surveillance. The objective of surveillance is to figure out exactly where cases are occurring. 'Contact tracing' is a central part of surveillance and involves identifying all the people who have come into contact with an infected person while they were contagious. These people need to be monitored so that if they start developing symptoms, they can immediately be isolated and treated before spreading the disease further. In this case, because Tewa Joseph was mobile, she had many contacts both in Lofa and from her long journey to Monrovia, including her taxi driver, food vendors and so on. So contact tracing was a huge task.

The other aspect of surveillance for a disease like Ebola is laboratory testing, since Ebola is often very hard to distinguish from other diseases. When the outbreak started in Liberia, there was no lab in the country that could test for Ebola and samples had to be sent to one that had just been set up in Guinea.

The second action in an outbreak is 'case management'. This means isolating and treating people who are suspected of being infected. Hospitals and clinics need to be able to take blood samples to send for testing and to provide appropriate medical care. Importantly, the virus can spread easily within healthcare facilities, so measures needed to be in place for strict infection control and staff need to have access to personal protective equipment (PPE) such as gloves and face shields. In addition, if a patient dies, either in an isolation unit or in the community, their body needs to be safely buried without putting relatives or burial workers at risk of exposure.

In this case, the Liberian Ministry of Health, with support from international partners, quickly set up an isolation unit where people who'd had contact with Tewa Joseph and had started showing symptoms could be treated. Understandably, there was a lot of fear amongst Liberian health workers about working in the isolation unit – two of the health workers in Lofa who had treated Tewa Joseph's sister had died of Ebola.[30] To help address this, the then eighty-year-old Health Minister, Walter Gwenigale, better known to us as 'Dr G', put on PPE and went inside the unit with the health workers. He told us about it the next day at a meeting, how he had "dressed like I was going to the moon". He felt it was important to show an example to other health workers: if he expected them to go into the isolation unit and risk their lives, he must be willing to take that same risk himself.

The third aspect of an Ebola response is communication with the public, often known as 'social mobilisation' or 'community engagement'. This communication must be regular and clear. People need to be informed about how to keep themselves safe, and what to do if they, or somebody they know, starts to show symptoms – critically, they should contact health authorities.

The catch with this messaging is that it presupposes that people have an entirely biomedical understanding of sickness and disease, rather than an understanding that combines traditional or spiritual beliefs. An example of this is the way a person might accept that their illness is caused by a virus, but question why the virus happened to strike them, of all people, at that particular moment, attributing this perhaps to other spiritual forces, such as an enemy seeking revenge. The social mobilisation messaging also presupposes that the population trusts the government and its international partners. If not, it is irrelevant how scientifically accurate the messages about Ebola are and how well-crafted. These issues were to come back to haunt us.

This communication step didn't go so well initially in Liberia. While the government put out regular radio ads and printed many posters and flyers, the initial messages focused on the fact that Ebola had no cure. One poster warned that "most of the people who catch it will die".[31] While this was technically accurate at the time, it was very problematic as it made people feel helpless. If there was no cure, why would you bother getting in touch with the authorities if you or someone you knew had symptoms? With the help of international partners, these messages improved over time.

Despite the problems, by implementing these actions and with international support, Liberia managed to bring its first Ebola outbreak to a close, with a total of twenty-one cases and ten deaths.[32] One senior CDC official said Liberia was "either good or very lucky".[33] Either way, by mid-April, things seemed to be under control.

Mind the (implementation) gap

With Liberia successfully dealing with its outbreak, and with no cases in Sierra Leone, I didn't have much engagement on Ebola in the weeks that followed. In those days in Freetown, we were swamped with the existing set of challenges in the country and very happy to let ourselves believe that the country had escaped Ebola altogether.

In addition, I was hearing encouraging noises from the Sierra Leonean Ministry of Health on their preparedness planning: a national taskforce up and running; daily teleconferences with the

Guinean and Liberian ministries and WHO offices; training of health workers; and awareness-raising of the public. Irish Aid were not centrally engaged in the health sector at the time. DFID were the lead donor in health and coordinated our donor group in the sector, so we agreed that they would attend the National Ebola Taskforce meetings on behalf of donors and report back to us.

Looking back, even with our indirect engagement, I should have been more wary of the reassurances from the Ministry. After three years in the country I had long since discovered that Sierra Leoneans were some of the best speech-makers that I had ever met – at any work or social event, you could call on practically anybody in the room without warning and they would be able to make a compelling speech or presentation off the top of their head. Some people could carry this over to eloquent and persuasive writing, and the country's ministries were often commended internationally for their well-crafted strategies and plans. However, on the ground, there was often a massive gap between a plan and its implementation, due to issues like lack of capacity, accountability problems or inadequate external support. And so it was with Ebola preparations.

In retrospect, the main point that reassured me in all of this preparedness work in Sierra Leone was the involvement of WHO. Everybody said that they had vast experience with these kinds of epidemics in other countries, even if the government of Sierra Leone didn't, so I assumed that they would provide the appropriate support. It was only later that I realised how naïve I had been.

OLIVER

First wobbly steps

The Sierra Leonean Ministry responded quickly to the news of Ebola. Within days of the Guinea outbreak being confirmed, they had established a National Ebola Taskforce. Meetings were usually held once or twice per week in the Ministry's main conference room and were chaired by the Minister herself. The Taskforce was attended by the senior directors of the Ministry, representatives of WHO and other UN agencies, donors and most of the health NGOs such as Save the Children and IRC, about thirty to fifty people in total.

When I got the invitation email for the first meeting, I was initially unsure if King's should even attend. Not only were we not experts in Ebola, but we were not a humanitarian agency and were not doing very much clinical work in the hospital, as we were more focused on improving management. In Marta, however, we did have a highly qualified infectious diseases specialist on our team, so we agreed to join in. The irony was that when we first recruited Marta I had been concerned that her infectious diseases skills would not be very useful to us, since our work at the time was mostly around emergency medicine and mental health – how wrong I was.

Marta and I became regular attendees at the Taskforce. Like most of the government meetings that I attended in Sierra Leone, the Taskforce meetings inevitably started very late, had little in the way of an agenda and went on incredibly long. As such, they were rarely useful for making decisions or coming up with concrete plans. At the time, however, they were pretty much our only source of information about what was going on. From a practical standpoint, these meetings did little more than bring all the relevant people together on a regular basis. They normally started with the Minister and WHO representative providing everyone with an update on the Ebola situation. After that point, we often found ourselves getting side-tracked and lost in the weeds. For example, we spent hours debating the exact wording of public messages on Ebola. Anyone in the room, regardless of their role or expertise, was able to interject and suggest changes. And despite the exhaustive discussion, critical mistakes were made.

Most significantly, we spent far too long creating messaging aimed at preventing humans from getting infected from animals. This was pointless, however, as it had been human-to-human transmission that had been driving the outbreak since the very first case in Guinea. This did not stop the Taskforce from spending a huge amount of time discussing the risks of 'bat mot', a Krio phrase meaning fruit (normally mango) that had been partly eaten by bats. The concern was that if a bat were to partially eat some fruit, and leave its saliva behind, then a human could pick up the same fruit and finish eating it. In doing so, they could ingest the bat saliva and become infected. So we had a long discussion on whether to advise the public that all fruit should be washed in chlorine before being eaten – something that would be a ridiculous idea even in a wealthy country, but was preposterous in rural villages where there was no running water and no chlorine for miles.

Underdog team

Marta and I also sat on the Case Management Pillar, which was one of the three sub-committees of the Taskforce, alongside surveillance and communications, and which was focused on the clinical aspects of the response. It was chaired by Dr Donald Bash-Taqi, an amicable paediatrician who was the Director of Hospitals & Labs for the country. In this role, he was responsible for overseeing the twenty-odd government hospitals, though his department consisted of just one secretary and one lab scientist. He had therefore been desperately understaffed and overworked even before being given this huge additional task.

We held the first meeting of the Pillar in late March at an office in Connaught, and it had a pretty good turnout from senior national doctors and medical NGOs. Our main priority was to develop a set of national clinical guidelines for how clinicians could safely identify, isolate and treat Ebola patients. These were adapted from existing WHO guidelines on Ebola that we downloaded from the internet. The guidelines were very helpful and included useful diagrams showing how to put on and remove the complex PPE that health workers would need for Ebola patients. They even showed how to tape plastic bags around your hands if you ran out of medical gloves.

We also made posters that could be put up around hospitals as a summary of the guidelines, although these included an embarrassing error on my part. We were using my laptop to design the posters and I just wasn't able to format them to fit onto one page. To make space, we decided to remove one of the symptoms from the list. I suggested hiccupping, since we thought it would probably be very rare and frankly, it seemed an absurd symptom to include. This just shows how ignorant we were about Ebola at the time, with hiccupping later proving to be one of the most distinguishing features of the disease. It had actually been the mention of hiccupping in a field report that led an MSF clinical team to suspect it was Ebola causing the outbreak in Guinea in the first place.

As that first meeting got underway, there was quite a lot of scepticism expressed by the senior Sierra Leonean doctors present. "These guys at Ministry will deliberately let this outbreak continue," the doctor sitting next to me muttered under his breath, "because they know the worse it gets, the more foreign aid money will come pouring in. After all, that's what they did with cholera in 2012." I scoffed at this and said I thought he was being far too cynical. But looking back on it, I have little doubt that some people saw the Ebola response as a lucrative opportunity right from the beginning.

Subsequent case management meetings were held at the Ministry, and Sierra Leonean clinicians largely stopped attending. The participants were usually just one or two people from the Ministry along with a handful of NGOs, with representatives from King's, Welbodi Partnership and the MSF office in Freetown. A couple of staff also attended from an Italian surgical hospital called Emergency, including a Ugandan paediatrician, Dr Michael Mwanda, who had previous training in Ebola and proved to be a great resource. I was very lucky that the King's team had an infectious diseases advisor who could input from London, Dr Colin Brown, who happened to be working at the Royal Free Hospital at the time, where the UK's Viral Haemorrhagic Fevers unit was based. Alongside Marta, he was a fantastic source of advice to call on during the many occasions when I felt out of my depth.

So it was just this tiny group that was working to prepare all of the country's hospitals and clinics for a possible influx of Ebola cases. Apart from MSF, we were all small organisations with very limited resources. Each of us, including our colleagues at the Ministry, had other full-time day jobs to focus on and so could only offer a limited amount of our time. WHO was almost never present in these meetings, perhaps because they had few people in their Freetown office with recent clinical experience. As with the broader Taskforce, these Pillar meetings were chaotic. Furthermore, the chairperson Dr Bash-Taqi was himself often unable to attend. This left the international partners present divided on whether to hold the meeting without him or to abandon it, since there was often no government representative, or even Sierra Leonean, present.

Although the Pillar came up with lots of plans on paper, very few of these were properly implemented. For example, having written the national clinical guidelines, we faced the challenge of physically getting them into the hands of doctors around the country. This ended up being a huge logistical difficulty. We soon discovered that the Ministry could not even provide a list of contact details for all the public and private hospitals, so we had to spend precious days compiling one from scratch. Even when we could get hold of an email address for a hospital manager and send the document to them, most were unable to download the guidelines and print them because of problems with their computers or internet. We asked WHO to help us distribute hard copies of the guidelines using their vehicles, but our request fell on deaf ears. In the end, we rang around friends working in the various provinces at different NGOs and begged them to print the guidelines at their local offices and use one of their vehicles to deliver them to the hospitals.

We were also concerned about the shortage of PPE. The limited supplies in-country were mostly sent to hospitals near the border with Guinea, leaving practically nothing for the rest of the country. Similarly, there were hardly any functional ambulances in the country, which would be essential for transporting Ebola patients for treatment.

Although the Case Management Pillar was responsible for formulating the plans, any decision involving money or resources for this Pillar was made separately by Ministry officials behind closed doors. We struggled to even find out what these decisions were, such as where supplies were being sent or how much money had been allocated for setting up isolation units at the hospitals, let alone contribute to the decision-making process.

What this all ultimately meant was that if the hospital managers were lucky, they might have received a hard copy of the Ebola guidelines by the time the country's first cases hit, but they were unlikely to have received much, if anything, in the way of PPE or any other on-the-ground support.

Lesson plans

One priority for the national Taskforce was to train health workers to prepare for possible Ebola cases.

Metabiota, a US company, volunteered to do the training. They were one of the partners in the Kenema Lassa Fever Centre, based in the government hospital in Kenema city, about a four-hour drive east from Freetown. This had been a regional reference centre for diagnostics and research on Lassa fever since 2004. Each government hospital was asked to send a senior nurse and a doctor there for a two-day workshop, where they were to be given training on the background and symptoms of the disease and how to wear PPE. While this was all well and good in theory, there were two major flaws to their approach.

Firstly, these trainings suffered from the 'per diem culture', which had a toxic effect on the health sector. Per diems were fees paid to people, including government staff, for attending a workshop or going on a day-trip out of town to visit health facilities.

Officially these per diems were intended to cover transport, food and accommodation costs, but they were often worth far more than that. With government salaries being so low, many health workers saw per diems as a vital way to supplement their income. One US-funded project I visited before the Ebola outbreak paid $100 per day for participants to attend a workshop that took place on a workday just a few hundred metres from the hospital.

These training sessions didn't have to be relevant to their work or of good quality, and people would drop pressing tasks just to ensure that they didn't miss a per diem opportunity. In addition, the staff selected to attend a training workshop would often be the favourites of someone higher up, rather than the most suitable person – the senior staff member could then expect to receive a cut of their junior's per diem. Finally, participants might only attend the part of the training necessary to get the brown envelope.

UN agencies and NGOs were often knowingly complicit in this per diem culture because it was in their interests as well. Their proposals for grants from donors might have targets, such as the number of people who attended a workshop, as a way of demonstrating that they had 'built government capacity'. The easiest way of reaching those targets, and therefore positioning well for future grants, was to pay high per diems and get excellent attendance.

Whilst some NGOs tried to resist this, it became almost impossible to compete with those organisations handing out large sums of cash, so the majority ended up following suit. In the spring of 2014, this system meant that many health workers were only interested in attending Ebola training for a per diem. Furthermore, those that were sent to the funded training sessions in Kenema were not always the most suitable people.

The second problem with the Ebola trainings was that they fell into the 'training the trainers' trap, another common fault of aid programmes. The logic here was that an expert, often an international consultant flown in for the task, could provide a brief training to a selection of local staff brought together from across the country. These staff would then 'cascade' this training to their colleagues after returning home. Whilst this may be effective in some specific situations, generally a few hours or a few days of classroom-based teaching simply does not give someone enough knowledge or hands-on experience of a complex real-world challenge for them to be able to undertake it independently or teach it to others.

The centralisation of the Ebola training in one location like Kenema made it much less relevant to the local situation in facilities around the country. Workshop attendees would return to their own facility only to find a layout and protective equipment that differed from what they had been trained in, or, even more commonly, no protective equipment at all. On top of that, these 'trainers' would often have no mandate or motivation to train others locally, nor the resources to pay their colleagues the expected per diem for a local training workshop.

When we raised concerns at Taskforce meetings that health workers were not adequately prepared, we were told that the training had already happened in Kenema. After weeks of requests, we were eventually able to get a list of the people from Freetown who had been trained there. It comprised just five people, only two of whom were hands-on clinicians. The only additional training put on was a classroom-based course for nurses that took place in Freetown. This goes a long way towards explaining why Sierra Leonean health workers were so poorly prepared for the arrival of the first cases of Ebola, despite two months of warning.

Connaught, the flagship

Apart from engaging in the Case Management Pillar, King's was helping Connaught to prepare for possible cases if the outbreak reached Freetown. We knew from previous outbreaks that Ebola could spread like wildfire through a rural village, but that these outbreaks often burned themselves out quite quickly. However, there was a widespread belief in the medical community at the time that the disease would not cause large urban outbreaks. I arranged to meet up with a former lecturer of mine, who was an infectious diseases specialist, in the café of a major London hospital on one of my regular trips back to the UK. I was keen to quiz him on this point: "Everyone keeps telling me this won't spread in Freetown, and I'm sure the experts must be right, but I don't understand why, can you explain it to me?" He couldn't give me a specific reason, and simply insisted that "Ebola does not spread in big cities", the same mantra I had heard repeated by many others as an article of faith.

This was despite the fact that some previous outbreaks, such as the Gulu outbreak in Uganda in 2000, had actually affected urban areas and everything we knew about the science of Ebola transmission suggested that urban transmission was not only possible but likely. This would presumably be particularly so in crowded cities like Freetown, where many families lacked adequate living space and 76% of the urban population lived in slums.[34]

But because of our lack of experience and despite our scepticism, we deferred to these experts. Our working assumption was therefore that whilst the outbreak might spread from Guinea into rural Sierra Leone, it was unlikely to spread much within Freetown. We thought we might see a small number of Ebola cases at Connaught, but that these would be patients who had travelled from rural areas to seek medical care.

Thus, as we set about helping prepare Connaught, we only planned for a handful of cases. This error helps explain why we got preparations so wrong in the early days. We were blinkered by the received wisdom, when really we should have been looking at the facts on the ground.

'Dodging the bullet'

I had discussed our role with the team, and with Andy back in London, and agreed we would allow our King's doctors to treat Ebola patients if they chose to. We all felt we should stand shoulder-to-shoulder with our hospital colleagues, and that refusing to put ourselves at risk would be abandoning them. At the same time, we wanted to maintain our usual role of supporting the hospital, rather than taking over, since we saw this as essential to achieving lasting change and promoting Sierra Leonean leadership.

With this in mind, Dr TB Kamara sought out volunteers amongst the doctors and nurses at the hospital to lead the preparations for Ebola. Recruiting volunteers proved extremely difficult, as not many of our Sierra Leonean colleagues, who were already overstretched, were interested in taking on a role that entailed extra work and no extra salary. Given all the politics within the Ministry, people were also wary of sticking their necks out by taking on responsibilities that might involve the management of resources, for things like procurement, as these could bring with them pressures from different quarters.

The doctors and nurses also saw dangerous implications of helping out with the preparedness efforts, with one intern doctor pointing out: "If I put myself forward now, I know I'll be the first person they send to treat any Ebola cases at the hospital, while everyone else gets to stay safe and refuse to go in." This was an understandable sentiment, especially given that health workers in Sierra Leone have no form of life assurance or health insurance as part of their jobs and are often the main breadwinners for their extended families.

These responsibilities weighed heavily on their minds. Stories were already starting to spread of doctors and nurses in Guinea and Liberia becoming infected. So the few staff we did manage to recruit were reluctant participants, and often did not turn up to meetings as they found themselves triple or quadruple booked alongside other responsibilities.

So, whilst on paper there was a flurry of activity in those two months after the first case in Guinea, in practice there were gaping holes. Initially, this seemed not be such a big problem as, by the middle of May, concern about Ebola coming to Sierra Leone had started to dissipate and preparedness planning slowed to a crawl. The news from Guinea and Liberia was that the outbreaks were almost under control.

The mood at the Ministry was self-congratulatory, with the Minister declaring to the Taskforce: "We've all done a great job, we prepared better than our neighbours and we've avoided a single case of Ebola as a result." Within my team, we felt it was more a case of good luck, given our obvious weaknesses in preparedness. Nevertheless, we were upbeat that we had 'dodged the bullet' and started turning our attention back to longer-term priorities.

SINEAD

Ominous silence

By mid-May, despite the problems we had heard about regarding the response in Guinea, things had gone quiet with respect to the virus. Case numbers there had declined every week since early April. When a country hasn't had any cases for forty-two days (twice the twenty-one-day incubation period) WHO declares the country as Ebola-free. The mood in Liberia was buoyant as they hit that forty-two-day mark on 22 May. MSF wound up operations in the country and made similar plans for Guinea, decontaminating their treatment centre in Conakry. Meanwhile, CDC pulled their people out of Liberia and Guinea towards the end of the month.[35]

However, just as the international organisations were commending themselves and the governments of Guinea and Liberia for the strong surveillance that had led to this defeat of the virus, a critical gap in that surveillance was emerging. Back in March, a Guinean surveillance team had gone to investigate the chain of transmission that had started with baby Emile and his family. On this trip, the team had been told about the death of a thirty-seven-year-old woman on 3 March who lived, not in Guinea, but in a nearby village in Sierra Leone. Villagers also told the investigators that the woman's daughter was now sick with similar symptoms. The investigators duly included this in their seventeen-page report to the Guinean health ministry and WHO.

There are different accounts of what happened after that. When the *New York Times* investigated, the Health Ministry in Sierra Leone denied receiving the information, suggesting that neither the ministry in Guinea nor WHO passed it on. This would be extraordinary given the daily teleconferences that were supposedly happening between the health ministries and WHO offices during this period.

The plot thickens further as MSF later said that they sent the information on the suspect cases to the Health Ministry in Sierra Leone and offered to come across the border to investigate. According to MSF, the Ministry denied them permission, stating that they had looked into the information but the surveillance did not find anything.[36,37]

So what really happened here? We still don't know. It would seem that the Ministry in Sierra Leone got the information, from MSF even if not from Guinea. After that it becomes blurry. Either they failed to act on it or they sent a surveillance team which somehow missed what was going on.

Regardless of the real story here, all three countries would pay dearly for this mistake as the Ebola virus, given at least three months to spread silently in Sierra Leone, was about to re-emerge with force.

THREE | Ebola emerges in Sierra Leone

SINEAD

A deadly funeral

On the afternoon of Sunday 25 May 2014, the first official case of Ebola in Sierra Leone was confirmed. Mamie Lebbie, a forty-two-year-old mother of two from Kailahun district in the south-east of the country, had tested positive. When we got the news at the Embassy, I found myself in the position of being the resident Kailahun expert, since I had visited a couple of times to monitor programmes that we funded. Admittedly, the bar was set low for resident expert status on Kailahun – few Sierra Leoneans, let alone internationals, had cause to go to Kailahun, which borders Guinea and Liberia and is one of the hardest of Sierra Leone's districts to reach from Freetown.

This difficulty was amplified by the road conditions at the time. While the main road to Kailahun had improved greatly in recent years, bringing the travel time from Freetown down to less than eight hours in the dry season (having been up to twelve hours in the past), the long rainy season that hit Sierra Leone each May could make other roads in the district completely impassable.

The origins of the first case in Sierra Leone are debated, as we now know that there was a suspected Ebola death in Kailahun as early as 3 March. However, there is agreement that Mamie Lebbie contracted the virus from a relative who conducted burial rites for a woman called Finda Nyuma.[1] Finda was a renowned traditional healer, and people infected with Ebola had crossed from Guinea into her village in Kailahun in the hope she would be able to treat them.[2]

Burial rituals are a central part of the spiritual life of many Sierra Leoneans, Liberians and Guineans. It is believed that if the right rituals are not performed in the right way by the right people, the deceased can be deprived of peace and rest and be doomed to wander eternally. For James Fairhead, an anthropologist who has been working in the sub-region since the early 1990s, this explains why people tried to stick with their burial practices during the epidemic: "To die of Ebola is one thing, but to be deprived of an afterlife is quite another."[3]

What's more, funerals are a key part of how communities function. They help to reinforce relationships between intermarried families that might be disrupted by the death of a spouse and to sort out potentially contentious issues like who owns what land.[4]

Precise practices vary from place to place, but if the deceased is powerful or famous, funerals can attract huge crowds coming to pay their respects. And so it was with Finda Nyuma. Traditional healers play an enormously significant role in the life of Sierra Leoneans, especially given the weakness and expense of the mainstream health care system.

The burial preparations for Finda Nyuma's funeral were elaborate. Many touched her body to say farewell the night she died – one woman removed her rings, while four friends washed her body using soap and a towel. She was then "washed again by four women from her family, according to local Muslim tradition. They removed her clothing. A cousin tied her hair tightly. Cupping tepid water in their hands, they doused her mouth, and nose and ears, then her feet, and bound her in a white cotton shroud."[5]

Such rituals demonstrate love, honour and respect. Unfortunately, they became extremely dangerous in the context of Ebola, with fourteen people said to have contracted Ebola from this funeral.

Within days of the funeral, Finda Nyuma's husband and grandson were dead, and several of the women who had prepared her body had fallen ill. One of these women passed the sickness to her mother, who then infected her daughter-in-law, Mamie Lebbie.[6] Mamie then travelled the five miles to the local clinic to seek treatment. Initially, the health worker suspected cholera and sent Mamie's stool sample to be tested.

Conspiracy theories

A week after Mamie Lebbie's Ebola test came back positive, the Ministry sent a team of surveillance officers to Kailahun to get a handle on the situation. The delay of a week was problematic, in part because Kailahun's District Medical Officer was new in his post. When the team did arrive, their vehicles were attacked with stones. MSF got the same kind of reaction when they arrived in Kailahun two weeks after that.

The reason for this was a lack of trust, which is hardly surprising. From the slave trade to corruption to the poor response of the national government during the early years of the war, the history of the region was littered with reasons for the local population not to trust the government or foreigners to assist them with this terrible new killer. Some people in Kailahun even felt these outsiders had brought the disease in the first place.

Conspiracy theories abounded. Some questioned the motivations of the government, which likely stemmed from the fact that Kailahun was in the heartland of the opposition party, the SLPP. The Ebola outbreak happened to coincide with the rollout of the national census process, with a population survey due to occur a few months later, in late 2014. One prevalent rumour was that the government was trying to depopulate Kailahun so that opposition supporters would not be counted in the census and hence the district would be allocated fewer government resources.[7] The leader of the first Ministry investigative team was from the north of Sierra Leone, the ruling party's heartland. He later told me his northern last name proved to be a major impediment on that first trip to Kailahun, as people were saying "the government wants to get rid of us to fix the numbers". Other rumours revolved around the belief that the government was using the Ebola crisis to 'eat money', a term commonly used in Sierra Leone for corruption.

There were also rumours that Ebola was a foreign conspiracy. Some said it was a US plot to kill Africans through bio-terror. Others claimed it was a foreign plot to steal the blood of Sierra Leoneans and harvest their organs. I later spoke to a survivor who described how he had initially refused treatment in an Ebola unit:

> I refused to take the injections of the medicine and the drip.
> They tried to force me. I knew a nurse, Rebecca, she was from
> my area. She asked me about the drip, she said it can help you.
> But I thought "the foreigners and government have gotten to
> you, you're on their side. You will remove my blood, give it to
> foreigners, those who don't have blood."

While these rumours might sound irrational, they usually had a linkage to facts, some historical and others contemporary. For instance, the national government did have a long history of marginalising people within this border region. And the US Army's Medical Research Institute of Infectious Diseases had been one of the partners in the Kenema Lassa Fever Centre for several years, involved in research activities which could involve blood samples. To a terrified population that had watched their loved ones die painful deaths from an unknown disease, it was not a huge leap to assign blame in these ways.

Compounding the lack of trust was a very bad start to awareness messaging. The early communications guidelines emphasised that the disease was fatal in an effort to ensure the population took it seriously. Unfortunately, as in Liberia, people interpreted this to mean that Ebola meant certain death – when a survey was done in Kailahun in June, 67% thought that Ebola could only lead to death. Therefore, people said, "Well, if I'm going to die anyway, I would rather die here with my family than look for treatment."

And they had a point. For the first month of the crisis until MSF set up their Ebola Treatment Unit (ETU) in Kailahun, anyone seeking care faced the prospect of a long, arduous and potentially very expensive journey on potholed roads to the ETU that had been set up at Kenema Hospital. Even assuming they survived that journey, the odds were that they would die in Kenema anyway, far from their loved ones and alienated from their traditional burial practices.

The tensions between community members and the response continued for weeks. A group of youths burnt a clinic's supply of medicines for children thinking they were part of the government plot to kill the local residents. Some families went to another clinic and removed family members awaiting their Ebola test results.

At the time, these incidents were described in Freetown and in the media as "community resistance", linked to the "stubbornness" of the people who refused to change their "backward cultures", such as burial practices. But things looked very different to communities in Kailahun. One WHO anthropologist in Kailahun described the population thus: "Angry, frustrated, scared of this disease that was killing them and of these recommendations that clashed with their belief systems, they felt misunderstood and abandoned by the whole world."[8]

OLIVER

A weak start to the response

We were both shocked and completely unsurprised by the news of the first confirmed case on 25 May.

We had found out about it from unlikely quarters. I was contacted by colleagues at Public Health England, a UK government agency, which had a young lab scientist based in Sierra Leone as part of a long-term project to establish cholera testing at the national reference laboratory in Freetown.

The lab had received some stool samples with a request to test them for cholera. These samples had been sent by a clinic in Kailahun, near the border with Guinea, and had been taken from a cluster of patients who were suffering from severe diarrhoea and vomiting. Fortunately, somebody had realised that these patients could in fact have Ebola, not cholera, and warned the lab in Freetown before the testing had started. It would have been incredibly dangerous for the lab staff to have done cholera testing on Ebola samples, since the latter disease is much more deadly and requires far greater infection control.

The laboratory staff were then left to find a way of disposing of these highly contagious samples sitting on the lab bench. The British scientist had asked her supervisors in London for advice, and they in turn had come to us. We advised digging a six-foot-deep pit outside the lab and using petrol to incinerate them. The cholera lab closed after that incident and remained so for the duration of the epidemic. Later the same day, the Minister organised an urgent meeting of her team and the outbreak was officially announced. It was a sign of how weak the preparedness efforts had been that health workers in Kailahun hadn't immediately suspected Ebola and that the correct protocols for handling suspected Ebola samples had not been followed. It wasn't a promising start to the response.

With Ebola now a concrete reality, we realised we would have to refocus our attention on getting Connaught prepared. We had previously found an empty office in the Emergency Department that we had designated the 'isolation room', in which we had put a bench and two 'cholera beds' left over from the last cholera outbreak. These were wooden beds, without mattresses, that had a large hole in the middle so patients with uncontrollable diarrhoea could defecate directly onto the floor.

Dr TB Kamara, the head of the hospital, immediately organised a meeting of senior hospital staff to run through the hospital's preparedness plan. All new patients arriving at the hospital were to be screened by a nurse to determine whether they met the criteria for a suspected Ebola case. The definition of a suspected case during the early stages of the response was any patient who had a recent fever, plus any three symptoms from the list of symptoms associated with Ebola, and a history of recent travel to an Ebola hotspot or contact with an Ebola patient.

According to the plan, if the nurse identified a patient as a suspected case, they should alert the designated Ebola Coordinator, a senior doctor in the hospital, to review the patient and confirm it. The patient should then be admitted to the isolation room and given initial treatment, such as fluids and paracetamol. Treatment for malaria should also be given in case this is the actual cause of their fever. Finally, a blood sample should be taken and sent for testing at the Kenema Lassa Fever Centre. It would then likely take a couple of days to get a result from the lab.

If the patient tested positive, they should be sent to Kenema by ambulance for further treatment. If they tested negative, they should be transferred back to the general wards of the hospital for standard medical care. In addition, Dr Sheik Humarr Khan, Sierra Leone's only virologist and head of the centre at Kenema, was to be called for clinical advice.

But in those early days, this system rarely worked according to plan. The nurses often screened patients improperly and, in any case, screening only applied to patients that presented to the Emergency Department, missing many patients who went directly to different clinics or sought 'off the books' private care in a doctor's office. There was no nurse on duty to perform night-time screenings. We had to keep the isolation room locked to ensure supplies were not stolen or that it was not misused as a staff changing room, and the key was often misplaced by the security guards.

The differences between a development and humanitarian approach

A few different Sierra Leonean colleagues had been nominated as the hospital's Ebola Coordinator at various times, but none of them had really had the time or commitment to do everything that was required.

We had agreed within King's that we should not take charge, but in reality we were having to sort almost everything out, from designing the screening protocol to setting up the isolation room and even doing the clinical assessments when Connaught doctors were unwilling or unavailable. This happened often and from the beginning it was a real stress for the team. On one particular occasion, Colin Brown, who was visiting from London, staggered into the office with one of our other volunteer doctors, ashen-faced and dripping with sweat.

Several hours earlier, they had been called down to the Emergency Department to assess a desperately ill young woman who had presented with a fever. They had isolated her and provided the best care they could in the circumstances, but she had quickly passed away. They thought it was unlikely that she actually had Ebola but had to take all the precautions, which included sealing her corpse in a body bag and scrubbing the floors and walls of the unit with chlorine to decontaminate it. The experience left them feeling fairly traumatised, and they headed off to a local bar after work to have a strong drink and recuperate.

Though we found ourselves responsible for much of the day-to-day work, we insisted the hospital management made the final decisions, which we accepted even when we disagreed, because we believed that our national colleagues knew better than we did about how to get things done in Sierra Leone. With hindsight, however, I regret not offering to take on the leadership of the Ebola unit at this stage, when it became clear that nobody from within the hospital was going to do so – I should have been quicker to recognise that Ebola would require a change in approach, and this hesitancy on my part helped contribute to the dreadful events that would follow.

To me, the question of how assertive to be in a situation like this is at the core of the distinction between developmental and humanitarian approaches to international aid. The development mindset tends to focus on supporting the country to better serve its population over the long term, and therefore recognises the importance of being led by the government. After all, it is the government that (usually) has the democratic legitimacy to make decisions about the country's future and is therefore best placed to run the services that aid agencies are looking to strengthen. Mutual respect and a collaborative relationship between the government and the aid agency are key in this kind of approach. As a result, timelines are usually slower than if aid agencies implement services directly.

A humanitarian approach can sometimes appear to be the exact opposite. The focus in an emergency situation is not on long-term improvements to government systems but on immediate relief for those in need. There is a strong sense of urgency, and aid agencies will sometimes take control, with only a token consultation with the government, so that rapid decisions can be made. Humanitarian budgets can be quite large, allowing the swift hiring of additional staff and the bringing in of supplies for the short-term effort.

Many of us on the ground in Freetown came from a more development-focused background, but we were increasingly finding ourselves in a humanitarian emergency. The transition to a different mindset was hard, and I was slow to realise how my role and approach would need to evolve. Having said that, I was also aware that, sooner or later, the emergency would be over and I did not want us to burn bridges with government colleagues, whose support would be critical again when we returned to development programming. More importantly, I knew our pre-existing relationships could be real assets to the response, and saw the potential to deliver the response in a way that would strengthen rather than undermine government systems. Nevertheless, the tensions between these approaches continued for the entire response.

Duty of care?

As a growing number of suspected cases started to arrive at Connaught, we grew increasingly concerned that we still didn't have the right PPE. We had already had extensive discussions in the Case Management Pillar about what we thought the minimum standards for PPE should be. From the beginning, the Pillar had decided to follow existing WHO guidelines about how to manage Ebola. These guidelines were relatively flexible about the exact specifications for the PPE, provided it covered the right parts of your body and was removed and disposed of in the right way. By comparison, MSF had developed much stricter and more specific standards, which required you to wear thicker PPE suits and more layers of material.

Our opinion on the King's team was that there were pros and cons to both of these options. Whilst the MSF PPE was more impermeable, it was also much hotter and harder to move around in. This made it more likely that you would get exhausted or make a mistake, which could be dangerous. It was also more expensive and difficult to get hold of. Although some argued passionately that the MSF-style PPE was safer, there was actually no evidence to support this claim.[9] In fact, we were told MSF had originally started using this particular PPE only because they had run out of stock of the lighter PPE they had been using prior to that.

With the national PPE shortages at the time, we had to do the best we could with the supplies we could find within the hospital. The storekeeper dug deep into the bowels of the old colonial buildings to pick out anything he thought might be useful. In the end, we cobbled together yellow surgical gowns, hair covers, shoe covers, some paper surgical masks and some surgical glasses that prevented splashes getting into your eyes but didn't protect them completely. This was far from ideal, but was probably enough to protect us until better supplies started to arrive a few weeks later.

Balancing the safety of the King's team with the need to scale up the response as quickly as possible was one my greatest challenges throughout the response, with different organisations in the health sector adopting very different approaches. Some groups said they would evacuate their international staff the moment any Ebola cases were confirmed in their district or hospital. Others put restrictions on their staff, banning them from clinical work and limiting them to administrative tasks.

This was a moral dilemma with no good options. Each organisation had a duty of care not to put their staff at unnecessary risk. It was widely thought at the time that there was an 80% chance of dying if infected, and it wasn't at all clear what treatment we would be able to access. Organisations also had to be mindful of reputational damage – many NGOs worried that if one of their staff died of Ebola, they would open themselves up to a law suit or having their funding withdrawn, thus damaging their wider efforts to help patients.

As health professionals, however, we also had a duty to our patients. Withdrawing from clinical activities not only harmed patients suspected of Ebola, but had enormously detrimental impacts on the care of other patients as well. For example, one NGO suspended their internationally-run outreach clinic, which provided the only health service available to many vulnerable people. Incidentally, this NGO reopened the clinic when one of their directors came for a visit with a press team, then promptly closed it again when the cameras left, much to the consternation of community members.

Most of the decisions made by international NGOs focused on the interests of their international staff – but what of Sierra Leonean health workers? As one senior official at the Ministry angrily pointed out, "It's like the civil war all over again, with all these NGOs packing up their white land-cruisers and abandoning us at the first sign of danger. They don't even bother to tell us their plans, they just leave and expect us to pick up the pieces. But what about us?"

Was it discriminatory to withdraw internationals whilst expecting national staff to stay at their posts and face the challenge alone – especially when international staff were often better trained and thus had a lower risk of infection? Faced with this decision, one NGO decided to close their hospital completely so national and international staff would be equally protected.

At King's, we tried to find a balance by allowing individuals to make their own choices. Although there had been no confirmed cases in Freetown yet, we never knew when the first one might walk through the door. Treating suspected Ebola patients and thereby putting their lives at risk was not what the volunteers had originally signed up for. I gave everyone time to think about it and asked them to opt in to treating Ebola only if they wanted to, but even so worried this still put some degree of peer pressure on them, since everyone in the group did ultimately decide to stay and treat suspected patients. I was concerned nobody wanted to be the first to say no, for fear of letting down their colleagues. As time went on and the risks grew, these questions would gnaw at me more and more.

SINEAD

The ghost town

In the early days after the first case was confirmed, the Ministry painted a positive picture of quick and effective action being taken in Kailahun. But one of our strengths in Irish Aid was that we were close to the NGO community, and it did not take long for our contacts in Kailahun to inform us that what was happening on the ground was far from what the official statements suggested. For instance, the Ministry asked MSF to build an ETU in Kailahun. However, when we discussed this with MSF in a meeting in early June they said there were delays in receiving the necessary paperwork from the Ministry. When they arrived in Kailahun in mid-June and tried to start working, they were hampered by a lack of information and transparency. The Emergency Coordinator recalled: "The Ministry of Health and the partners of Kenema Hospital refused to share data or lists of contacts with us, so we were working in the dark."[10] This immensely complicated their early efforts at surveillance and community engagement.

MSF were horrified when they got to Kailahun: "we realised we were already too late. There were cases everywhere."[11] In addition to concerns about those who were infected, our partners there started to tell us about those left behind. Save the Children called me one day to say that they were increasingly coming across orphans who were not being taken care of. This was highly unusual in Sierra Leone, where extended families commonly care for their orphaned relatives. But some terrified people in Kailahun were reluctant to take in a child whose parents had died from Ebola. In other cases, whole extended families were being wiped out by Ebola, with the exception of a few children. A nurse at the MSF centre spoke to one such child: "[He] told me he doesn't remember how many members of his family have died – he thinks about 13. All he knows is that he is now alone."[12]

In some of the villages first struck by Ebola, large proportions of the village lost their lives. The most affected village at the time was called Njala. A nurse who had treated Mamie Lebbie had died and been buried in Njala, which started a chain of transmission there.[13] A WHO anthropologist describes his arrival in the village:

> Njala was a ghost town. Ebola had killed more than 40 of its residents, nearly a third of the village. Most of the remaining people had fled. Houses were closed, there were a lot of orphans and there was nothing to eat. No one wanted to bring them food, too scared of this unknown, deadly disease.[14]

At this time, we also started hearing of what we began terming the 'secondary crisis' – people being indirectly affected by Ebola. Some frightened, untrained and poorly equipped health workers at local clinics abandoned their posts for fear of catching Ebola from their patients. This meant that people such as those with malaria or women about to give birth had no one to take care of them.

Naturally, with these kinds of reports, our scepticism about the positive noises coming from the Ministry grew rapidly. As a result, my colleagues and I decided we needed to get more involved.

My wake-up call on WHO

On 12 June, I emailed the donor group and a few key diplomats and said that I thought we urgently needed to do two things. Firstly, we had to get together with UN agencies to ask WHO for a frank analysis of the situation and a clear assessment of needs so we could all help. And secondly, we needed to go above the level of the Ministry and meet with President Koroma to express our concerns and offer our support. At the time, based on my experience in Sierra Leone, I didn't see either as a particularly challenging task. I thought the WHO meeting with donors could happen within a few days and the meeting with the President perhaps a week or so later, given the urgency of the crisis.

In my naïveté in those early Ebola days I thought, "Right, health crisis, WHO are here. They know what to do. They are a big global organisation; they will bring in the people they need. And if they have resource gaps, they will tell us and we will help them." I soon found out that not only could we not rely on WHO to sort the response out or give the international community a realistic assessment of needs, but that we donor partners could barely get a meeting with them.

When we did, we discovered that the presence of the WHO representative was not sufficient to gain a better understanding of what was going on with Ebola. In the first meeting of this kind, the WHO team gave a presentation on Ebola, but it focused on the overall numbers of infected cases and deaths, which we already knew. It didn't tell us where the cases were in the country, didn't utilise WHO's previous experience with Ebola to analyse what the data really meant, and, crucially, didn't tell us what we donors and diplomats could do to support the response. The presentation was intended to reassure us, but when I asked a half a dozen questions afterwards, including where could we direct funds, the answers were vague and unsatisfying. This left me so frustrated I texted a diplomatic colleague sitting across from me and requested he congratulate me on the fact I hadn't yet gotten up and hit the presenter over the head with my chair. The response shot back: "You'll have to beat me to it!"

I have often asked myself why I felt so dependent on WHO to coordinate the international community. One obvious factor was my concerns about the Ministry. In March 2013, just over a year before the Ebola crisis started, twenty-nine staff members of the Ministry, including the then-Chief Medical Officer, had been fired for corruption involving the disappearance of over $1 million of international funds meant for vaccination campaigns.[15] The current Minister was not implicated as she had only assumed the role in January 2013. Nevertheless, for this and other reasons, we at Irish Aid simply did not have confidence in the Ministry's systems when Ebola hit. In particular, we wanted WHO to give us an independent view on whether the plans and budgets proposed by the Ministry were covering the right priorities at the right cost.

However, we got none of what we needed or asked for from WHO. And because this was my first time working with them in any in-depth way, I was too slow to realise that we were not going to. This point harks back to the discussion on the development versus humanitarian approach. One of my own personal learnings from Ebola is that I was overly hung up on mandates in the early days. I saw WHO as the global organisation with the mandate on this issue. I was reluctant to bypass them for fear of there being 'too many cooks', which I thought would create chaos and waste valuable time. I still think this is a valid consideration. But looking back, I wish I had gotten sooner into 'emergency mode' and realised that WHO were simply not up to the task and that we needed to find other ways to get things done.

When we realised that WHO's performance on country-level coordination was unlikely to improve, I worked at the international level with DFID and the EU to send messages to WHO in Geneva that they needed to ensure that the organisation's performance in Sierra Leone was massively ramped up.

Meeting the President

When I said in my emails to donors that I was "increasingly thinking the Ebola response needs to go above the Ministry" and that we should meet the President, I had a bit of history in this area. Two years previously, I had seen the State House work quickly and decisively on a health crisis when the Ministry had not stepped up.

In August 2012, about a year after I had arrived in Sierra Leone, the country had a particularly bad cholera outbreak. I say 'particularly bad' because Sierra Leone generally has at least a small number of cholera cases every year. But in 2012, cholera killed 298 people.[16] However, for various reasons, including the fact that the then-Minister of Health was phasing herself out of the role to take up a role with the UN, and the fact that most international actors were on holidays in August, there was a lack of strong leadership in the cholera response. The President had also been out of the country at international meetings when the outbreak had escalated.

On a Sunday night, just after the President returned, I ran into an advisor from his office whom I had been planning to track down at, of all things, a reception for the closing ceremony of the Olympics. The poor guy missed the entire ceremony as I barraged him with information on the cholera situation and the Ministry's inadequate response. He was very concerned and asked me for the statistics, which I emailed to him later that night. Within seventy-two hours, the President had called an emergency meeting of international partners and declared cholera a National Emergency. This declaration enabled some partners to release additional funds, and the coordination of the response improved hugely after this. So, when I saw what seemed an inadequate response to Ebola by the Ministry, it seemed obvious I should take the same approach. I assumed it would work again. I was wrong.

I tried fruitlessly for several weeks to get the President to hold a meeting with international partners on Ebola. I first went to the rest of the diplomats and donor partners and suggested a joint approach, which was agreed upon. We made a formal request, and I and others made informal requests as well. I emailed, called and texted my usual contacts. Nothing worked. It was odd; in terms of meeting diplomats and donors, the President was usually very accessible.[17] I couldn't figure out why he was not getting publicly and deeply engaged in the crisis

Meanwhile, the situation on the ground was getting worse and worse, and not just in Sierra Leone. The Sierra Leone outbreak had reignited the Liberia outbreak, and when I travelled to Liberia in mid-June for meetings, Dr G., the Minister for Health, pointed angrily at me every time he talked about "the outbreak from Sierra Leone". There was a feeling that Sierra Leone had failed to act promptly enough, which had led to Ebola spreading across the border. Given the inadequate response that we were hearing about in Kailahun, it was difficult to disagree.

OLIVER

Too many meetings and not enough action
Alongside getting Connaught prepared for the possibility of Ebola cases, I continued to attend the national Taskforce meetings

after the announcement of the first case. However, I grew increasingly frustrated with how things were going. There were too many meetings and not enough action. One senior Ministry official later summarised the situation as: "WHO were working from a position of weakness. The Ministry were working from a position of darkness." I saw three major problems at the time: the general dysfunction of the response, a lack of transparency about what was going on and the Ministry's insistence on painting the outbreak in a positive light.

Some of the dysfunction at this stage was almost beyond belief. We had one extraordinary situation where the blood sample of a suspected case at Connaught went missing. After hospital staff had collected the sample from the patient, a Ministry team was supposed to transport it from the hospital to the laboratory in Kenema. It was important to keep these samples secure at all times, and the protocol was that they be taken directly to the lab in a special vehicle.

A couple of days after this particular sample had been collected we still hadn't received the result. So we called up the lab, who denied having received it. We tracked down the surveillance officer who had picked up the sample and, after a great deal of denial and obfuscation, he admitted he had taken it home on a public bus. Before leaving for Kenema Hospital, he had then somehow lost the sample in his house.

We couldn't believe that this critical task had been botched in such a dangerous way. After I failed to get assurances from my usual channels at the Ministry that these errors wouldn't be repeated in future, I decided to raise the issue publicly at the next Taskforce meeting. All hell broke loose and the Minister reprimanded the relevant Ministry official. Immediately after the meeting, this official tracked me down. "If you ever embarrass me in public again," he warned me through clenched teeth, jabbing his finger into my chest, "I'll make sure you regret it." This was part of a pattern. When NGOs raised concerns directly in the Taskforce meeting, they were generally shut down aggressively by anyone at the Ministry who might be exposed by it.

This was far from the only example of the dysfunction of the early response, and we were constantly getting reports about how it was playing out on the ground. One Friday in early June, a colleague from an international NGO phoned me to tell me about a friend of hers who was working at a large Catholic mission hospital in Makeni, the regional capital of the north of Sierra Leone.

The story was that a patient had arrived that morning in a taxi with three family members. They were coming from Kailahun and had first gone to the government hospital, where the staff told them to go to the mission hospital instead. By the time they had arrived at the mission hospital, the patient had died. Given the symptoms, the hospital manager was afraid this person might have had Ebola and was anxious to protect her staff, who lacked sufficient equipment or training. She tried to call the Ministry and the district health team but was unable to get hold of anyone. So she refused to take the body, and the taxi left with the corpse and the family members to take the deceased to be buried in their home village.

Every part of this story was a disaster. A patient with symptoms matching Ebola and coming from an Ebola hotspot was being moved around the country, meaning that their family members, the taxi driver, unprepared health workers and participants in the subsequent funeral were potentially being exposed to the virus. And nobody from the Ministry at district or national level could be reached, at 11 a.m. on a Friday morning. These were all the ingredients you would need for Ebola to spread quickly and widely, which was, of course, exactly what happened.

Another issue plaguing the response in those early days was the lack of transparency from the Ministry. In order for doctors in hospitals to identify which patients might be suspected Ebola cases, we needed to know not just their symptoms, but also whether they had come from an Ebola hotspot. We therefore needed to know exactly where any new confirmed Ebola cases were, so we could immediately isolate possible cases.

The Ministry, however, dragged their feet, and for a long time refused our requests to be given access to the laboratory and public health data on new cases. This put us one step behind the outbreak just at a time when we might have been able to get it under control.

When NGOs were finally given access to the daily updates, the data inside them was in complete disarray. These reports were the foundation of the entire response, mapping where new cases were emerging and therefore where the resources should go to stop the spread. One NGO colleague's note to me from a Taskforce meeting was indicative: "The official report was saying we had 163 positive patients: 46 of them had died, 45 were [undergoing treatment] in Kenema, 15 had been discharged. Where were the others?" At this critical phase, when every single person with Ebola needed to be traced and isolated, more than a third of the total were unaccounted for.

We thought the secrecy might be because the Ministry was desperate to put a positive spin on the scale of the outbreak, just as was happening in Guinea. And it was not only the Ministry that was attempting to look at the crisis through rose-tinted glasses. In one particular meeting, an international epidemiologist stood up to proclaim how well we were all doing. "Madam Minister," he said, "Sierra Leone is one of the best-prepared countries on the continent for Ebola thanks to the Kenema Lassa Fever Centre." He assured her that with the country's laboratory testing capacity, and with the resources his team was flying in, she could be confident that everything would be okay. And this was, naturally, exactly what the Minister wanted to hear.

Based on the experiences that they were having in Kailahun, as well as across Liberia and Guinea, MSF put out a statement on 21 June saying that "[t]he epidemic is out of control."[18] With patients emerging in sixty separate locations across the three countries, they found themselves completely overstretched. Once again, they were accused of alarmism, and the Minister was absolutely livid with them for speaking out. In the next Taskforce meeting, she accused them of scare mongering and creating public panic. She asked the MSF Country Director to stand up, but he was absent from this particular meeting, with only a junior colleague there to represent him. The Minister carried on regardless, dressing down the man for the MSF statement and warning others not to speak to the media if they were not 'on message'.

I was so worried about the state of the response that, on 20 June, I decided to write a letter to the Chief Medical Officer at the Ministry, which I later sent on to the Minister, outlining our concerns. Although I did this partly in the hope they would take action, I also wanted to put these issues on the record. All sorts of thoughts were going through my head. What if we ended up getting staff infections at Connaught and people tried to blame King's? Or even sue us? What if we were being seen to endorse the Taskforce budgets or were accused of being complicit if any money went missing?

In the letter, I did my best to be diplomatic but explained that "we have a number of significant concerns, which we believe create a risk that this outbreak will continue to spread in Sierra Leone." I listed nine major areas where we thought the response was not working. There was no reply.

Trying to scale up

After weeks of raising the alarm, the NGOs on the Case Management Pillar were finally given permission to assess hospitals around the country for Ebola preparedness. We divided up the country so that key partners – MSF, King's, the Kenema Lassa Fever Centre and the Ministry – each took responsibility for assessing a different cluster of hospitals.

For King's, this was a huge challenge because we were so under-resourced, and because we only had my car to share between us, we had to hitch a lift or borrow a vehicle from other NGOs in order to do our set of hospital assessments. Although these assessments were never completed, the ones that were done showed that most hospitals around the country were failing on practically every aspect of the preparedness checklist.

I experienced this first-hand when I travelled up to the north of the country for a conference. Marta was due to fly back to Sierra Leone that morning, having gone on leave to New York. I had agreed to pick her up in a town called Port Loko, which was near the airport. For convenience, I suggested we meet outside the town's hospital, since it would be easy to find, and joked that whichever one of us arrived there first should set up an isolation unit while we were waiting.

Sure enough, I arrived to find Marta's suitcases abandoned outside as she, straight off an overnight flight, had taken me at my word and was putting the finishing touches to an improved isolation unit! Staff at the hospital looked bemused but grateful for the help. Looking back on it, I wish we had taken that opportunity more seriously, as that was perhaps the main practical support the hospital had before being overwhelmed with Ebola cases a few months later.

It was clear that the hospitals desperately needed much more hands-on support. MSF were telling us that they were already overextended from their work in Guinea and Liberia, and could not commit more resources to Sierra Leone. The other big health NGOs were nervous about doing hands-on work with Ebola patients, since they had no previous experience and it seemed so risky. Thus, even though we had no Ebola experience ourselves, we began to realise we urgently needed to scale up our role.

We therefore put together a proposal to bring out two infectious diseases specialists from the UK for a month as volunteers, to go and spend time at each hospital helping set up the appropriate screening and isolation facilities. They would train the hospital staff on-site, as well as provide the additional basic equipment (such as buckets, stretchers and signs) needed to make the units function at a basic level. We estimated that we would be able to prepare at least a half-dozen hospitals over four weeks, at a cost of $12,500.

After the next Taskforce meeting, I approached the health advisor from DFID to ask if they would be able to fund us for that work. "$12,500 is too small for DFID," she told me hurriedly as she headed towards the stairs, "we just don't give out that sort of tiny grant." She suggested I try asking UNICEF and WHO instead, which I did, but I had no luck there either.

Not knowing where else to turn, I ended up asking my mother for a donation, which at least helped us get the Connaught unit better established. But we were unable to get funding for the preparedness work in other hospitals, and most were poorly prepared when their first Ebola cases arrived. This led to a total catastrophe a short time later. Looking back, I should have done whatever it took to get the resources we needed, but I underestimated how significant a role our small organisation could, and later would, take.

SINEAD

Aid donors and (in)flexibility

The King's funding request raises a much broader point about the aid sector. The sum of $12,500 was absolutely tiny compared to what we donors ended up spending on the response in Sierra Leone. The US government estimates that US$3.6 billion was spent on Ebola across all three countries so we could conservatively estimate that Sierra Leone's response cost well over US$1 billion.[19] Relatively minuscule amounts, such as the King's request, could have been extremely effective in preventing the spread of the outbreak if they were available early in the response. Why weren't they?

Two reasons: Firstly, we donors did not always know about these requests because of poor coordination, as discussed. Secondly, even if we did know about the requests, our systems did not always allow us to act on them.

It is a broad issue across many governmental aid donors that staff numbers have been cut in recent years, as part of broader cuts in government numbers in many Western countries.[20] This is part of an attempt to increase the efficiency of the civil service and reduce 'bloated government'. As a result, we have fewer and fewer people managing the same amount of money.

Having a low ratio of staff to funds is very problematic in countries like Sierra Leone, where there are high rates of corruption and major issues around capacity shortages in partners such as the government. These factors mean that donors actually need *more* people to understand the context and to be able to develop the best strategies. In addition, in countries like Sierra Leone, the most effective donor role is focused on more than just appraising, spending, and monitoring the use of funds – the 'traditional' donor role. It is also assisting government with our staff and expertise. Otherwise, our taxpayers' money may be spent in a way that does not bring the expected benefit to the population. This broader donor role obviously requires enough quality staff within the donor organisation. This is the hard part!

With lower-than-optimal ratios of staff to funds, many donors have resorted to giving out fewer but larger grants. This makes sense in that if you have fewer grants, staff can focus their limited time on fewer different partners and projects, and thus support and monitor them better. Fine in theory. But problems arise, as in this case with DFID and King's, when donors lose the flexibility to make relatively small strategic and timely investments.

It is a difficult issue, but I think we have two options as donors. By far my preferred option in a context like Sierra Leone, where there are vast needs and real gaps in human resources, is for donors to lobby internally to get more staff. Maybe instead of one health advisor for Sierra Leone, we need three, in order to support the government and provide small or large grants as the context dictates. If that fails, the second option is for donors to reflect on what budget can realistically be spent well, given the available human resources in our field offices, and then lobby for that budget, and no more. The notion of lobbying for smaller budgets is counterintuitive for bureaucrats like myself, as increasing budgets is generally seen as 'success' in bureaucracies, but increased budgets will be counterproductive if we don't have the people to decide how to spend the money for maximum benefit.

In Irish Aid, one of the ways that we mitigate this, to some extent, is by having what we call 'micro-project' funding in our country programmes which can be disbursed quickly. These grants are usually less than $10,000.[21] In my five years in Sierra Leone and Liberia, I found this fund absolutely indispensable. We used it to help partners with urgent issues, such as Ebola-related needs, or to fund a strategic first step towards a larger goal of a policy process. Other donors often called us to ask us to fund something that they believed was important, but didn't have the flexibility to fund themselves.

Having said that, our fund was by no means perfect. We still found that micro-projects took up a lot of our time – it was still Irish taxpayers' money being spent, meaning we needed to monitor each individual expenditure even if the total amount was far less than our other grants. Even so, I would still highly recommend a flexible and quickly administered small-grants fund as one tool in any donor's portfolio.

Obviously, there was also a vital role for the big investments in the Ebola response, and DFID, to their credit, made plenty of those later on.

The beginnings of a response in Kailahun

As we entered the second half of June, three weeks into the outbreak, ninety-one people from Kailahun had been confirmed as Ebola-positive. With the severe resource shortages at the time, it was impossible to keep track of what happened to all of them but, from the cases that were known about, the average fatality rate was 74%.[22] Even worse, many other cases fell outside the system as rumours continued to circulate and people avoided the response. Tensions grew further in late June when the government ordered schools to close in Kailahun and Kenema districts, preventing children from taking their exams and progressing to the next year of schooling.

MSF would normally have had significant community outreach to help with these dynamics, but they were completely overstretched and didn't have the resources to do much else in June other than build their ETU. Despite the desperate situation, the ETU took them longer than usual to build. Apart from the bureaucratic delays from government, there was a huge debate over where the ETU should be built as nobody wanted it near them.

Fortunately, an experienced Ebola hand, Dr Yoti Zabulon, arrived in mid-June to lead the response in the district for WHO. A gentle but resolute Ugandan epidemiologist who worked at AFRO, Yoti showed us that WHO did have high-quality people who could tackle a crisis like this. He had vast experience with the East African outbreaks. When he arrived in Kailahun, unlike most people in Sierra Leone at that time, he could clearly see the big picture and knew what needed to happen next.

Yoti first engaged the local leadership and asked them to assist MSF with the ETU location. Fortunately, local leadership was influential and helpful in Kailahun, led by a popular District Council Chairman. The decision on the MSF ETU was finalised and it opened on 26 June with an initial thirty-six beds. It was a start, but that same week, a month into the outbreak, there were more than eighty new cases reported in Kailahun, and many others under the radar.[23]

Yoti knew there were two key ingredients needed to defeat Ebola: communities changing their behaviours, and a major infusion of resources. Working with a District Taskforce that was established with Ministry staff at district level, the small Ministry team from Freetown, local leaders and some international organisations, Yoti set about guiding these tasks. Awareness-raising sessions started with communities.

The chiefs also set up by-laws to monitor and control movement between villages, and to try to ensure that people both sought treatment if they had Ebola symptoms and reported dead bodies for a 'safe burial'.

A safe burial was intended to avoid the kind of infections that occurred after Finda Nyuma's funeral. The plan was that trained burial teams would bury all corpses in a sanitised manner, in a central location, wearing PPE and using special equipment such as chlorine and body bags. But this was enormously difficult for communities to accept, as it robbed them of the rituals they needed to perform. In addition, community members viewed these burials as "something demeaning and associated with garbage – the plastic [of the bodybag] was seen to be similar to that of a garbage bag and . . . caused relatives to think their loved ones were being 'thrown away like rubbish'".[24]

This issue became the source of one of the greatest cleavages of understanding in the response. Not being well-informed about the context, some international responders could not comprehend why people were so reluctant to undertake a safe burial, since the risks from performing a traditional burial were so high. Couldn't people see that? However, international responders were not alone in displaying a lack of empathy.

Some Sierra Leoneans, particularly those who were more elite or urban, reacted in the same way. One WHO international staffer told me of a meeting where the issue came up:

> We talked about the fear of improper burials leading to relatives haunting them from the grave, which young Sierra Leonean doctors in Freetown laughed about – but if it's the reality of people at community level then this is what we have to deal with. Death is not the worst thing that can happen to people in Sierra Leone.

This is also a lesson for international aid workers. We sometimes assume that if nationals of a country tell us something about a community, that they must be right because they are 'locals'. In actuality, we can't assume that even members of a certain village represent all voices in that village. Instead, we need to exercise our own understanding and empathy.

So, some communities continued to do traditional burials, as well as block access when responders wanted to do surveillance or contact tracing that might lead to more loved ones being taken away. Despite the positive early steps of the District Taskforce, community engagement was set to be a long and difficult road.

Too little, too late

Yoti's second major priority was resourcing. When he arrived, he estimated from his past experience that they could end the Kailahun outbreak if they had $286,000 and sixteen cars for surveillance, complementing the resources being deployed by partners such as MSF. He worked with the District Taskforce to write a proposal for this amount to the WHO office in Freetown. They eventually received $86,000 and one car donated from a UN agency (the Food and Agriculture Organisation). It was not nearly enough.

When I learnt, long after the fact, that Yoti had asked this of the WHO Freetown office in June 2014, I was gutted. I remembered sitting in those meetings in Freetown, along with other donors, pleading with WHO to tell us how we could help. Meanwhile, WHO's own Ebola lead in Kailahun was urgently requesting money, and not getting most of what he needed. As a donor group, I believe we could quite quickly have produced far more than the amount that Yoti had asked for, if only we had known that he was asking. Sometimes talk about things like 'improving coordination' in an emergency response sounds a bit mundane and relatively unimportant, but this was a clear example of just how critical it is.

Resources were also not forthcoming from the Ministry. Their team in Kailahun requested that the Ministry in Freetown send more surveillance officers and were told that there were officers available but some didn't want to go. They were also told that there was no financial support for officers to go, even to put fuel in a vehicle. Yet the Ministry wrote in their situation report of

26 June that the government had allocated US$1.8 million to the Ebola response.[25,26]

A senior Ministry official later told me that there had indeed been money available, but that "Nobody wanted to take responsibility for it. We had money but use of money was a different thing. This is where we did not function. There was no trust. When it comes to money there is no trust." The dysfunction in the Ministry at that time was such that people feared that if they signed off on expenditure, other colleagues would steal the money and they would be held responsible.

All this led to a huge disconnect. This was the observation of one WHO staffer when he arrived in Kailahun:

> At the national level, you could see that people were trying to organize a response, even though it was rather limited. But at the district level, I was so surprised. There was almost no one, except for the district medical officer and a few staff. There was no one from the national level and hardly any partners. There was a real disconnect between the national and district level. The districts were not really supported.[27]

Others, such as Save the Children and UNICEF chipped in to help with the Kailahun response, but it was only a fraction of what was needed. By the end of June, there were 199 confirmed Ebola cases, that we knew of. Though Kailahun had the lion's share of the WHO and MSF Ebola expertise in Sierra Leone at the time, the baseline level of mistrust by the population, early mistakes in community engagement, and under-resourcing of the response meant the critical moment when Ebola could have been contained was missed. This was all too evident when Ebola reached the neighbouring heavily populated district of Kenema, which everybody recognised as the gateway to the rest of Sierra Leone.

SINEAD

Trouble in Kenema

As June turned into July, I started getting alarming phone calls from NGOs in Kenema, a city of 200,000 people located within the district of the same name. I decided to make a visit there on 10 July to see what was going on. The relatively new tarmac road meant you could get from Freetown to Kenema in just four hours, provided traffic wasn't bad.

I made the trip with the British High Commissioner, Peter West, who was a close colleague and good friend. Peter had great political judgement, as well as a dry and often mischievous sense of humour. We were both tall, but other than that we were pretty different. Peter, in his mid-fifties, looked the quintessential diplomat with his salt and pepper beard, navy suits, and (what I considered to be) posh English accent. As a woman in my mid-30s, on the other hand, I didn't fit in with many people's stereotype of an ambassador. At one meeting with visitors from the UN, the organiser of the meeting, who was new to Sierra Leone, assumed I was the Irish Ambassador's personal assistant, holding the fort until 'he' arrived. I couldn't resist playing along, citing "traffic".

Our Embassy was next door to the British High Commission, so Peter and I often shared a car to meetings, although there was usually a tussle over whose car we would take. My car was bigger, making it the practical choice, but that meant Peter had to sit behind the Irish flag flying at the front of the vehicle, which he always complained bitterly about!

We left Freetown at 5 a.m., reaching Kenema just in time to sit in on the morning meeting of the Kenema District Ebola Taskforce at the UNICEF office. To get to UNICEF, we had to pass through the centre of the city and the shops of the Lebanese diamond merchants, which always seemed incongruous to me. Living in Freetown, you could easily forget that the country had a profitable export-oriented diamond industry in the east with significant foreign investment. Then again, you could also forget this in Kenema town as you bumped along its potholed, unpaved roads, given that most of its population lived below the poverty line.

The Kenema District Taskforce meeting that morning, chaired by local government leadership, consisted of about thirty people around the UNICEF conference table, including UN and NGO staff who were helping out with the response. The meetings had started in late June. One of the WHO staff told me about the first meeting:

> It took place at the town hall. But there was a giant thunderstorm
> halfway through the meeting which, given we were under a
> tin roof, made listening and providing technical advice almost
> impossible. A decision was reached to hold District Taskforce
> meetings every day at UNICEF, something I wholeheartedly
> supported, though would soon regret with the amount of time
> they would take.

Indeed, the meeting we attended that morning ran way over time. The issues being discussed were daunting. The Ministry was reporting 315 confirmed cases so far in the outbreak, with sixty-seven new cases in the past week.[1] None of us thought that even these figures reflected anything close to the real numbers on the ground. But even with the questionable data, the District Taskforce could see that more and more cases were originating from Kenema itself, rather than coming over from neighbouring Kailahun. The meeting included candid discussions on the gaping holes in the response.

For instance, seventy-eight contacts of confirmed Ebola patients had not been visited for several days. This meant that some of these people could have developed symptoms and be passing on the infection to others. In one case, a man had been diagnosed with Ebola after spending several days in a private clinic, which proceeded to operate as normal, even though there was a high chance that staff might be infected and contagious. The health workers from Kenema Government Hospital were supposed to go there and check if the staff had symptoms, but were too busy at the overwhelmed ETU. There were similar difficulties to Kailahun in engaging with communities; the District Medical Officer said he had recently shown up at an awareness-raising event in a village but that "only goats were met in the meeting venue."

It was an incredibly difficult situation. The District Taskforce came up with action points, but only a small fraction of these were implemented from one meeting to the next. We observed a lot of very senior, well-intentioned and worried people in the room, but they ran into two big problems that were outside of their power to fix: not nearly enough resources, and poor coordination.[2]

The gap was in both financial and human resources. The financial gap was similar to the situation in Kailahun. But Kenema had an even bigger gap in technical expertise – Kenema didn't have MSF and had fewer WHO experts than Kailahun. The few WHO staff in Kenema at the time were so busy at the ETU and with surveillance that attending these long Taskforce meetings put them under huge pressure.

This links to coordination, which was a vital skill-set missing in this meeting. Like its national counterpart, the District Taskforce would get bogged down in details. Peter and I witnessed a twenty-minute discussion about the need to get raincoats for people working at the checkpoints the government had set up on the main roads to monitor people for Ebola symptoms. This was an important need given the daily monsoon-like rains, but didn't require twenty minutes of the time of the entire District Taskforce. What's more, as was often the case in meetings in Sierra Leone, everybody would get to say their piece; in non-crisis times, this was often an endearing reminder of how relatively non-hierarchical Sierra Leone was, but in this kind of situation it just wasted precious time.

The media often portrays emergency responses as incredibly exciting, with responders dashing around refugee camps in the middle of the wilderness or jumping onto helicopters in flak jackets to get to the latest inaccessible conflict. However, most emergency response work is a lot less sexy, taking place in planning and coordination meetings and requiring skills such as meeting management, minute-taking, mapping out who is doing what, and writing situation reports.

These skills have been recognised as so critical in the humanitarian response world that there is an entire UN agency called the Office for the Coordination of Humanitarian Affairs (OCHA). After seeing this meeting in Kenema, I started calling for OCHA to be deployed in the Ebola response.

Having said that, excellent coordination would not have been enough in Kenema without more resources – there were not nearly enough ambulances, not nearly enough burial teams, not nearly enough contact tracers to get the job done.

Sierra Leone's first ETU

After the District Taskforce meeting, Peter and I drove to the hospital, passing through the market where traders lined the streets with their makeshift stalls, selling bananas, soap, rice, second-hand t-shirts from Europe and a multitude of other wares. Kenema Government Hospital was the main hospital in the east of the country and had a catchment population of over 650,000 people.

I knew the hospital well from previous visits to monitor programmes that Irish Aid funded.[3] It was home to the district's main treatment unit for malnourished children, and housed International Rescue Committee's (IRC) 'Rainbo Centre'– one of only three centres in the country where a girl or a woman could go for support if she had been sexually assaulted. I had probably been to the hospital close to a dozen times over the years, but I had never seen it like it was that day in July.

We entered through the large gates, manned as usual by security guards trying to find a reprieve from the sun as midday approached. Normally, despite the security, the town spilled into the hospital, with street traders roaming around the compound selling snacks to people waiting for treatment. But, that day, the whole place felt eerily deserted. People had developed such a fear that they would catch Ebola at the hospital that many preferred to stay away, no matter how sick they were.

The hospital was a large sprawling compound with various white-painted buildings linked by covered concrete walkways and separated by patches of grass or open spaces where cars and motorbikes were parked. These buildings were in various states of repair depending, in part, on whether they had a donor-funded project going on inside.

An energetic young American from IRC showed us around what had become the Ebola section of the hospital. The IRC, led by a Sierra Leonean friend of mine, Saffea Senessie, were working like Trojans, trying to plug the many holes in the response in Kenema, and we were providing them with some funding for this effort.

We first went to the Lassa Fever Centre. It might seem strange that the government chose to set up the first lab and treatment unit for Ebola in Kenema, rather than in Freetown, which had a disproportionate number of the country's hospitals and health workers. The reason for this was the presence of this centre, led by Dr Sheik Humarr Khan. Although less infectious and deadly than Ebola, Lassa fever was from the same family of viruses.

The centre was supported by Tulane University and a private company called Metabiota, both from the US. We spoke to some of the busy lab scientists from Tulane, who explained how they had adapted the Lassa testing protocol to test for Ebola, which involved detecting genetic material from the virus in a patient's blood.

When I asked about their challenges the lab staff said their main one was preventing infection while handling the samples. They were fortunate to have highly trained staff who had experience of testing for Lassa, but they were being inundated with samples from different parts of the country, since they were the only government lab that was advanced enough to do this testing. The only other lab in the country at the time which could test for Ebola was a Canadian lab set up next to MSF in Kailahun to test suspected cases from their ETU. The previous day, in addition to testing thirty-five patients from Kenema and Kailahun, the Kenema lab staff had tested eight patients from the southern districts of Bo and Moyamba, the northern district of Port Loko, and Freetown. From these forty-three samples, twenty-seven (63%) patients tested positive, including five from outside the hotspot areas.[4] Despite the impression being given by the Ministry, Ebola was on the move.

We then walked the short distance to the ETU and saw the makeshift tents and tarpaulin which had been set up to separate the suspected patients from the confirmed patients. Having unconsciously built an Ebola Treatment Unit up in our minds as something highly sophisticated, Peter and I were amazed at the simplicity of the set up. While we were looking around the outside of the structure, a group of suspected Ebola patients arrived in the back of a Toyota Land Cruiser ambulance from a nearby village. Staff in PPE suits guided three men into the suspect ward to be tested.

The Ministry was running the ETU with WHO support. Similar to the decision that Kenema should be the national referral lab for Ebola, the national Taskforce decided that Kenema Hospital's experience on Lassa fever would make it the best referral centre for patients too. They said that staff were more prepared to treat Ebola patients, and would be able to provide better medical care and maintain higher safety standards than others could.

So it had been decided that as soon as anybody tested positive for Ebola, they should be moved by ambulance to Kenema. As a result, the ETU, like the lab, was completely swamped with patients, mostly from Kenema but increasingly from other districts too.

Naturally, we were not permitted to enter the 'red zone' for confirmed Ebola patients, but we were able to speak to some of the recovering patients through a fence around the back of the confirmed tent. This setup was an excellent idea, as it enabled family members to visit and speak with patients who were well enough to go outside. It was a simple adaptation to the design of the ETU, but a huge psychological boost for patients and families. I spoke to a woman named Hawa who was going to be discharged the following day. She was so radiant at the prospect I didn't want to dampen her mood by asking her about her experiences, so I could only imagine what harrowing times she must have gone through.

A wing and a prayer

We then met with District Medical Officer, Dr Mohamed Vandy, the head of health for Kenema, who I knew from previous visits. Dr Vandy was a good guy doing his best, but he was completely overwhelmed. He seemed delighted to see Peter and me that day, albeit surprised, and I felt a bit guilty for not telling him in advance we were coming. But I had my reasons. I knew from experience in Sierra Leone that if a government official knows a couple of diplomats will be visiting, there is a very good chance they will drop other plans in order to receive us, even if they are in the middle of a crisis. So, to avoid this, I snuck around the country during the Ebola outbreak, trying to minimise the amount of the practitioners' time I took up. I just needed enough time to grasp the key issues so that I could relay these to higher levels and then I would get out of their way.

What was evident from speaking with Dr Vandy was that the ETU was operating very much on a wing and a prayer. As at Connaught, Sierra Leonean doctors were reluctant to treat Ebola. The small number of WHO doctors that had been seconded there, who were supposed to be mentoring Ministry staff, were instead having to spend most of their time treating patients themselves, with the support of Ministry nurses.

Although these health workers were making huge efforts, the national response was so weak and case numbers were climbing so fast that the work in the ETU was completely unsustainable. Critical gaps were emerging all the time. Two days before we arrived, the hospital had run out of chlorine, with fifty-three confirmed patients in the ETU. They had to borrow some from MSF in Kailahun, a four-hour drive away. There is probably nothing more critical to the operation of an ETU than chlorine, save perhaps gloves for health workers, and shortly after our visit, Kenema ran out of those too. Again, they had to be bailed out by MSF, who of course also needed their limited gloves and chlorine supply.

Our meeting with Dr Vandy that day provided us with a concrete example of how the weak coordination at national level was manifesting itself. When Peter asked him how he found the support from the Ministry, Dr Vandy said, "Oh, yes, it's very good. The Minister is very supportive. I just text her. Even at 4 a.m., I can text her and say 'We don't have any gloves left', and she will send me gloves." While it was of course positive that the government's top health official was deeply engaged with the response, the fact that the district-level representative was texting her directly to put in supply requests for the ETU spoke to a total lack of proper systems in the response, six weeks after the start of the outbreak.

Ministry battles

To understand why the Minister was answering text messages from Dr Vandy at 4 a.m, it is important to understand a bit about the political dynamics within the Ministry at that time. These politics were hindering the coordination agenda and undermining the possibility of a strong response. Within the Ministry, there were two camps: the Minister's camp, and the camp that was keen to see her fired.

The Minister, Miatta Kargbo, was tall and striking, and alternately described as passionate or domineering depending on which camp a person was in. The 'pro' camp contended that the Minister was trying to enact reforms that would reduce endemic corruption in the health sector. The 'anti' camp claimed she was inexperienced and arrogant, and that she refused to listen to senior staff of the Ministry. The 'pro' camp argued the reason she didn't listen was because she knew they were out to sabotage her. And so on. Within all this, it was probably not insignificant that she was a relatively young woman in a government, and a society, that was very male-dominated.

One example of how this battle manifested itself was when the Minister announced a plan to send one of the deputy ministers to Kenema to help with coordination. I remember being keen on this idea, as there was such a gulf between the national and district-level discussions. But the deputy refused to go as agreement could not be reached on his housing arrangements.

The country is facing a huge health crisis and a decision at the ministerial level falls down over housing arrangements? As with so much of the early response, even these seemingly minor issues were unresolvable given the politics in the Ministry.

Firefighting

In Kenema that day, Dr Vandy knew things were bad but, like most of us, it was his first Ebola outbreak and he didn't have anything to compare it to. It was only later in the day when we spoke with British epidemiologist Chris Lane, a volunteer with WHO and veteran of other Ebola epidemics in Uganda and Democratic Republic of the Congo, that we started to understand how meagre the valiant efforts in Kenema were compared with the need.[5] As Chris explained to us, we were way behind the virus. He noted that there was essentially no district-level plan – everybody was just firefighting. Ebola would only be stopped at the community level when people believed Ebola was real (not just a government or foreign conspiracy), and when they changed their behaviour by avoiding contact with people who might have Ebola, making sure that these people went to the ETU to be tested and cooperating with the new policy of safe burials for all deaths (the government had recently decided not to limit safe burials to suspected Ebola deaths).

Of course, this was all far easier said than done given how few resources there were to support communities, with people often waiting several days for dead bodies to be picked up and buried. Chris stressed that the response needed many more "boots on the ground" to do awareness-raising and surveillance. But, for this, WHO needed far more international staff with the right experience in the field to guide and supervise this work.

We left Kenema sombre. While there was a great deal of commitment and goodwill, it was clear what was happening was only a fraction of what was needed to get ahead of the virus. Things were bad and getting worse.

Complacency

Back in Freetown, I was struck by how little sense there was of what was going on four hours down the road. There was no feeling of alarm or urgency. That same week, we diplomats were invited to a meeting with the Ministry of Foreign Affairs, who had begun holding quarterly update meetings with diplomats on key current issues. I was happy to see this meeting was on, until I noticed Ebola was not on the agenda as a 'current issue'. What could have been more important for us to talk about with the government of Sierra Leone at that moment in time? It felt like a parallel universe. I emailed a group of donors and diplomats to indicate my incredulity about this and one colleague wrote back, agreeing that it was strange but saying "I think we should not impose" by suggesting it be added to the agenda. I thoroughly disagreed! I contacted the Ministry to request it and they put it on the agenda and, in the end, it was actually all we talked about.

But it was not just the government that seemed slow to grasp what was going on. Ebola was not much of a topic of conversation in Freetown at all, with most headlines in the newspapers about other issues. Many of my Sierra Leonean friends saw a parallel with the early years of the civil war, before it hit Freetown: "Here we go again. Until it comes to our doorstep we will just live with our head in the sand." They said it was not that people didn't know what was going on, it was that they didn't *want* to know.

While donors were still having no luck meeting the President, we managed to get a meeting with some cabinet ministers, chaired by the Minister of Finance. I welcomed it at least as an opportunity to get an update on the data from the Minister of Health. They had stopped the daily updates on case numbers, due to what the Minister called "misuse of data by unscrupulous journalists."

Before leaving for the meeting, I got a call from the UN to say that the Assistant Director-General of WHO, Dr Keiji Fukuda, was in Freetown on a trip from Geneva. He was to meet with President Koroma that day, having visited Kenema the day before. This was great news. Maybe hearing about these issues from such a high-ranking WHO official would be the wake-up call President Koroma needed. I called a friend in Kenema to ask how the visit had gone. "Great", he said. Apparently, Dr Fukuda had been so struck by the situation in Kenema that he had extended his stay, originally scheduled for just a few hours, and spent the night so that he could have more discussions. "This is excellent," I thought. "He will have heard plenty of substance to report to the President."

I drove to the meeting with Peter, who I had asked to attend. Normally, the British High Commission wouldn't have attended as such meetings were more for donor agencies than diplomats. But DFID was going through a period of leadership transition and it was also a time when staff were starting to take summer holidays. There had therefore been gaps in who had been attending Ebola meetings on behalf of DFID over the previous couple of weeks. I would sometimes find myself texting people in DFID at the start of meetings to see if anybody was coming. This worried me because we needed the UK – they were the lead donor in health and the largest bilateral donor to the country. I thought maybe the High Commission could help provide some consistency.

Peter and I made our way to an air-conditioned conference room at the Ministry of Finance, and sat down at the glossy oval conference table, behind the placards bearing our country names.

The Minister of Health spoke first, reeling off an enormous shopping list for the Ebola response. "There is a need for gloves, PPE, ambulances, fuel, chlorine, mobile phones for contact tracers, body bags, beds for the centres . . .". I didn't disagree with any of it, but it was totally un-prioritised. Given how few resources we had and how severe the outbreak was becoming, we needed to know what the most pressing needs were in order that we could support them. We were disappointed, although not particularly surprised, that the Minister did not provide any kind of serious analysis of what was going on.

Clearly irritated, the Minister called for donors to do more. She talked about commitments made by donors that "were not yet seen". This is often a valid point – donors can make commitments on paper, especially in emergencies, that they often take a long time to meet, and sometimes don't meet at all. But in this case, there were also other sides to the story. For instance, one donor had given the Ministry authorisation to reallocate their funds, which had already been transferred to the Ministry's bank account, to Ebola. But the Minister refused. The donor recounted: "I told the Minister, you need to restructure the health portfolio, you won't be able to do most of this other stuff anyway. But she said we want new money." And then of course there was the issue of trust which was always underlying our interactions with the Ministry.

Next, it was our turn as donors to talk. I talked about the huge gaps in Kenema. I also reiterated a call that many of us in the donor community had been making for weeks, for a 'command and control' centre at the national level which would focus on the technical aspects of the response. This was also a veiled way of saying we needed the Minister and other politicians to stay out of the day-to-day operations. Other donors made similar points. The Minister was not happy with us speaking so negatively, but even so I thought the meeting was going okay.

Then Keiji Fukuda came in, straight from his meeting with the President. I hadn't known he had been scheduled to attend and was encouraged. I scribbled a note to Peter saying, "Nice! He'll give the Minister a reality check about Kenema."

Dr Fukuda took the floor and started off stressing the need for a prioritised plan by the Ministry and better coordination. So far so good. But then he concluded by saying: "The Ministry is doing all the right things. The situation is not out of control as some people are saying." I couldn't believe my ears. How was this possible, after what he must have seen in Kenema?

Later, I would come to understand that this was not necessarily Dr Fukuda's individual view based on what he had seen – WHO staff in Kenema told me he really 'got' the severity.[6] Rather, this was a high-level representative of WHO verbalising the agreed institutional position. This position reflected WHO's prioritisation of their relationship with host governments over, it seemed to me that day, alerting the world of an impending crisis. I later found out that, a few weeks before, a memo had been sent to the WHO Director-General advising her against declaring Ebola a global emergency, known as a 'Public Health Emergency of International Concern'. The memo noted that there was a risk that if

WHO made this declaration, the governments of Sierra Leone, Guinea and Liberia could interpret it as a "hostile act".[7]

But that discovery came later. When the meeting was wrapping up at the Ministry of Finance, I was livid and frustrated. How could the rest of us make the case for how bad things were and how much improvement was needed if the global health experts in WHO were saying things were moving in the right direction?

OLIVER

Riot at Connaught Hospital

Seeing suspected cases at Connaught was no longer an exception; it had become the norm.

One day, we got a call from a director at the Ministry about an elderly man in a coma admitted to our intensive care unit, who the doctors thought was suffering from a stroke. The patient was an acquaintance of his and, it turned out, was the storekeeper at the government hospital in Kailahun, the epicentre of the outbreak at that time. The director advised us to isolate the patient immediately. We did, and he died overnight.

His family members were outraged, convinced that we had taken him to the isolation unit in order to kill him. About twenty more family members arrived at the hospital. They didn't think Ebola was real, and thought that we had murdered him with a poisonous injection. Early efforts to calm them only made matters worse, and when they were told they could not take away the body until the results from the Ebola test had been completed, they became aggressive. As a throng, they stormed through the hospital towards the administrative building, where the King's office happened to be situated.

The first I heard of it was a huge commotion approaching on the pathway outside. As I headed out into the corridor to investigate, I was astonished to see one of the hospital's most esteemed doctors scrambling up the stairs on all fours and yelling to a secretary to lock the door to her office behind him. We heard the angry cries of the relatives getting closer, and the five of us in the office had a quick discussion on what to do. Some of the team thought we should lock ourselves inside our office as well, but I pointed out that if we did this we would be trapped, as this was the only exit. I was worried that locking the door might only make the crowd more confrontational, and could enrage them into smashing down the door or setting the building on fire. We decided that we would stay seated at our desks with the door open, in a totally nonconfrontational posture, in an effort to deescalate the situation.

At that moment, Dr Eva Hanciles dashed into our office, having been chased by the deceased patient's relatives through the building. She was a formidable woman, so if she was afraid, it meant that things were really out of control. She insisted that we lock our door and, after an awkward moment where my team looked to me to decide whose orders they should follow, I agreed to follow her judgement. We remained holed up there until the chaos outside subsided.

As it turned out, the late storekeeper had not had Ebola. But the incident panicked many of the senior doctors and made them even more reluctant to engage with Ebola for fear of being infected. Several of them had cared for the patient without the precautions that would have protected them from Ebola had he been infected. The risk of attack compounded their fears, and many doctors therefore decided to stay away entirely from Ebola matters from that point forward.

Dr TB Kamara discussed the risks with the senior management of the hospital and decided to request a permanent police presence. A team of police officers was dispatched to secure the main gate where the Ebola unit was located. This was the start of a security presence at hospitals nationwide, one that would only grow in the months that followed.

It also became clear to me that day that we would never be able to control the outbreak if communities did not believe the disease was real and had no trust in health workers. The current situation of distrust left us as sitting ducks, sandwiched between a flawed government strategy and increasingly hostile patients.

Expanding the Connaught Ebola unit

A few days later, Marta called up to the office from the wards to tell me that she had referred a suspected Ebola patient to the two-bed isolation room. Before long, I got another call saying a second patient had been admitted and that both beds were now occupied. A third suspected case was identified in the Emergency Department and had to be left on a bed in the general ward as there was nowhere to put them, which of course was unsafe. Marta and I hurriedly searched for senior colleagues to tell them we needed to radically scale up our isolation room, as we had clearly underestimated the number of cases we were going to be seeing in the coming weeks.

As a group, we toured the Emergency Department and decided to shut down half of it, an entire wing of the building, to set up a nine-bed isolation unit. It was already 5 p.m., but our team and hospital staff, including Dr Martin Salia (the head of department), Sister Cecelia Kamara (the nurse in charge), Dr Hanciles, and the maintenance team got to work. I sent our office assistant out with a bundle of cash to buy as much plastic sheeting as he could from the local market, whilst the hospital put in an urgent request for essential equipment. Two young male cleaners volunteered to scrub the place clean, even though they had not received their salary for months. The maintenance team put up fans overhead and removed the dirty ripped curtains that had separated the beds for years, replacing them with plastic sheets to help stop Ebola from spreading between beds through projectile vomit or other means.

I worked with Dr Terry Gibson, a retired consultant physician from London who had joined us as a long-term volunteer, to find the most intact mattresses we could from around the hospital. Most had their foam sticking out, which absorbed any fluids that touched them, a huge problem when it came to Ebola infection. Even the quasi-intact mattresses that we did find needed to be wrapped in plastic.

The unit wasn't perfect but it would do, and we were proud of our handiwork. It was an extraordinary moment of camaraderie and teamwork, and showed what is possible when a committed group of people comes together with a common purpose, even within a government hospital that is dysfunctional in other ways. Little could we have predicted that over 1,000 patients would be isolated in this unit over the coming year, of which over 500 would test positive for Ebola.

At about 10 p.m., just as we were putting the finishing touches to the new unit, a nurse from the other side of the Emergency Department came to tell me there was another patient she was worried about and wanted me to see. I told her that, surely, we couldn't have four suspected Ebola patients in one day, but she corrected me – it wasn't Ebola she was worried about, but cholera. A young boy had been carried up from Kroo Bay, the slum on the waterfront just below the hospital, with acute watery diarrhoea. When I saw him, he was collapsed listlessly on the examination couch.

It was almost too much for me to take in, because our contingency plan for a cholera outbreak had been to close off the other half of the Emergency Department as a cholera unit. The thought of having to manage two separate infectious disease outbreaks in the hospital at the same time pushed me close to breaking point, and I had to take a moment to steel myself. We got lucky – it turned out that the patient did not have cholera, and that nightmare scenario never came to pass. But others would.

Ebola reaches Freetown

On 10 July, we got confirmation of the first Ebola case in Freetown, but as usual this information came through informal networks rather than from the Ministry or WHO. A friend had received an email forwarded from one of the big NGOs in Freetown, who had received a forwarded email from their headquarters in London, of an email sent by a UN team in Senegal describing their briefing from the WHO representative in Sierra Leone. Just to recap, this was how we, at the main hospital in Freetown, got news of the first confirmed Ebola case in Freetown.

The patient was a young man from a village in Kenema, whose mother and brother had died. He had then travelled to Freetown and spent nine days sick in a house with his relatives, before going to Macauley Street Hospital just up the road from Connaught, where he spent five days on the general wards without being screened for Ebola. Eventually, as his symptoms progressed, the staff decided to contact the Ministry's disease surveillance team, who transferred him by ambulance back to Kenema for Ebola treatment. Shortly after that, he died.

The first case in Freetown had also shown us the huge risk that health workers on the general wards in hospitals were facing. Alongside our efforts to set up the isolation unit at Connaught, where we now had a small supply of PPE, we were working hard to improve infection control measures across the rest of the hospital. We ran refresher courses on hand washing and helped nursing staff do audits of broken sinks and shortages of gloves or soap on the wards. We scrambled around for supplies, but every plastic apron in the Ministry's central stores had already been deployed to health facilities around the country. At King's, we still had no money for our Ebola work, but my colleagues in the UK had approached Guy's & St Thomas's Hospital in London, who stepped in to donate over a tonne of supplies. We were able to convince Gambia Bird Airlines to ship them over to us for free.

Within twenty-four hours of the first case in Freetown, we had our first confirmed case at Connaught. A disease surveillance officer brought in a young man from Kenema who had a fever and had been sick for a week. When he had gone to a local clinic in Freetown, the staff had become suspicious because of his links to Kenema and had called the Ministry. The Connaught junior doctor, who was on the duty roster for the isolation unit that day, was called to see the patient but refused to go inside until Marta agreed to accompany him.

That night, the lab results came in that the patient was positive, and an ambulance was called to take him to Kenema for treatment. The same thing happened the next day when another suspected case arrived – the junior doctor on call refused to treat the patient until Marta went in with him. It became even clearer that our plan at King's to take a backseat, and support the Ministry doctors in taking a lead on Ebola, were not working. We were going to have to step up our role.

Hazard pay

Whilst the doctors at Connaught were increasingly unwilling to go inside the isolation unit, we were having a bit more success with recruiting nurses, cleaners and lab technicians, some of whom needed the extra money. The matron and her colleague, Sister Cecilia, had appealed to the nursing staff and managed to cajole four nurses from the Emergency Department to help us.

Susan Mohammed and Lovetta Jawara worked on the morning shift together, whilst Tamba Senessie helped with the afternoon shift. The hospital was normally quite deserted at night but one older male nurse who worked in the trauma ward, Joseph Lahai, had agreed to supervise the unit during his usual night shift. For suspected cases, the nurses' job was to give the patients their medications each day, which was a mixture of tablets and injections, and to ensure they had enough food and water. They also helped counsel patients and relatives, remove corpses if the patient died, and ensure that the unit was clean.

Just as important for the unit were our cleaners, who became known as 'hygienists' during the Ebola response. They would make up the chlorine solutions for cleaning and decontamination, mop the floors and help sterilise the beds between patients by spraying down the walls, plastic curtains and the bed itself. Preventing the virus from spreading between suspected cases in the unit, infecting staff, or getting out of the red zone and contaminating other parts of the hospital was a top priority, so their role was critical.

Two of the hospital cleaners had volunteered to work in the unit early on, Abdulai Sesay and Mohamed Sillah. The two men were chalk and cheese. Abdulai was short, elderly and very hard to communicate with. He was, however, tireless, and once he set off on a task he was unstoppable, vigorously scrubbing everything in sight. Mohamed was young, tall and handsome, and had a natural charisma and intelligence that made him Abdulai's interlocutor and a very safe pair of hands.

The security guards based at the front gate also had an important role in stopping people from accidentally walking into the unit and in preventing patients from leaving. The latter was easier said than done and normally involved a lot of shouting. While we had made the space work for us, the way the unit was laid out was a real problem. For suspected Ebola patients to get into the unit, or for confirmed cases or corpses to be brought out, they had to travel down the same corridor the staff used to get to the office and PPE dressing room. We did our best to manage this by having the cleaners spray the corridor with chlorine regularly, but we did occasionally have suspected cases trying to wander into our office by accident, forcing us to back away into the corner while we hurriedly redirected them. Normally, though, the security guards prevented these kinds of incidents.

Another key role for the cleaners and security guards was disposing of waste, which had to be incinerated, as it was highly dangerous. The hospital had no suitable incinerator, so we arranged for a big hole to be dug, where we would pile up the rubbish and incinerate it with kerosene. Unfortunately, the only space we could find was halfway down the cliff face at the back of the hospital. Because it was rainy season we had real trouble keeping the fire lit, so we build a zinc roof over the pit, although this was soon stolen by a couple of guys from the shanty town below.

Safely getting the sewage-filled bags of leaking rubbish from the patient buckets in the unit to the pit was a nightmare. In the end, we took an old patient gurney to a welder and built a watertight metal box on top that resembled a coffin. Once a day the rubbish would be piled into the box and wheeled slowly through the hospital, with an escort of security guards, and cleaners in full PPE spraying chlorine in front and behind, like a bizarre funeral procession. It was far from ideal, but it worked.

We also needed lab technicians from the hospital laboratory on the floor above us. They would come down twice a day to take blood samples from the patients and package them for collection. With the lab technicians, we were faced with the opposite problem to that we had with the doctors. When we asked for three lab techs, one for each shift, we were given a list of thirteen by the head of the lab, who refused to edit the list down. Every one of the hospital lab techs wanted to be on the team.

The main reason for the enthusiasm from all these staff was simple: money. The moment we had admitted our first confirmed Ebola patient, the staff who worked in the unit had become entitled to receive a weekly hazard pay, also known as risk allowance, from the Ministry. This had been agreed by the Taskforce early in the response as a national programme and was initially set at 100,000 Leones per week, which was about $25. For doctors, this allowance was pitiful compared to their overall income and did little to incentivise them to work in the unit or put themselves at risk. But for other staff, this amounted to a significant salary top-up.

A few months later, the amount was quadrupled to $100 a week, making it an extremely lucrative job for staff who might usually have only received that amount as their monthly salary and who were struggling to make ends meet. Mohamed soon recruited his two younger brothers to join him as cleaners, which meant that between them they were due to earn $1,200 per month, which they hoped would allow them to save enough to finish their education and start their own small business.

These staff thoroughly deserved this extra pay for doing such arduous and risky work. Indeed, they deserved a lot more, especially when you compared what they were earning to the eye-watering sums we heard many UN staff were being paid as 'risk allowance', despite sitting in air-conditioned offices far from the actual danger. Whilst many of the staff in our isolation unit were motivated by compassion for our patients and a sense of patriotic duty to Sierra Leone, the hazard pay was a major reason why they came to work each day.

But in spite of the hospital sending off the appropriate letters and paperwork to the Ministry, the staff complained that they weren't receiving the money they had been promised. Before long they started going on regular strikes, which was a disaster for the patients and left the King's team covering shifts in a desperately short-staffed unit.

My first patient

I wouldn't normally have come in to work over the weekend, but, towards the end of July, with Ebola taking hold in Freetown and the staff strikes, I had woken up knowing that I wouldn't be able to relax until I'd checked that everything was okay. Stepping through the front entrance of Connaught, I was confronted by a restless crowd of nurses, porters and onlookers anxiously staring at the gate of our isolation unit. In their midst was the stocky and assertive hospital matron. At the centre of her gaze, beyond the gate, were two middle-aged men dressed up to the waist in white suits of personal protective equipment, their hands half-jammed inside ill-fitting medical gloves. They were sprayed with blood, and unconscious at their feet was the young boy who would turn out to be my first Ebola patient. As we caught sight of each other, they froze, and so did I.

The crowd of staff and onlookers turned towards me expectantly, looking reassured that I'd be able to sort out the situation. I really had no idea. I hadn't done any clinical work since medical school three years before, and I had never been taught how to handle Ebola or wear protective suits. As King's country director, my role was in strategy and management, so I had not attended any of the trainings on Ebola that my team had put on for the staff at the hospital. Someone had to do something, though, so I had little choice but to get involved.

The gate was a rusty swing door, barred prison-style, in a dingy corridor that connected the isolation unit to the main entrance of the hospital. The gate was usually barred with an iron chain and a padlock which the security guard held the key for.

A few health facilities had seen Ebola patients leave and go back into the community, putting themselves, their families and the entire country at risk. Indeed, the previous week I had come to work to find one of our suspected Ebola patients dead on the street outside the hospital, after he had left the unit at night while it was unsupervised. Ideally, we would have had enough nurses to actively supervise the patients around the clock, but with a total of only four nurses willing to go inside, this wasn't possible. Our safety depended on having total control over which parts of the hospital were contaminated, called the 'red zone', and which were safe, or 'green' – a patient walking out of the unit could have put us all in danger.

During case management discussions at the Ministry in the previous months, I had argued against locking up patients as I felt it would create a confrontational and dangerous environment, and that we should ensure our patients remained in the unit by convincing them and their families that it was better for them to stay. In reality, this approach just wasn't working.

Technically our patients weren't under arrest and, as far as we were aware, there was no law that permitted us to lock them up. It felt to us a violation of their human rights. But we believed the city was facing an unparalleled threat, and that if the chains of transmission got out of our control, the outbreak could become virtually unstoppable. So, we decided to keep the unit gates chained shut at night. It was one of the many difficult decisions we would need to make during the outbreak that pushed us to the very limit of our moral boundaries.

That morning, the matron explained what had happened. The boy was our only patient at the time, and he had spent the night in the unit completely alone. We were still waiting for his Ebola test results but, from his symptoms, we thought he was highly likely to be positive. He had woken up early, agitated and confused, a common occurrence with Ebola patients who get neurological symptoms as the virus attacks their brain. He had walked to the main gate of the unit and tried to leave. Finding it locked, he had cried out, before vomiting onto the floor and then pulling out the cannula in his arm that supplied him with intravenous fluids. This had caused him to hose blood onto the walls and floor before collapsing onto the ground, leaving the entire area highly contagious. A new male nurse and one of our security guards had taken it upon themselves, bravely but foolhardily, to go into the unit to try to help. But they didn't know how to wear the protective suits properly and looked unsure about what to do next.

I went to help, but the logistics were challenging. At that time, our entire stock of PPE was stored in the changing room inside the unit, and the patient was lying directly in the only path to that room. The situation wasn't ideal – I was wearing a t-shirt, shorts and pair of raggedy Toms espadrilles.

Stepping over the visible blood and vomit on the floor, treading carefully over the patient's splayed limbs and threading my body between my two frozen colleagues like I was doing three-dimensional Twister, I made it to the changing room. By this time, more supplies had arrived and the array of equipment was dizzying: face masks; body suits; rubber boots; short gloves; long gloves; visors; goggles; hair nets; shoe covers and aprons.

I started dressing whilst calling out to my colleagues. "Stay there, just stay there, don't move an inch." The nurse held his nerve, but the security guard lost his and pulled off his PPE, throwing it on on top of the boy, whose condition was rapidly deteriorating. Face mask off, gloves off, suit off, all in a panic. The secret of staying safe with Ebola was all in the undressing – you can wear whatever expensive bodysuit you like, but if you take it off wrong and scrape just a sliver of infected material against your inner clothes or skin, then you're at high risk of infection. I'd known this security guard for over a year. In that moment, I believed he would infect himself, and there was nothing I could think to do to stop him.

My own life was at a crossroads. I had to help, but I was way out of my depth and I knew it.

There was the sound of an engine at the main entrance, and I was overwhelmed with relief. My colleague Marta had arrived on the back of a motorbike taxi, her long brown hair blowing behind her, dressed for the beach in a cream-coloured dress and sandals. She'd had the same thought as me and had decided to stop by on her way out of town for the weekend. Her timing was impeccable.

Marta is, without a doubt, the reason why I, and many hundreds of others, are alive today. She came to my rescue as I stood there in that changing room. We hugged, as always, but exchanged few words. She taught me how to dress quickly, and we headed together to the corridor. Marta has a supremely reassuring presence, and she quickly helped the catatonic nurse in the corridor, leading him through to the undressing room to help him to decontaminate.

I was left to help the patient as best as I could. I knelt down next to him, feeling the liquid cool of his blood pressing against my skin, which was protected only by the thin white Tyvex suit. Pulling the sleeve and gloves of the security guard's discarded suit from the boy's face, I looked for signs of life – breathing, a pulse, any kind of movement. He looked so healthy and strong, as if he had been playing football yesterday, not anything like the patients I was used to seeing back in the UK, who normally died after months or years of chronic illness that left them weak and emaciated. I tried to remember the proper steps to declare someone dead from when I was a student, but it had been a long time. There was not much doubt here, though.

Marta re-emerged and together we unwrapped and unzipped a black body bag next to the boy. First, we had to douse him with chlorine; the spray bottle reminded me in a painfully ironic way of the plant sprays my mother used to water the flowers at home. It felt completely wrong, against all my instincts, to spray this sleeping boy in the face with such a toxic chemical.

Marta helped to rinse his body by splashing solution with her cupped hands, like a baptism. Together we heaved and dragged his body onto the body bag – he was heavy and slippery and it felt awkward and indecent, especially with so many people watching. We hauled it onto a trolley to await the burial team and got to work spraying and mopping the corridor to make it safe.

Marta guided me through the decontamination process to take off my PPE suit, step by step. First wash with chlorine. Take off first set of gloves and apron. Second wash. Body suit. Third wash. Face mask. Fourth wash. Goggles. Fifth wash. Second gloves. Sixth wash. Boots. Seventh wash of hands and arms and we're out. I was dripping with sweat and my clothes were clinging to me. Even after decontamination, I didn't dare wipe my face or rub my eyes, just in case my hands still had a particle of the virus on them that had survived. We walked out into the dazzling sunlight.

There wasn't much to say. Job done for the day and I was reeling and speechless, and still fearing for the security guard who had been exposed (he turned out to be fine). I hoped I'd never have to do that again, but I had no idea what would be coming our way over the next few months. This was just the beginning.

SINEAD

Balcony advocacy
On 18 July, we at last got some good news from the national level. As the confirmed cases climbed to 399, the Ministry announced

the creation of the Ebola Emergency Operations Centre (EOC) in collaboration with WHO. This was supposed to be a hub for the response, to be open 24/7. One of its most promising features from my perspective was that the Minister was not supposed to be involved in chairing the daily meetings of the EOC, rather it was to fall to one of her senior directors. This was in line with the lobbying we had been doing for more technical, less political coordination.

The EOC got off to a promising start. One of our UN partners called after two days to say that the EOC had made more decisions in its first two meetings than the national Taskforce had made in two months. More international support arrived in the form of a new team from the US Centers for Disease Control and a small contingent from Public Health England. Things seemed to be looking up.

Unfortunately, the situation in Kenema had continued to deteriorate since our visit. Peter and I had tried to call attention to what we had heard and seen, writing a report on my laptop in the car on the way back and circulating it widely. I raised the issues in interactions with my colleagues in Dublin, Brussels, Geneva and New York, as well as in meetings in Freetown and contacts with the State House and in the international media interviews I was starting to do.

One opportunity arose when I got a call from Chris Lane, the WHO staffer who Peter and I had met in Kenema, to say that he was passing through Freetown on his way back to the UK. I hurriedly organised a reception in my apartment and invited about twenty donors, diplomats, UN and NGO representatives, and private sector friends who had expressed an interest in helping, so they could hear directly from Chris what was happening in Kenema.

This was a major tactic of mine in the first six months of the response from May to November – because coordination during the work week was so bad, I would strategically invite over people I thought should be collaborating or sharing information, but who might not otherwise do so. Generally, my goal was to bring frontline implementers like Chris together with people sitting at the policy table or making funding decisions. I usually didn't tell people this explicitly for fear of putting them off, I would just say "Come over for a glass of wine" and, lo and behold, there appeared various people I wanted them to meet. Attendance was generally very good because there was so little else to do socially at that time.

Organising these events wasn't always straightforward. Some people were nervous interacting with people working on Ebola in any way. So I hired a security guard to stand at my apartment door with a big bottle of hand sanitiser. Not exactly the casual feel I was going for but needs must. It was also tricky to get catering as a lot of businesses had stopped functioning normally. One on occasion, I had ordered from an Indian restaurant near my apartment, but they had to cancel at the last minute because their Indian kitchen staff "ran away".

At that particular reception, Chris didn't let me down. He was completely exhausted from weeks of sixteen-hour days at Kenema but was still energetically informing people about the situation and how they might help until 1 a.m. on my balcony. Quite a few people told me as they were leaving how struck they were by what he had said, although one or two also admitted to me they found themselves keeping a nice safe distance from him!

I really wish I could say we saw some improvements in Kenema as a result of this lobbying, but as July wore on, things only got worse and worse.

Kenema explodes

Because there still weren't enough resources for proper community engagement and because a lot of what was being done was more instructions to communities than dialogue with them, conspiracy theories had continued to flourish in Kenema. And, just as in Freetown, there was a riot at the hospital with residents demanding that the ETU be closed.[8] As one nurse described it to me later:

> I was walking back to the hospital after lunch. There was banging on the hospital gates. There was a mob. It was like a football crowd when the results went the wrong way. Most staff left the hospital. They were all told to evacuate. Lena from Tulane stuck around – loads of patients were waiting for results. I stayed and one of the other nurses, Nancy Yoko. Lena and Nancy strong-armed a lab guy and they worked on getting the results. Nancy sat there, she was in charge and refused to leave, she sat there indefatigably – in the nurses' area. We were there for a few hours. We didn't go inside the unit as it would have been harder to escape and in PPE you would have gotten a beating. We fully expected the hospital to be overrun. It was a few hours before order was restored by the police. It turns out that a former nurse who was mentally ill had gone to the market saying that we were harvesting organs and taking blood and this confirmed people's beliefs.

But this riot was just the tip of the iceberg.

There were huge problems in the lab. When eight tests were double-checked by staff from the Public Health Agency of Canada, "worrying discrepancies" were found in four of the eight tests and another assessment showed that up to five people had been incorrectly diagnosed with Ebola. This obviously had enormous implications for efforts to gain the trust of the community.[9] In particular, questions were raised about the role of the US company Metabiota in the lab. Their role supporting the government on surveillance also came in for severe criticism by MSF and WHO.

What's more, in the two weeks since my visit with Peter, the ETU reached its breaking point as more and more patients arrived from all over the country. The unit could have up to 100 patients at a time. To deal with this they usually had three or four WHO international doctors, a handful of Sierra Leonean nurses and a British nurse, Will Pooley. Given the high physical and mental demands of caring for Ebola patients, including the time-consuming process of donning and doffing PPE, these ratios were ludicrous.

Despite the staff being so overstretched and short of resources, they were still determined to use aggressive therapy whenever possible, including intravenous drips, to try to give every patient the best chance of survival. One WHO staff who worked in Kenema told me: "The kind of commitment that the doctors displayed – it was ridiculous. At one point, Ian Crozier was the only doctor for a weekend with eighty patients."

Not only were there very few nurses, but none of them had any experience in dealing with Ebola. Some were fresh graduates without any nursing experience at all, and they had received little Ebola training. But they were keen to be put on the Ministry's payroll and, in a speech he had given on the radio on 1 July, President Koroma had said: "I hereby instruct the immediate absorption of these brave volunteer nurses and health workers in Kailahun and Kenema into the civil service."[10] While they were still waiting for this to actually happen, there was no question that this promise was hugely motivational for the volunteer nurses who would normally have to volunteer for months or years before getting a government job.

But these courageous nurses who worked on Ebola got infected and died at an unprecedented rate. One of the surviving nurses later told me:

I remember when the first patient came to Kenema. She was in the minor theatre. I was one of the first nurses, we were eight. We were told that it was very infectious but I volunteered. Four of these nurses are dead and four are alive. Then in the second batch we were fifteen nurses, out of these seven are alive.

The ETU was overwhelmed by the sheer volume of patients and the few health workers became exhausted and demotivated and had to constantly deal with interruptions in critical supplies such as chlorine. Tim O'Dempsey, a WHO doctor there, described infection prevention and control standards at the ETU as "catastrophic".[11] An extraordinary example of this was when one of the senior nurses got infected and some other staff would visit her in her private room without wearing PPE. What's more, according to one of the other nurses, "She held the [hospital] keys in her purse – her brother would come in and out of the red zone and pick up and drop off the keys."

This insane situation at Kenema was thrown into sharp relief when MSF visited to monitor infection prevention practices at the ETU. As one health worker described it:

It's not that MSF were not trying to be helpful, but Kenema was a state. It was a hellhole. So, they were obviously very critical. I remember somebody passed me a blood sample through a window. I washed it in a bit of chlorine and brought it down to the lab – MSF were there. I was caught in the act! They said: "You should have double containered that sample. You should have had it in ice, used a special vehicle". But we had a different set of safety levels and expectations – we were getting hit every day with blood and vomit. Every staff member in Kenema felt every day, "maybe I got Ebola today". So carrying a blood tube! I was not going to think twice about it. That MSF person was an advisor on infection control but probably never did a shift in as dangerous a situation. Their attitude to risk – it was not

comparable to the levels of risk we were facing – MSF had a
different set of expectations.

The central point here is that staff in Kenema were between a
rock and a hard place. They knew that they were overwhelmed,
but sometimes patients would be dumped outside the gates by a
taxi driver with no indication where they had come from. The
ETU staff could either take these people into the crowded unit or
leave them outside to die and possibly infect others. The Kenema
ETU was serving a vital role for the entire country on isolation
and treatment, but it had enormous costs for the health workers
inside.

A WHO doctor from the US, David Brett-Major, describes a
period of a few days where only he, the nurse Alex Moigboi and
the hospital matron M'balu Fonnie, a co-founder of the Lassa
fever programme, were working in the red zone, with up to eighty
patients at a time:

> Alex and Sister M'balu almost certainly were infected in that
> week. I wanted to stop their exposure risk and even close [the
> ETU], but this was their community with [Ebola] and they were
> going to support the patients that came for care regardless of
> what anyone said or tried to do to intervene. The patients had
> to go somewhere. They had adopted the ethics of conjoined
> risk with the members of their community, particularly their
> co-workers.[12]

Alex and Sister M'balu died shortly thereafter.

Around 20 July, the Ministry finally acknowledged how bad
the situation was and asked MSF if they would take over the management of Kenema, but MSF responded that they were completely stretched already and even though they could see how
bad it was, they couldn't intervene beyond making recommendations. PPE supplies dwindled. Major water supply problems

plagued the hospital. Four more nurses died. The entire hospital staff went on strike over the conditions and the delays in their hazard payments, leaving only a few expatriates to work in the unit. On 22 July, it was announced that Dr Sheik Humarr Khan, head of the Kenema Lassa Fever Programme and Sierra Leone's only virologist, had tested Ebola-positive.

Dr Khan

Despite everything that preceded it, Dr Khan's infection was really what sent shockwaves through Sierra Leone and around the world. Unassuming, friendly and in possession of a captivating smile, Dr Khan was highly respected in the medical community in Sierra Leone and with international colleagues. He had studied abroad, but had come home to lead a successful battle against Lassa fever. He had been profiled by the *New York Times* and had become a symbol of Sierra Leone's resistance to Ebola as literally the only Sierra Leonean to have the technical capacity to deal with this epidemic. And now he had Ebola. International newspapers rushed to cover the story.

While Sierra Leone was on tenterhooks about whether Dr Khan would make it, international panic rose even further when Kent Brantly, an American doctor working in Liberia for the NGO Samaritan's Purse, was confirmed positive for Ebola.

Dr Khan went to the MSF ETU in Kailahun for treatment. Two options were considered for him there that had not previously been considered for other Sierra Leonean health workers: use of an experimental treatment (ZMapp) and medical evacuation.

The first question was whether Dr Khan should be treated with ZMapp, which had never been tested on humans, but which was considered to be a very promising treatment of Ebola from its initial trials. MSF happened to have access to two doses of ZMapp, out of only about five doses in the world at that time.

This was because ZMapp was a Canadian drug and the laboratory next to the Kailahun ETU was run by a Canadian team. They had these doses in their fridge, in case they got infected testing Ebola samples.

The MSF medical team treating Dr Khan faced a difficult dilemma: "Would the drug, known as ZMapp, help the stricken doctor? Or would it perhaps harm or even kill one of the country's most prominent physicians, a man considered a national hero, shattering the already fragile public trust in international efforts to contain the world's worst Ebola outbreak?"[13] MSF staff were also deeply concerned about the ethics of offering the drug to Dr Khan and not to other patients, and some staff even threatened to resign if he were to receive the drug. Tim O'Dempsey, the WHO Clinical Lead from Kenema who was consulting on the case, requested that MSF administer the drug, but they ultimately refused.[14]

Hopes then turned to med-evac. To put this in context, practically every expatriate who was diagnosed with Ebola in the subregion was ultimately evacuated to Europe or the US. In-country treatment was never considered to be the preferred option for any international health worker. But Dr Khan was a Sierra Leonean health worker, so his prospects were very different. Although WHO Geneva initially refused to consider med-evac since Dr Khan was not a WHO staff member, they later agreed to do so.

However, the plane took seventy-two hours to reach Freetown, and then the med-evac company refused to take him. They said it was because he was vomiting and had diarrhoea, and that they did not have the capacity to evacuate an Ebola patient with these symptoms, even though these are two of the most common symptoms of Ebola.

Dr Khan died in Kailahun on 29 July, aged thirty-nine.

Ultimately, eighty health workers in Kenema district died of

Ebola, including Dr Khan, Alex Moigboi, M'balu Fonnie and the indefatigable nurse Nancy Yoko.[15] Meanwhile, Kent Brantly was evacuated to the US. He received one of those same two ZMapp doses that had been in the fridge in Kailahun. This time, nobody seemed to express doubts about the inequity of using the drug. Dr Brantly survived.

FIVE | Armageddon

SINEAD

The nemesis on the move

On 25 July, three days after the announcement of Dr Khan's infection, and two months to the day after the confirmation of the first case in Sierra Leone, President Koroma held an emergency meeting on Ebola with diplomats, donors and the UN. About fifteen of us sat around the conference table at State House, with about twenty others in chairs lined up along the side. As the meeting began, I was relieved that, despite his near public silence up until then, the President seemed to really 'get' the urgency. In his opening address, he said that this "nemesis" that Sierra Leone was facing was clearly not under control.

I couldn't have agreed more. We had had 450 confirmed cases of Ebola by then and while they were mostly in Kailahun and Kenema, there had been cases in nine other districts too, meaning that the outbreak had now spread to the vast majority of the country.[1,2] The President announced the creation of the Presidential Taskforce on Ebola and said that a revised national Ebola plan would be launched a few days later.

As the meeting concluded, I was feeling quite upbeat. Finally, some momentum. Then my phone started lighting up with several text messages arriving in quick succession. I took a surreptitious glance. An Ebola case had been confirmed in Lagos, Nigeria. Patrick Sawyer, a Liberian diplomat, having contracted Ebola in Monrovia, flew to Nigeria and died soon after arriving. My first thought was, this could be catastrophic.

I slid my iPhone across to Peter, who was sitting to my left. He had spent four years in Nigeria. The alarmed expression on his face confirmed my initial reaction: this was on another level now. Lagos had a population of twenty-one million, around the same population of Guinea, Sierra Leone, and Liberia combined.[3] The city was also vastly more connected to the rest of the world. And this meant that a person infected with Ebola had travelled on a commercial airline, opening up a new dimension of international panic.

Unsurprisingly, the announcement from Lagos amplified the media storm that had started after Dr Khan's infection, and had reached fever pitch when Kent Brantly had become the first white Westerner to test positive. A couple of days later, a headline from the satirical news website *The Onion* started to do the rounds on social media in Freetown: "Experts: 'Ebola Vaccine At Least 50 White People Away.'" It certainly appeared that the increased proximity to the Western world massively ramped up the global level of concern on what many had previously considered an African problem.

State of Emergency

After that first meeting, President Koroma kept his focus strongly on Ebola, making his first trip to the affected areas of Kenema and Kailahun on 28 and 29 July. On 30 July, he made a statement mourning Dr Khan's passing and declaring a national State of Public Emergency.[4] As part of this, Kenema and Kailahun would be quarantined, meaning the districts would be cut off from the rest of the country, using checkpoints manned by the military and the police. Any movement in or out would require a special pass issued by the government.

The President also announced another level of quarantine for households anywhere in the country in which Ebola was found. If anyone in the household was diagnosed with Ebola, then military or police personnel would stand guard at the house for twenty-one days, the length of the incubation period, to ensure that nobody left and that only authorised surveillance personnel entered. He also stressed the need to root out the denial of Ebola and announced that there would be house-to-house searches for infected people. He banned public gatherings (generally interpreted as any group of more than ten people) through-out the country, with the exception of meetings related to the Ebola response.

As I listened to the speech on the radio with my colleagues, I was a bit perturbed by the emphasis on the police and mili-tary, but this was overshadowed by my relief. Here was Presi-dent Koroma finally coming to terms with the severity of the situation and taking very serious steps. However, I would soon see that this emphasis on the security dimensions was a fun-damental problem, the emphasis being on restrictions, rules and punishment, rather than dialogue and cooperation with the population.

The next day, President Koroma decided to pay a visit to the supposedly '24/7' EOC at the WHO office, but didn't find any-body there. He was livid and didn't waste any time communi-cating this to the Ministry and to WHO. State House put out a press release saying: "Unfortunately, when the President visited WHO this morning, the centre was closed with no sign that there is an emergency in the country right now."[5] This incident was so poignantly representative of the lack of urgency and the chaos that we had been seeing for the previous two months that I have to admit that my first reaction to hearing about the debacle was to burst out laughing. But of course, it was no joke.

Departures

In the days after the Patrick Sawyer and Kent Brantly news, we started hearing from colleagues and friends that they were being told by their organisations to leave Freetown. For some, the catalyst was the Peace Corps' announcement on 30 July that they were pulling their volunteers from Guinea, Liberia and Sierra Leone.[6] But we soon started seeing a domino effect whereby people were leaving because other people were leaving.

I was due to go on annual leave on 1 August. It was to be my first proper holiday in six years, as I had finished my part-time PhD in April 2014. But there was no way I could leave. For one thing, the sheer volume of work to do on the crisis was enormous. I also felt I needed to be around to make continuous judgement calls about the safety of our staff in the rapidly evolving situation.

On top of this, as an Embassy, we had to be constantly thinking about our travel advice for Irish citizens who were living in or thinking of travelling to Sierra Leone. Paula and I agonised over the wording we were recommending to our headquarters for the website. On the one hand, we were determined to issue advice that was reflective of the situation on the ground, rather than of the rising panic which seemed to be increasingly colouring people's judgements. We felt a responsibility to Sierra Leone not to just jump on the bandwagon. On the other hand, an even greater concern was not to give Irish citizens a false sense of security. The main issue we were worried about was not actually Ebola, but the ability of our citizens to get non-Ebola healthcare. Getting quality health care in Sierra Leone was not easy even at the best of times, and with Ebola it had become far more difficult – some doctors were shutting their practices and others were not accepting any new patients as they feared getting infected. One of my Sierra Leonean friends called me in a panic one day when he couldn't get his pregnant wife accepted into the main private hospital in

Freetown even though he could pay. In a country with one of the highest rates of maternal mortality in the world, he was understandably freaked out. Fortunately, I knew the head of the hospital and he agreed to allow her in as a favour to me. But clearly this was not remotely sustainable. If one of our citizens had a car accident or caught malaria, would they be able to get treatment in a hospital in time? It was definitely not the period for tourism to Sierra Leone.

We had the same concerns for our staff. Paula and I agreed we should give the Embassy staff a briefing on health and we wrestled with what to say given the limited options. I opened by saying, "Don't get sick." We all laughed, but it was uneasy laughter, as we all knew that there were actually no other good options.

Our headquarters back in Dublin were, understandably, not thrilled with the situation and worried about us, not least because of the alarming media coverage they were reading. They called us every day to check in and frequently asked us if we thought we should leave.

Fortunately, my small international team was united on this point. None of this bedlam going on or the increasingly hysterical media coverage meant that the facts on the ground had changed or that it had become any more likely any of us would contract Ebola. And precisely because the Ebola situation was getting worse and we were working on it, the very last thing we wanted to do was leave. Until the world woke up and sent in the cavalry of people who actually knew how to deal with this crisis, people like us needed to stick around and do whatever we could. The one exception was my colleague Lorna Stafford in Liberia, who was six months pregnant at the time. When her doctor was quarantined for having contact with an Ebola patient, we knew she needed to get on a plane.

For our Sierra Leonean and Liberian staff, prevention of infection was much more complicated, since they had far less control over their home environments than we internationals did. One day, when I was on the phone with my mother, she came up with an idea. I had told her previously that all the offices and businesses had started to have security guards outside with thermometers to check that no visitors had a temperature. My mother said, "Why not give your staff thermometers for their houses so they can monitor anybody coming in?" It was a great idea.

There was only one problem: people had been panic-buying thermometers, chlorine, hand sanitiser, gloves, anything they thought might protect them from Ebola, so pharmacies in Sierra Leone were completely sold out. We could ask our colleagues at headquarters, but our procurement system would have taken weeks. So, my mum just went up to the local pharmacy in Dublin, bought the thermometers and sent them over with somebody travelling from one of the NGOs. These kinds of things were small measures but meant a lot to our staff.

Airline watch

Unfortunately, many other developments were outside our control. Compounding the growing sense of panic, two regional airlines suspended flights to the sub-region after Patrick Sawyer flew to Nigeria. We had been on daily 'airline watch' ever since. Friends working for airlines admitted things were shaky as airline crews were reading the newspapers and getting nervous.

Every day, we would get calls from Irish citizens asking whether their flight would still be leaving, and we would text around our friends in the airline industry. Paula and I would shout over to each other across the hallway separating our offices. "Brussels, business as usual but the crew are having a meeting tomorrow . . . Royal Air Maroc, all good . . . Air France okay for now, but check back tomorrow because they have a conference call with Paris this evening."

When Air France cancelled a flight because two of their crew refused to fly to Sierra Leone, we started to get worried about British Airways. But then their CEO went on the news saying that they would maintain flights. We breathed a bit more easily.

So, it came as a shock when British Airways announced on 5 August that they were suspending flights to Sierra Leone and Liberia due to the "deteriorating public health situation".[7]

This announcement caused pandemonium. British Airways was not just another airline to Sierra Leone. The Freetown–London flight was by far the most significant international connection to the country. Outside of its immediate neighbours, Sierra Leone's closest bilateral ties were with the UK. Harking back to colonial times, thousands of Sierra Leoneans were UK citizens and many Sierra Leonean families had relatives or friends in the UK. However, this flight cancellation was not just a practical inconvenience. More importantly, it symbolised that Sierra Leone was becoming isolated from the wider world and it had a deep psychological effect on many Sierra Leoneans and expatriates alike.

In the hours and days after the announcement, the trickle of departures that had started in late July turned into a flood. Individuals and organisations wrestled to get the last seats on flights. Our phones at the Embassy were hopping with calls from citizens and sometimes even their families back in Ireland. Because there were no landlines in the country and my mobile phone number was on the web, I would sometimes get calls at night or on the weekend from a worried mother somewhere in Ireland, who was usually taken aback at getting straight through to the Ambassador! We also got frequent calls or texts from friends working for NGOs or private companies telling us they were on their way to the airport. Some were barely given time to pack a suitcase.

The British Airways decision had very tangible impacts for us at the Embassy. Our colleague Emma had gone home for annual leave and now her flight back had been cancelled. Our headquarters decided she should stay in Ireland, and that a new staff member for our Liberia office should not come out either, given the growing uncertainty. We also had to suspend recruitment for two other vacancies. This left us severely understaffed at a time when the Ebola workload was increasing every day. And we weren't the only ones. For all the organisations trying to stay, the British Airways decision made it so much harder, both in practical terms and in terms of making our case to concerned headquarters. At one of our donor meetings, somebody asked the question: should British Airways be held accountable for its contribution to the panic and hysteria, or do private companies get off the hook?

We didn't really have time for these kinds of discussions however. Every day brought more questions we could not answer. Would the few remaining international airlines also cancel, leaving Sierra Leone completely isolated? How would we fly in urgent Ebola supplies like PPE and chlorine, which were already in short supply? Would shipping companies be next? Sierra Leone was totally dependent on imported fuel; would that dry up too? What would we do then? We really had no idea.

Nigeria quashes Ebola

While all this was going on, we watched in wonder as Nigeria conducted its own fight against Ebola. Nine health workers had contracted Ebola from Patrick Sawyer. But the response was impressive. We heard they had contact tracers with master's degrees – we were struggling with some contact tracers who couldn't read (due, in part, to politicians trying to get jobs in the response for people they knew). The Nigerians had set up websites, social media pages, hotlines, mobile apps to communicate with the population – we still wrestled with getting any data whatsoever from the Ministry. They had a stronger health system overall and were able to build on an existing surveillance structure, originally designed for polio, which kicked into action.

In addition to domestic capacity, they also had international support. The notion of Ebola in Lagos completely freaked out the public health community and some of the world's foremost experts from organisations like WHO, CDC and MSF flew over to help – the kinds of experts we were crying out for in Sierra Leone. And, despite some big initial challenges, it was working. In the end, the Nigerians quashed Ebola with nineteen cases and eight deaths.[8] So, the world was capable of responding quickly. But, somehow, we were still waiting.

On 8 August, WHO finally declared Ebola a "Public Health Emergency of International Concern".[9] This seemed a little obvious to us from where we were sitting: more than a thousand people had died across four countries. But nevertheless, we assumed it had to be a good thing. This was only the third such announcement since this trigger mechanism was created in 2005, the first two having been for swine flu and polio. Surely the cavalry would be coming now.

OLIVER

Stopping a chain reaction

At the start of August, the shock and fear induced by Dr Khan's death was continuing to reverberate throughout the medical community in Freetown. He had been a contemporary and close friend of many of the senior doctors at Connaught, who felt his loss keenly and personally.

It was really only after Dr Khan's death that I think many of us realised how bad things had become in Kenema, as it had started to overflow as the referral centre for patients that had tested positive elsewhere in the country. I also realised how unrealistic our expectations had been that this one man would be able to sort out the whole clinical side of the response. Although we had been talking regularly in the Taskforce and Case Management Pillar meetings about setting up a lab and ETU in Freetown, we just hadn't been able to find anyone willing and able to take this on.

By this time there were stories coming in daily of suspected cases being identified across Freetown and in several other major towns in the country. Hard facts were difficult to come by, but the national picture as a whole seemed increasingly alarming, with the number of confirmed cases over the 500 mark and rising fast.[10]

We still hadn't managed to convince a Sierra Leonean doctor to lead the Ebola unit and I worried that if King's took over it would set a terrible precedent for our collaborative approach and would also leave us exposed to the fraught politics within the Ministry, which as outsiders I knew we would struggle to navigate.

Above all, we knew that the scale of Connaught's response would soon have to expand. We needed the help of Sierra Leonean doctors, since the King's clinical team by this stage was just Marta and Terry. Since my first case a couple of weeks before, I had started to occasionally help out with coordination when nobody else was available. This mostly involved logistics, such as making sure lab samples had been sent, and putting corpses into body bags. It meant I could still be useful because the role didn't require me to have a medical licence, even though it did involve direct physical contact with patients.

If we couldn't find a Sierra Leonean to run the unit and more national doctors to work in it, we were worried that we might not be able to keep it open, resulting in a chain reaction with terrible consequences. The general wards in the hospital would become exposed to Ebola, with nowhere to safely isolate suspected patients. In that event, we predicted that staff across the hospital would soon start to become infected and the hospital would inevitably close, just as the main hospital in Monrovia had closed in July.[11] This would deprive many people in Freetown of access to essential medical care.

But the psychological damage could be even greater. If staff at Connaught Hospital, the country's flagship healthcare facility, thought it was too dangerous to stay open, then how could health workers at smaller facilities across the country be expected to stay at their posts? Our main fear was a ripple effect, whereby the closure of Connaught would trigger the closure of all health facilities in Sierra Leone.

So, I developed a dogged mantra, that Connaught Hospital had to remain open at all costs, regardless of the risks. It could not be allowed to fall. And the first step in keeping it open was convincing a senior doctor at the hospital to take the lead.

To my surprise, Dr Modupeh Cole, one of just three senior Sierra Leonean physicians at the hospital, volunteered to take over this role in mid-July. I say surprised because in my eighteen months at the hospital, Dr Cole had seemed uninterested in hospital management affairs.

Dr Cole had a somewhat quiet management style, but what mattered for us was that he was one of the few brave souls who would go to assess suspected Ebola cases himself. But on the morning of Friday 1 August, he didn't turn up at the unit's morning meeting. When I eventually tracked him down, he told us that, with Dr Khan's death, he felt it was just too risky to carry on as Ebola Coordinator and would be stepping down from the role. I convinced him to at least meet with us to discuss it, and after lunch Marta and I went to meet him at his private office.

We started by trying to convince him he was safe, that if he followed the protocols, there was very little risk. We also offered him more training and reminded him how important the role was to the hospital, promising him that we would be there to support him. But I could tell we were getting nowhere.

So I decided to be much more forceful, to use every argument I could think of to convince him. I painted the scenario of what would happen if he quit. How the hospital would close and the response would collapse. How Ebola would sweep through the city unchecked. How his country needed him desperately and was calling out for his bravery. I asked him how he was going to feel when his family members started to get sick and die, and he knew it was all because he had run away.

I could see that Marta thought I had crossed a line. As we walked back to our office, the two of us had a blazing row. Marta thought I had emotionally manipulated him and downplayed the risks. She felt it was his right not to see Ebola patients if he felt that doing so was too dangerous. I argued that we were facing catastrophe, that he had a duty as a doctor he could not hide from, and that if we were unable to strong-arm people like Dr Cole into remaining at their posts, then many vulnerable people would die.

Once again, we faced the tension between the rights of an individual and the good of the population as a whole. I was not certain if I had done the right thing.

For the time being, though, it worked, and Dr Cole reluctantly agreed to carry on in the role.

A contest of wills
Whilst the situation in the hospital might not have changed much, the world's attention to the outbreak had increased dramatically

since late July. For the media, Ebola had all the ingredients of the perfect story, with graphic descriptions of a gruesome disease, heroes dressed in space suits and the fear that Ebola could be coming to a home near you.

We had originally decided not to speak to the media, since we felt that it should be Sierra Leoneans, not someone from King's, who explained their country's situation to the press. The Ministry had also made it clear they did not want anyone speaking out of turn.

But the situation had become so desperate on the ground that I felt we now had to speak out. After doing one radio interview for the BBC World Service, I was suddenly flooded with interview requests from most of the major news channels and newspapers. By then, the media seemed like one of the few tools available to try and influence the response. By telling the world how weak the response was, and warning of an impending catastrophe, I thought we could create public pressure for a bigger international response and communicate directly to the decision-makers in London, Geneva and Washington who might be listening. In addition, after I started doing interviews, we saw a surge in donations and volunteer applications at King's, at a time when we still had no money for our Ebola work and were severely short-staffed.

I quickly learnt that a media interview is really a contest of wills between you and the presenter. You go in with a set of key messages, but the journalist usually has their own agenda. With Ebola, they often wanted to focus on the blood and gore of the disease or the risks back in the UK, neither of which I was interested in discussing. The presenter gets to choose his or her questions, but you get to answer however you want. Somehow, though, you have to make sure you make it interesting enough for them so that they give your interview prominence and ask you back in future, whilst they have to make sure they do not frustrate you so much you refuse to speak to them again. It was a dance that took me practice to learn.

I remember an interview with the UK's Channel 4, who were otherwise very good, where the interviewer asked me to "tell the public what an Ebola patient looks like, how gruesome is it, how horrible is it?" I replied that Ebola patients usually looked just like any other patient as their initial symptoms were like the flu. Not satisfied, he said, "That's great, but let's try that one more time. How gruesome is it, how horrible is it?" Holding back my frustration, I declined to answer again.

We also received many messages of support from members of the public who heard me on the radio or saw me on TV and took the trouble to look up my email address. These were often beautiful sentiments that I would read out to the team, and they gave us a great deal of encouragement.

Others were hilarious. My favourite email came in with the subject line "Balls" and read: "Oliver, You've got some. I'm sure you can rationalise it all away, but nonetheless, thanks. All the best, David." I forwarded the message on to Will Pooley, who was a friend, saying that I thought the message was intended for him, given how he'd jumped on his motorbike and ridden down to Kenema when he'd heard about the challenges there, and volunteered to join the national nurses on the wards.

London starts to worry

The flip side of this high-profile media exposure was that it drew attention to our risky work on Ebola amongst the powers-that-be back at King's in London. At the end of July, I had written an email to my bosses at King's, saying:

> I believe there will be a major outbreak in Freetown. I think
> we should stay but I think we should acknowledge that there
> seems to be a significant risk to staff who are involved. I think as

individuals we are all aware of that risk [of us becoming infected] and stay by choice – but I think that King's needs to be prepared for that possibility.

I wanted to be sure that King's would stay the course and keep supporting Connaught even if one of us did test positive.

But a week after Dr Khan's death, and the ensuing media bonanza, I received an email from London that hinted at mandatory evacuation. So, a second front of the battle opened up for me. I was now not only fighting the disease but also fighting a rearguard action, trying to ensure we would not be forced to leave.

It was easy to understand why King's would be concerned. We were a university, not a humanitarian agency, and the team weren't even supposed to be doing much clinical work in the first place. Whilst Ebola had started to seem, in a surreal way, like a part of daily life for those of us who had been in Sierra Leone over the previous few months, the way the disease was suddenly and graphically portrayed by the media was terrifying to my colleagues back home.

Whilst their anxiety was partly linked to issues like legal liability and reputational damage, there was also genuine concern about our safety. We had been trying to get assurances for the previous couple of months from the UK government that we would be med-evaced to London for specialist treatment if one of us got infected, which we knew would significantly increase our chances of survival. This had historically been standard practice for UK citizens infected with a viral haemorrhagic fever. But in mid-July I had received an email from the British High Commission, after they had consulted with London, that said: "in the case of an epidemic of this nature we would not assist with repatriation of UK nationals back to the UK (including [Her Majesty's

Government] staff), but would be supporting you where we could to get the best care in-country." Knowing what the best care in Sierra Leone looked like at that time, this was hardly reassuring.

To make matters worse, I got a mortifying email from my boss in London informing me that my parents had phoned a senior director at King's, demanding that I be recalled home immediately. In hindsight, I had not been doing the best job at calming my parents' nerves, and, understandably, they were desperately worried about my safety. After receiving a couple of despondent emails from me, and hearing how stressed and irritable I had started to sound on the phone, they were convinced I wasn't coping. Although I was furious with them at the time for undermining me at a crucial moment, this was of course completely unfair of me. It's just one example of the ordeals all of our families were going through back home.

The following Tuesday, British Airways pulled out, and the response from King's was swift. Within hours I had been instructed to fly back to London with the King's team, in case we became trapped. Only Marta, because she was an infectious diseases specialist and trained to handle an outbreak like Ebola, would be allowed to stay.

This created a terrible dilemma for me. Of course, part of me wanted to get my team to safety. But I also knew that leaving Marta on her own without support would put her in jeopardy. Sierra Leone had become my home and I wanted to stand with my colleagues at the hospital as they faced the growing threat. I also believed that I had a duty as a doctor to care for our patients.

London sounded resolute, however, so I decided that the best I could do was to play for time and hope I'd be able to change their minds. In a rapid-fire exchange of emails over the course of the day, I proposed a phased withdrawal of the entire team that would start with our students. I would only leave once all the others had been safely evacuated. Fortunately, this did the trick and I was granted a reprieve whilst this was arranged.

Ironically, months previously, I had booked a plane ticket for that very same Tuesday night, as I was due to go on leave for a few weeks. The previous eighteen months in Sierra Leone had been intense and I had become increasingly burned out. I feel ashamed to admit it now, but going on leave did not seem so ridiculous at the time, and I was still considering it right up until the last minute. I had even packed my suitcase, which was sitting in the back of my car outside. But with the panic caused by British Airways, I felt there was no way I could leave now, and we scrambled to change the name on the ticket to evacuate our first student, who was anxious to get on the plane that night.

The mood was ominous, and every hour that day would bring news of another friend or colleague joining the exodus out of the country, making us feel more and more isolated. Our continued presence felt like it was on a knife's edge.

Squeezing in more beds as the caseload rises

The following day, we had to plan what to do in this suddenly altered reality. The number of patients in our isolation unit was continuing to rise, and we were receiving three or four more suspected cases each day. It was taking a week to get lab results, so Marta and I decided to reconfigure our unit to squeeze in another five beds.

In a room at the back, we would put those patients whom we thought were most likely to test positive and had symptoms that would make them the most contagious, such as diarrhoea and vomiting. This reduced the risk that any patients who tested negative for Ebola could be exposed to the virus during their time inside the isolation unit.

Only Marta, the cleaners and I were willing to go inside, as by this time Terry was focusing on the general wards. We desperately needed more staff. Fortunately, a newly qualified King's nurse called Andy Hall, a former British Army paramedic, volunteered to come to Freetown and help us. He had agreed to come independently, rather than through King's, since I knew I wouldn't be able to officially add anyone to our team at the same time as London was trying to evacuate us.

I was looking into all sorts of contingency options to see if a humanitarian organisation, such as MSF or the Red Cross, would be willing to take over operations at Connaught and absorb us onto their staff, in case King's went ahead with the instruction to evacuate. After initial enthusiasm from several humanitarian agencies, they all balked at the level of risk involved in our work at the hospital.

Marta and I took a walk together in the hospital grounds, both of us admitting to the other that if we were instructed to evacuate, we would stay on independently anyway. "I really want to stay," I told her, "but I'm worried about the risks you're taking. I know how far you go for your patients and how hard you work yourself, but I can't let you get sick." She was quick to suggest that the same was true for me. We knew we would take risks with our own lives that we would never allow for each other, and agreed to take responsibility for each other's safety.

I also knew, however, that Marta and I could only hold on for so long before we got exhausted and overwhelmed. If that happened, we would start making mistakes and ultimately get sick, at which point it would be game over, not just for us but for our whole cause of keeping Connaught open.

Our only chance was if I could convince King's to not only let us stay, but also let us expand. We needed more clinicians and support staff, and ultimately to open more Ebola isolation units beyond Connaught. As it happened, it looked like we might finally have enough funding to do this. My friend Laura Miller at IRC had pulled together a consortium of NGOs to apply for DFID funding and, after seeing how desperate things had become for us on the clinical frontline, had invited us to join.

I reckoned the only way I would be able to convince King's to agree to an expansion would be to go to London and show them in person that I was okay and that we had a feasible plan. Most of the rest of the team, including Terry, would be leaving in the meantime, however, and our new nurse, Andy, would not be arriving for another few days. It was a very risky move, because I knew I would be leaving Marta alone. What I didn't realise was that we were about to get news that would further compromise our chances of remaining.

News about Dr Modupeh Cole

Dr Cole had been absent from work that whole week. Word reached the hospital that he was sick at home and afraid to tell anybody. Terry went to check on him, and found Dr Cole lying under a fan on the sofa in his house, being cared for by family members who were kitted out in makeshift PPE. His symptoms were non-specific, but Terry wanted to test him for Ebola just in case. Two days later the result came back positive.

A short investigation traced the probable cause of his exposure. Hours after Marta and I had tried to convince him to continue as Ebola Coordinator, Dr Cole had gone to assess a suspected case in our unit. The young man was quite sick already, and Dr Cole had struggled to insert an intravenous line. He'd become covered in blood and, when he went to undress, found the chlorine in the decontamination room had not been prepared. It was then, as he removed his PPE without using chlorine, that he most likely got exposed.

An ambulance was hastily arranged to take him to the MSF unit at Kailahun, which we believed offered him the best chance of survival. I felt huge guilt about the infection of our colleague, particularly given I had pushed him so hard to continue in his role. And I knew immediately this would have a devastating effect on confidence and morale in the hospital.

This incident also spurred King's to issue me with an ultimatum. They booked me a flight on Gambia Bird Airlines out of Freetown for the following day, and said that if I failed to get on it, they would close the King's programme.

The situation in that moment was so volatile, and we were so short-staffed in the isolation unit, that I knew I couldn't just leave. I Skyped my boss Andy and explained the situation. "This probably won't surprise you," I said, "but I won't be getting on that plane tonight. I know that means King's will close us down. So I'm going to resign and stay on independently, for as long as I can." He wasn't happy about it but he understood.

But later that day, news came in that Gambia had closed their airspace to flights from Sierra Leone and Liberia. Gambia Bird would be suspending operations, effective immediately. Although from a wider perspective the further cancellation of flights was a disaster for the country, it bought me the extra few days I needed to calm everyone's nerves, recruit a team to support Marta and get key systems in place for while I was away. Fortunately, my formal letter of resignation hadn't yet been sent and my boss was gracious enough not to bring it up again!

Confidence collapses at Connaught

The impact of Dr Cole's infection on Connaught was enormous. The junior doctors immediately went on strike, and the senior doctors largely absented themselves from the hospital premises. A long meeting was held in a medical school classroom, led by the

Deputy Minister and the Chief Medical Officer, in which they did their best to convince the junior doctors to go back to work. The demands of the doctors seemed reasonable: they wanted training on Ebola and the necessary protective gear. Their nominated rep. was particularly animated, taking to the floor to say "Why should we be the ones to see Ebola patients when we only just graduated? How can you expect us to work while our seniors, who are the experts, are not coming onto the wards at all anymore and instead are just sitting in their offices?"

Marta and I did our best to reassure them, offering additional training and a guarantee that there would be adequate infection control measures across the hospital. This wasn't enough, so at the end of the meeting we also agreed to their demand that they should no longer be expected to treat suspected Ebola patients. In doing so, we helped ensure the hospital as a whole could remain open, but at the cost of having no national doctors to support us in the isolation unit. It worked, however, and by 8 p.m. the next day, the junior doctors had mostly returned to their posts.

While this had been going on, all of the isolation unit staff, apart from two of our cleaners, had also gone on strike as they had still not received the hazard pay they were due from the Ministry. Despite multiple calls to the Ministry, this issue had not been resolved.

This left the unit desperately understaffed. I explained the brutal new reality to a colleague in London: "I was chatting to a suspected case just after she arrived last night in the isolation room. She was found dead on the floor at 11 p.m. No staff had realised until 10 a.m. this morning – the other patients were freaking out." This was the fourth time a corpse had been left unnoticed overnight on the floor of the unit in the last couple of weeks.

So we decided to introduce our own system of performance-based pay. Each week, every staff member in the isolation unit would be assessed on their attendance, performance and safe practice. They would receive a bonus each week depending on their score, with written feedback on how to improve next time. Although the maximum bonus was just $35 per week, it worked like a charm. Staff immediately returned to work and there were noticeable improvements in professionalism. With Marta and I now in charge of the isolation unit, we redoubled our efforts to improve the safety of the unit and make sure better systems and checks were in place.

With that aspect of the crisis averted, we set about raising standards of infection prevention across the hospital. In addition to screening at the gate, every patient on the wards would be assessed for symptoms of Ebola each day. We set up checkpoints at the entrances to the hospital, where an infrared thermometer would check the temperature of anybody trying to enter. Nobody, even the Minister, could enter without washing their hands with chlorine.

I also did my best to put contingency measures in place for my departure. The valuable support team who had been managing the supplies, the bonus payments and the office would be leaving with me, so we began to look for others in Freetown who would be willing to take over these tasks. We found a number of courageous volunteers. One of them was Amar Kamboz, who a few months previously had taken a year off from her career as a stage manager for West End musicals in London to teach at a school in Freetown. When the outbreak started to get serious, she volunteered with the Red Cross and joined a team of Sierra Leoneans that went door-to-door with megaphones to raise awareness about Ebola. I thought I could put her significant organisational skills to better use. Just as with our incoming nurse, Andy Hall, I had to keep her off the King's books so she did not get caught up in the evacuation. Such volunteers showed great courage in stepping in at a critical moment to keep us afloat.

The following Wednesday, we received news that Dr Cole had died in Kailahun, a profound loss to all of us. It was not a surprise, however, since almost nobody we knew who had become infected with Ebola had survived. By Friday, more than 800 patients had tested positive nationally and it was clear the prediction I had made at the end of July of a major outbreak in Freetown was coming to pass.[12] Connaught had thirteen suspected cases with no empty beds, and one corpse in the Emergency Department with nowhere for it to be safely stored.

On Friday 15 August, with enormous trepidation, I headed to the airport with the rest of the team, hoping against hope that Marta would be able to hold things together on her own while I was away.

SINEAD

Devastation in Monrovia

On 16 August, I was on my way to a meeting at WHO when I got a panicked call from my colleague Teta in Monrovia. "There are riots going on in West Point", she said. "Nobody believes in Ebola even though patients are everywhere. The city is exploding".

The Liberian capital and its one million inhabitants had been at the epicentre of the disease from early on in the country's second outbreak. With nowhere to put the many people who were infected, the government had set up an isolation unit in a school building in the middle of an urban slum called West Point. Angry residents, who hadn't been consulted beforehand and many of whom didn't believe Ebola was real, stormed the centre on 16 August, carrying out seventeen patients who were probably infected with Ebola. They also looted bloody mattresses and vomit-drenched towels. Journalist Helene Cooper described it as "an act so monumentally counterproductive that only raw panic and a profound distrust of government could possibly explain it."[13]

In an attempt to regain control over the situation, the government imposed a twenty-one-day quarantine on the 120,000 residents of West Point, enforced by armed police with helmets and riot shields. As Cooper describes it, "what happened next is a case study in the inadvertent creation of panic, the sort of stampede that inevitably arises when healthy people are told the government is quarantining them with the fatally infected. West Point residents went insane with fear." A riot ensued and police shot a fifteen-year old boy, Shakie Kamara, who later died from his wounds.

I was planning to travel to Monrovia on 23 August to support Teta who was, by then, alone in our small office. My headquarters understandably weren't keen on me going, and there were no longer any flights to Monrovia anyway so it became a moot point.

The updates Teta was sending us showed that, outside West Point, the situation was equally catastrophic. MSF had set up their largest Ebola Treatment Unit ever – 120 beds – but it wasn't even close to being enough to deal with the mass of infected people.[14] The latest estimate talked about 1,082 cases of Ebola and 624 fatalities, but nobody believed this was even remotely accurate. There were 232 new cases in the second week of August and this more than doubled in the following two weeks. The epidemic was so overwhelming that cases couldn't even be counted.[15] Safe burials became logistically impossible so the government ordered mandatory cremations, much to the horror of the population.

The scene outside the huge MSF ETU in Monrovia became a symbol of the world's neglect as scores of patients lay dying outside the gates trying to get in. As one MSF staffer described it:

By the end of August, [the ETU] could only be opened for 30 minutes each morning. Only a few patients could be admitted to fill beds made empty by those who had died overnight. People were dying on the gravel outside the gates. One father brought his daughter in the boot of his car, begging MSF to take her in so as to not infect his other children at home. He was turned away.

For the 'lucky' few who made it in, conditions inside were terrible. One MSF staffer recalled: "We could only offer very basic palliative care and there were so many patients and so few staff that the staff had on average only one minute per patient. It was an indescribable horror."

Quarantine

Ten days into the planned twenty-one-day quarantine of West Point, President Johnson Sirleaf cancelled it. It had been a complete failure, eroding what little remaining trust residents had had in the government.[16] From this point on, the President would change the way her government interacted with communities. Instead of a punitive approach, she started to promote community leadership in defeating the disease, backed up by government and international support.

Unfortunately, Sierra Leone went in the opposite direction.

This issue of the punitive approach first came to my attention in mid-August, when I had approached MSF for a meeting. None of us really knew MSF because they hadn't had a big presence in Sierra Leone pre-Ebola. I was keen to get their field perspective from Kailahun and their general Ebola expertise to inform my advocacy. For any other NGO – keen to have donors raise issues on their behalf at higher levels – such collaboration would have been a no-brainer. MSF, though, were different. They were well known globally for jealously guarding their independence so that they could serve affected populations first and foremost.

This independence was often critical in war zones, but the insular internal culture did mean that they often didn't coordinate very well with others, even in less sensitive situations. So, I wasn't really sure what to expect from my first meeting with their Italian country director.

We met for a ginger beer at a local restaurant one humid evening. My apprehensions were quickly allayed after I outlined why I wanted the meeting. "Look, I get it", he said. "We don't have a strong presence here in Freetown. We need donors like you to help us communicate how bad things are in Kailahun." We were on the same page. I asked him what specific issues he wanted me to raise and one stood out above all: "Household quarantine is a disaster", he said, "it's only making things worse". As he spoke about the negative effects of quarantine, I became more and more alarmed. I organised a meeting at my office for a few days later so that MSF could share their experiences with a wider group, and I invited donors, the UN and other relevant experts, including the CDC.

There was a lot of interest in hearing directly from MSF and, in the end, we had to remove the tables from our small conference room at the Embassy to squeeze everybody in. As it happened, Oliver's colleague Marta from King's was at the meeting as I was also trying to use the meeting to raise awareness of the horrendous situation there and seek donations of supplies for their unit.

MSF gave a damning assessment of how the 21-day quarantine for households of confirmed Ebola cases was operating, arguing it had huge implications for people's lives and livelihoods. Most immediately, while food was provided to quarantined households, it was often not enough. There were also no provisions made for medical care if someone in a quarantined home got sick of a non-Ebola illness. Added to that, people could lose their jobs if they didn't show up for work for so many days. If people were self-employed farmers or traders, which many were, they were likely to lose income.[17] All this on top of the terror of being cooped up with others who might have Ebola.

The fear of quarantine was a big factor in worsening the already huge problem of people avoiding the response. If someone thought they had Ebola, they might avoid showing up at the MSF ETU in Kailahun for fear of their family being quarantined. If somebody died and the community thought it could be Ebola, they might hide the body for the same reason. In other words, rather than being incentivised to cooperate with the response, they were being incentivised to hide and flee.

A final problem with quarantine was that, while it took up huge financial and logistical resources, it was often implemented poorly. Sometimes security forces took bribes to let people out. Around this time, I was trying to contact a woman in Freetown to give her a letter. I called her and asked if she could come to the Embassy the next morning to pick it up. "No, I can't come in the morning", she said, "I'm in quarantine. But I can come at around three." In countries with endemic corruption like Sierra Leone, often when you introduce a rule or restriction, you open up new avenues for bribery.

The MSF presentation in my office became the basis for our policy recommendations on quarantine, and over the following months we pushed for it to be reviewed with a public health lens. We recognised, however, that this was a very difficult issue for the Sierra Leonean government. For one thing, restricting movement in an Ebola outbreak had always been and was always going to be necessary; it was not an option to leave Ebola-positive patients free to move around and potentially infect others. The key issue was *how* to restrict movement, while minimising the negative side-effects on the population. The experts told us it could be done but that it required deep community engagement, and this is where we fell short for most of the response in Sierra Leone.

Screaming continues in Kenema

Unbelievably, despite the outcry after Dr Khan's death, things only got worse in Kenema in August, with the Ministry seeming to be operating on another planet. On 11 August, they sent out a situation report saying that the Kenema ETU was "fully functional". At the next Presidential Taskforce two days later, the Minister stood up and, despite mentioning "challenges", gave a broadly positive picture of an improving situation: "There is good news from Kenema. Within the timeframe of 60-90 days, I am confident that the outbreak will be under control."

I then went up to the podium, as I was to speak on behalf of the donors. Without actually saying, "The opposite of what she just said," I basically said the opposite of what she had just said, based on the information I was receiving daily from Kenema. Amongst other issues, I mentioned that over 10% of the clinical staff in the hospital had died of Ebola in the previous six weeks and yet salaries and hazard pay were still not being regularly received by the remaining health workers, while the volunteer nurses still hadn't been put on the payroll.

The entire time I spoke, the Minister, who was sitting in front of the podium, scowled at me. I also got the distinct feeling that many in the room just wanted me to just sit down and shut up. I was not 'on message'. It was uncomfortable, and even though I only spoke for three or four minutes, it felt like forever. I had promised our NGO partners that I would convey their messages, though, and hoped that the gaping discrepancy between the Minister's account and mine would cause the President to ask her some questions after the meeting.

To be fair to the Minister, I later learnt there were sometimes contradictory messages emanating from Kenema. One
international health worker in Kenema told me: "I once heard
the [senior hospital official] on the phone at the hospital, I heard
her say 'Minister' and then say that 'Things are under control, no
problem.' And the numbers of patients in the ETU she was giving
on phone to the Minister were misleading."

But within WHO, by all accounts the messages emanating
from Kenema were clear and unambiguous. One nurse there
told me:

> One night in August, I remember opening an ambulance and
> bodies and patients just fell out the back and I said to [WHO
> doctor], "This is the end of the world." The doctor replied, "They
> just won't listen to us." I said, "We should be shouting about it,"
> and the doctor said, "It's being done but not listened to."

Another WHO staffer told me that they were "screaming" to their
superiors in Freetown and Geneva, but it was like banging their
heads against a brick wall.

Enter the Red Cross

It was widely agreed that there was no solution to the clinical situation in Kenema other than a new ETU, properly designed and
with enough trained staff. But who would run it?

It was an enormous relief when the International Federation
of the Red Cross volunteered, and even more so when I found
out who they were sending to run it. Amanda McClelland was an
Australian humanitarian expert and nurse, as well as being an old
friend of mine from our time in the same village in South Sudan
ten years previously.

With a situation as intractable as Kenema, I felt Amanda was a
great fit; she got things done and didn't take any prisoners. She

also had practical experience on Ebola from Uganda, and when we spoke over the phone she helped me to better understand some of the issues that would feed into my advocacy. In exchange, I would send her Diet Coke and other supplies from Freetown. On receiving an SOS one night that she had ripped her last pair of jeans and couldn't find any replacements her size in the market in Kenema, I sent her a pair of mine. They were my favourite jeans but, not really thinking it through, I sent them to a woman who would be building and then working in an Ebola treatment centre, naïvely expecting I would one day get them back!

With the help of the Kenema Taskforce, Amanda found an excellent site for the new ETU, just outside the city on a disused airstrip, nice flat land that would be easy to build on. However, she was then told that government officials had denied the Red Cross permission to build on the site, apparently because it was too close to town, and she was shown another site about ten miles out of town. Amanda strongly resisted this new proposal – the land was essentially jungle and would take weeks longer to clear. She kept pushing back until she got a direct call from President Koroma himself on her mobile phone, saying that the Red Cross could either build on the new land, or not build at all. So that was that. Changing the location of the ETU added an extra month to the building process.

It is clear that President Koroma was under a great deal of public pressure to ensure that the ETU was kept far away from Kenema city. After all, the issue of relocating the ETU had caused the riot at the hospital in July. As in Monrovia, this pointed to the need for the political leadership to engage early and appropriately with communities. Unfortunately, the failure to do this in Kenema had enormous consequences. The delay in the Red Cross ETU meant the existing unit at Kenema Hospital, overwhelmed with patients and failing to ensure the safety of its health workers, remained one of only two in the country until the new ETU opened in mid-September.

OLIVER

Recruiting despite the risks

My flight back to London was surreal. To avoid a repeat of the incident when Patrick Sawyer flew with Ebola from Liberia to Nigeria, Lungi Airport had been transformed into something between a fortress and a field hospital. An obstacle course of repeated temperature checks and hand washing stations had been laid out between the entrance and the plane itself, to make sure nobody with a fever could leave the country.

The chaotic situation with the flights meant our journey to London was desperately convoluted, with stops in Dakar, Las Palmas and Madrid along the way. I was surprised at how liberated I felt leaving Sierra Leonean airspace, now that I no longer had to worry about being exposed to Ebola. And I think all of us felt emotional as we reflected on the enormity, exhaustion and horror of the previous few months.

I spent much of the next few days sitting at my laptop at my parents' dining room table, trying to support the team from afar whilst catching up on sleep. The payoff for my decision to return to the UK was that we had received a provisional green light from King's to bring out more clinicians for the team. They were reassured that I had followed their instructions to return and was able to present a clear plan going forward. So we went on a recruitment frenzy, sorting through CVs.

I nearly ruined everything, however, when I accidentally mentioned in an interview on the BBC that I would be flying back to Freetown "in a few days' time." This was news to King's, and within minutes, a curt message arrived in my inbox, kindly requesting that in future they hear about my travel plans in person rather than through the media.

In the middle of my week home, I was stunned to be forwarded an email circulated by an MSF doctor who was currently working at their ETU in Kailahun. In the email, he advised people not to volunteer with King's. His message was in response to a recruitment advert we had sent out to a group of tropical medicine doctors. He said he had felt compelled to reply and that King's "must be either joking, be irresponsible, blinded by good intentions, or have no clue about an Ebola epidemic." He went on to state that

> I know for a fact that in the whole country there is no single
> health facility that can handle Ebola suspects or confirmed Ebola
> patients adequately and safely other than [the MSF ETU] . . .
> MSF rightly keeps as much distance as possible from any health
> facility it has not full control over. These places are a public
> danger . . . Flying into the country to work purposively in such
> uncontrolled environments would be nothing heroic but totally
> stupid and constituting a real danger for colleagues, patients and
> themselves.

With friends like these, who needs enemies? He was not alone in holding these views, however, and there were certainly factions within the medical and humanitarian communities that saw the risky work some of us were doing in government hospitals like Connaught and Kenema as irresponsible.

On the one hand, they had a point. There was likely a greater risk if you worked in a government health facility where, as an NGO, you did not have complete control. That said, it was hard to know for sure that Connaught, now under Marta's expert supervision, was actually less safe for staff than an MSF ETU. We were operating according to the WHO guidelines, after all.

But even if you did accept that the King's team was at greater risk than our MSF colleagues, the question for me was whether that risk was worth it. How much were the lives of our Sierra Leonean patients worth? What would have happened to Connaught if we had left? How would our Sierra Leonean colleagues have fared without our support? Did we not have the right as individuals to put ourselves at risk, and did we not have the right as an organisation to recruit other volunteers who fully understood the dangers they would face?

I respected the professionalism and expertise with which MSF were running their ETUs in the region. They were one of the few organisations that had deployed quickly, they had had the courage to speak out when the outbreak had first spiralled out of control, and they had scaled up to the point where they had a central role in the response. But they were also admitting publicly that they were stretched to capacity, and were unable to open more ETUs.[18] So, in the face of this worsening crisis, what were the rest of us supposed to do?

As my colleague wrote to the MSF doctor in reply:

> A balance must be struck between risk-mitigation for volunteers and the dire needs of the local population. If you take the line taken by the MSF author, then you have struck the wrong balance – trying to control the risks to international volunteers so much that you are unable to mount an effective response that the population needs . . . MSF cannot be everywhere that Ebola is at the moment. As MSF admitted themselves they have drained their pool of volunteers and have no more capacity to expand further. Therefore there is an imperative to work with and improve the nationwide and international response, not just have a few good MSF facilities.

It was a contradiction that they acknowledged themselves when MSF-Belgium later published a report that noted: "On the one hand we were sounding the alarm but on the other hand we were saying to other NGOs: 'Let the professionals do the job' and 'Be careful, don't come into Ebola, we know how to deal with that.' That was the double discourse at the very beginning."[19] This comment was specifically about the June and July period, but my experience showed it was still a view being expressed in private by MSF staff later in the response.

MSF played a vital role in the response and should be recognised for their bravery, dedication, and, later in the outbreak, for providing support and training that many organisations found invaluable. At the same time, when the outbreak grew beyond their capacity to respond, I believe they contributed to the delays in opening up more Ebola facilities by discouraging other NGOs from stepping up. In doing so, they made the situation worse than it might have been.

Meetings in London

One of my key aims whilst I was back in the UK was to raise the alarm with the British government as loudly as I could. My media work helped with this, but I was also able to secure a meeting with a team at the Foreign and Commonwealth Office (FCO). We met around a polished mahogany antique table at the bottom of a grand staircase in the heart of the FCO building, and for over an hour I poured my heart out about the crisis we were experiencing, making a series of pleas for a dramatic scale-up of the response.

I pointed out a number of major gaps. Funding was not reaching a lot of the organisations on the ground. Coordination was extremely poor. In addition, we urgently needed to find agencies to provide clinical support to enable new isolation units to be set up in Freetown. My final recommendation was the one I made most forcefully: "You guys have got to deploy the British

Army, the situation is desperate and I don't see how anyone else can set up quickly enough. The NGOs are too scared and don't have the muscle. We need field hospitals, staffed by a disciplined medical corps and with the backup of a massive supply chain." On that point they wouldn't give me a straight answer, but from their body language I guessed it might already be on the cards.

I spent my last few days in London getting rested and ready for my return. On Friday 22 August, as I was walking out of the gym, a BBC News alert flashed up on my phone. A British health worker had been confirmed positive for Ebola in Sierra Leone. For a split second, I thought it must be me, ridiculous though that sounds, and I was puzzled how the BBC knew before I did. Then I realised. It was Will.

All hell broke loose. The public gorged on the story and the press worked themselves up into a frenzy. Dozens of emails came flooding in from news organisations. Was it me that was infected? Was it someone from King's? Did we know who it was? We put out a press release stating that it wasn't anyone from the King's team and otherwise remained silent.

After farewells to my extremely tearful parents, I set off for Freetown. By this stage, Will's name was all over the news.

As I was at Heathrow waiting for my plane, Will was headed in the opposite direction. It appeared that UK citizens who contracted Ebola would be med-evaced home for treatment after all. I watched the TV screens in the departure lounge as he was wheeled in a plastic Drexler tent off the RAF Hercules plane, and then live-filmed from a helicopter as an ambulance sped him through London with a police escort to the Viral Haemorrhagic Fever Unit at the Royal Free Hospital. Knowing Will, I was aware how much he must have hated all the media attention, although I suspected he had other things on his mind at the time.

On arriving back at Connaught on Tuesday morning, I saw

that the situation had deteriorated considerably in my absence. Marta explained that our beds had filled up rapidly, and the patients had become understandably restless and angry at being locked up inside. And the challenge went beyond Connaught. I heard how during the previous week, fifty-six new Ebola cases had been confirmed on just one day, enough to fill our isolation unit several times over. Many of these had only been identified as Ebola cases after their deaths in the community.

We also had a young child in our unit who had been referred from the Ola During Children's Hospital, having spent two days in their Emergency Department before being identified as a suspected case. Fearing their staff had been exposed, the hospital decided to close indefinitely. International doctors from the two NGOs based at the hospital were amongst the only voices calling for the hospital to remain open, and were left with the task of sending 125 sick children back home without treatment. It was a devastating blow that left the country without any specialist children's services, a situation described by one senior Sierra Leonean doctor as "very shocking and pathetic." The hospital would not reopen for months.

SINEAD

Dispensing with protocol

On 20 August, we got news that the WHO representative was being replaced. Finally! Three days later, the new representative Daniel Kertesz arrived. Daniel's arrival happened to be on the same day as a reception was taking place at the Radisson hotel for David Nabarro, the UN Secretary-General's recently appointed Special Representative on Ebola, who was making his first visit to Freetown.

Meetings at the Radisson hotel had become a daily occurrence for many of us during the crisis, as most of the VIPs and visiting responders from WHO and CDC stayed there. A crisp white rectangular building flanked by coconut trees and set inside a compound with a pool and tennis courts, the hotel was located on the far end of a long stretch of beach, a few miles from the city centre. It was Sierra Leone's only brand-name hotel and had opened just a few months earlier.

Spending so much time at the Radisson was productive for me. I was constantly in the business of seeking and passing on information and requests. I would have these scrawled in the notebook that I carried everywhere, organised by the name of whoever I thought needed to know or could help. "WFP: warehouse" meant I needed to tell World Food Programme that my friend Eric had warehouse space in Kenema that he was happy to let them use for the food supplies they were bringing in. "CDC: quarantine" meant that I needed to ask the CDC head at the time if they would write up their public health assessment of quarantine so we could use it in our lobbying. If I sat in the lobby coffee shop on my laptop for long enough, almost inevitably, whoever I was looking for would walk by. Over time, this became well known and there would be frequent groans of "Oh God. What's on my list today." My bugbear at the Radisson, though, was the ice-cold air-conditioning, since my body temperature had, by then, kicked in to tropical West Africa, so I kept a fleece scarf and gloves in my handbag for the less formal meetings.

As we were waiting for David Nabarro to arrive in the restaurant that evening, Daniel Kertesz, a soft-spoken Canadian who looked to be in his late thirties, tapped me on the shoulder. "Are you Sinead?" he said. "I heard I have to ask you what I can do to improve coordination." It was music to my ears.

I liked Daniel immediately. He was calm, competent and experienced. Most importantly, I was relieved to see that he got it.

Unlike his predecessor, he openly acknowledged just how much trouble we were in. He had quite a job ahead of him so, having been tipped off by colleagues that worked with him in Mozambique, I sent him a bottle of whiskey on his first Monday morning in the office. He texted me his gratitude, but I warned him that with the situation he would be dealing with, I would be surprised if the bottle lasted him past Thursday.

David Nabarro himself arrived at the reception shortly after I had spoken with Daniel. David, a Brit, was a distinguished-looking UN veteran in his 60s who had previously been head of the Scaling Up Nutrition movement, for which Irish Aid was one of the lead donors. I had intelligence from my colleagues at headquarters that David was a great guy. On another occasion, with a VIP like that, I might have been a bit hesitant about marching up and pulling him aside before he even had a drink in his hand, but things were so bad I didn't really care about protocol anymore. I grabbed Peter, who was also there, and we went off to a corner of the terrace with David. Dispensing with small talk, I said, "We're delighted you're here. Now, there are six things we need you to push for . . ."

David took a pen and paper out of his bag and wrote everything I said down. My kind of guy! The most important thing about David, as the epidemic progressed, was that he always insisted on talking to people at the field level, regardless of hierarchy. Between David and Daniel, my evening was going extremely well. Things continued to look up when, a few days later, Tom Frieden, Director of US Centres for Disease Control (CDC), arrived and announced a major ramping up of their support.

The Irish PPE scandal

At the national level, changes were also afoot.

One improvement was on the issue of supplies. Up until August, the system for Ebola supplies had been run out of the

Central Medical Stores. It had been a weak and leaky system even
before Ebola, and now with a huge influx of emergency supplies,
it just wasn't working. At Kenema, Connaught and elsewhere,
there were often shortages of critical supplies at the frontline.
UNICEF and World Food Programme approached me and said
that they could take over the supply chain if requested by the government, and I added that to my list of lobbying points. However,
the Irish Embassy may also have helped this point to move forward in a rather unexpected way.

The previous month, we had naïvely thought there would be
no harm in having PPE for the office in case somebody came down
with Ebola symptoms. In retrospect, this was not a smart idea as
it would likely have only endangered our staff further if one of us
had tried to use PPE without training. Nevertheless, one of my
colleagues went into town to try to buy PPE. He managed to find
some, but the circumstances smelled fishy. He had enquired in a
pharmacy and had been sent to a doctor's private office. The doctor said he had an excess in his "personal supply" of PPE. We took
one look at the label in Mandarin and surmised that they had probably 'fallen off the back of a truck' from the Chinese PPE supplies
that had just been sent to the Ministry. We reported this to the Ministry and the UN and didn't think much else of it. Later, I found
out that 'the Irish PPE scandal' had become a big issue within the
EOC, symbolising the total mess of the system and the enormous
leakage of supplies. The UN told me it was helpful in leading to the
change in the system. I told them they were welcome.

But the big change that donors on the ground and the international VIPs were all lobbying the President for was strong, non-
politicised, transparent leadership of the national response.

Interestingly, it was not only internationals who were questioning the national leadership. At one Presidential Taskforce
around this time, we listened as usual to the presentations on the

Ministry's data. It had become standard practice by this stage in the response for one of us to put up our hand to question the data, as there were usually major holes in it. For instance, in one meeting, the data said there were only three contacts who hadn't been followed up in the entire country for the entire outbreak. Given the challenges in contact tracing we had heard about, we all knew this to be ludicrous.

That day, I started making eye contact with the other donors around the table to see who wanted to intervene on the data but, much to my surprise, it was not another donor who raised this issue first, but the Deputy Minister for Health. Dressed in an immaculate flowing white tunic, Dr Abu Bakarr Fofanah stood up and declared, "I don't believe this data." He then went on to give an explanation as to why he thought the data was completely flawed. Just to recap, this was his boss's data. I was stunned – this never happened. How much of this was about Ebola and how much was politics?

A few days later, on 29 August, I was at a reception at the Radisson when I got a call to tell me Miatta Kargbo had been fired as Minister for Health. In her place, President Koroma had appointed the very same Abu Bakarr Fofanah.

OLIVER

Sister Hajara Serry

At the end of August, I was working in the unit when the nurse in charge of the Emergency Department, Sister Cecilia, asked me to come quickly. She led me across the corridor into the resuscitation room, which the inspiring young nurse Hajara Serry had recently helped us to establish.

As I stepped through the door, my heart sank. Sister Hajara was slumped in a chair behind the nurses' station. Her usually meticulously kept hair was unkempt and she had a look of resignation in her bloodshot eyes as she stared at me across the room. She had the 'Ebola look', a particular expression of red-eyed exhaustion that we had learnt was a tell-tale sign of an Ebola case. The second I saw her I knew it, and I could see that she knew it too. Several of her colleagues were gathered around her, holding her hand and pressing their faces against hers. I wanted to hug her. I wanted to cry. But I knew I couldn't, so, feeling empty inside, I went to work.

Doing my best to appear calm, I asked Sister Cecilia to take the other nurses next door so they could wash their hands and faces with chlorinated water to decontaminate. With the room to ourselves, and wearing an apron and gloves, I crouched down next to her and tried to find out what had happened. She was so exhausted she could hardly even lift her head, but slowly she explained to me that she had started feeling feverish and unwell on Monday, so she'd stayed at home. Sister Cecilia, realising she was sick, had insisted she come to Connaught for medical care.

We decided to move her to a single room in the women's ward of the hospital's private wing, rather than the isolation unit. This was partly due to a widespread professional convention not to treat health care workers alongside their patients, but also because conditions in the unit just felt too undignified for someone we cared about so much. It was, for us, a window into how the loved ones of other patients must have felt when leaving them at the unit, and another reminder of how terribly degrading the conditions were. We were able to spare Sister Hajara that misery at least.

To my surprise, after Marta assessed her, she said it might not be Ebola but a kidney infection. But we would do a blood test for Ebola just in case. We convinced ourselves that there might just be another explanation.

The next day I was alone on the afternoon shift. The responsibilities were already overwhelming with so many new patients to be admitted, so many blood samples to be collected and a number of corpses to be decontaminated and removed. And for each death, I had to go with the nurses to break the terrible news to the family outside.

Amidst all of this, I saw on my phone that the lab results had come back from Kenema. I immediately rushed up to our main office on the other side of the hospital, where we had internet, to check the spreadsheet. Scanning the list of names, I found the one I was searching for. Hajara Serry. Female. 22. Positive.

Deep down, I had always known it would be, but reading the cold truth on the spreadsheet felt like drowning.

I went downstairs to break the news to Susan, who was the nurse on duty with me that day and one of Hajara's closest colleagues. There was nothing we could say – we just hugged. The matron and I dressed in PPE and went to tell Hajara. She had gotten a lot sicker overnight and had pulled out the cannula in her arm. Blood was everywhere. She did not speak, but we could see from her eyes that she understood. We promised her the best treatment, that she would get better and be back here soon, but all three of us knew it was a lie.

In addition to Hajara, I had four other positive cases and just two ambulances, with a queue of new patients needing a bed. So I decided to put two patients in each of the ambulances and called my WHO colleague at Kenema, Dr Ian Crozier, who promised he would be able to find beds for them. The fifth patient, an elderly man, was unconscious already and I doubted he would survive the journey, so I decided to keep him in the unit for the night. We dispatched the first ambulance with two patients before turning to Hajara.

The female ward was on the third floor of a tall old colonial building and the lift had broken decades before, so Susan and I had to carry and bounce the gurney to the top. After strapping Hajara in, we wheeled her into the corridor, where a group of her colleagues was there to watch. I felt overwhelmed with emotion and could hardly talk. As we wheeled her towards the stairs, I saw one of her colleagues take out a phone and start to video Hajara.

I lost it. Maybe I was unfair – it seemed culturally acceptable in Sierra Leone to video people when they were sick in a way that completely offended my Western sensibilities. When Dr Khan had died, there had been videos circulating of his dying moments that the senior doctors would huddle together to watch, which I never understood.

I bounded over to the videoing nurse in a rage, even as I was dressed in full PPE and covered in Hajara's blood. I shouted at her, my words muffled by the fabric mask pressed against my lips. How dare she? How could she humiliate her friend like this? What did she think she was doing? She did not understand my words, but she got the message and put her phone down.

Carrying Hajara down the stairs took an age. Moving a stretcher down stairs with just two people is hard at the best of times, but now we were in full PPE, facing awkward angles at every turn, and were both beyond upset. We eventually reached the bottom and wheeled Hajara through the courtyard towards the waiting ambulance. People in the hospital knew something must have been up because it was unusual to wear PPE in the private wing of the hospital, so a crowd had gathered in the courtyard between the buildings to watch in silence.

After struggling to manoeuvre the gurney into the ambulance, we eventually got her inside. Susan then stepped away, too upset to continue. I climbed up next to Hajara, holding her hand as we stared into each other's eyes. I knew I would never see her again and that whatever I said next would probably be the last words she would ever hear. When I spoke, it would have to be for all of us, and it felt like too much responsibility.

I told her she was a hero. I told her I loved her, that we all loved her.

And I stepped back out again.

I could not see and I could not breathe. She was the best of us and I had failed to keep her safe. With the whole crowd staring at me silently, I broke down. I didn't just cry, I wept uncontrollably, the kind of deep sobbing that hurts and leaves you hunched over. All this in PPE, with my goggles steamed up and my mask soaking wet. I couldn't bear to be watched, so I ran back out into the courtyard where it was now dark and raining.

After a couple of minutes, as I began to regain my composure, I remembered that I still had work to do, and with Susan gone I would have to do it alone. With tears still pouring down my face, unable to speak, I went back into the unit and silently ushered the other confirmed patient, a woman of a similar age to Hajara, into the ambulance, and laid her down on the narrow padded bench opposite the stretcher. I watched as the ambulance pulled away.

The next morning, on Sunday 31 August, I called Kenema to check on how Hajara was doing. Ian explained that the ambulance had arrived late at night, and that when he had opened the doors he found the two women dead inside, their bodies collapsed together on the floor. Unable to work out which woman was which, the burial team had decided to inter them both in graves labelled 'anonymous Freetown cases.'

SIX | The long wait for action

SINEAD

The world wakes up

On 2 September at the United Nations in New York, MSF called for military intervention, the first time the organisation had done so in its forty-three-year history. In her speech, MSF International President Joanne Liu was categorical:

> To curb the epidemic, it is imperative that States immediately deploy civilian and military assets with expertise in biohazard containment. I call upon you to dispatch your disaster response teams, backed by the full weight of your logistical capabilities. . . . Without this deployment, we will never get the epidemic under control.[1]

Next day, the World Bank President, Dr Jim Kim, hosted a high-level meeting on the crisis at the Bank's headquarters in Washington, DC. As it happened, Dr Kim, a physician, had co-founded the organisation Partners in Health with Harvard Medical School's legendary doctor and anthropologist, Paul Farmer, and had experience working on infectious diseases in developing countries. By all accounts, the meeting was fraught. A *New York Times* article later reported that Dr Kim had said to the WHO Director-General, Dr Margaret Chan: "You have the authority to act in this emergency. So why aren't you doing it?"[2] It was agreed that Dr Kim and the UN Secretary-General Ban Ki-moon would reach out to the leaders of Guinea, Sierra Leone and Liberia over the following two days to determine how the international community could support each affected country's response plan. It seemed at long last there was a sense of urgency at the global level.

On 9 September, President Johnson Sirleaf helped raise the global temperature even further by sending a letter to President Obama, which quickly got reported in every major news outlet.[3] In it, she wrote:

> I am being honest with you when I say that at this rate, we will never break the transmission chain and the virus will overwhelm us . . . Only governments like yours have the resources and assets to deploy at the pace required to arrest the spread . . . Without more direct help from your government, we will lose this battle against Ebola.

I remember feeling that this increased global activity must relate to the fact that August holidays in Europe and the US were over. A lot of people were back at their desks looking at this crisis anew.

Bailing out a leaky rowboat with teaspoons

This global momentum could not come a moment too soon for us in Freetown. In the first week of September, we had 157 new cases in Sierra Leone, bringing the total number of people infected in the outbreak to 1,276, that we knew of.[4]

We started hearing that the countries would be carved up as per their colonial and historical linkages: the US would help Liberia, the French, Guinea and the UK, Sierra Leone. This prediction was supported by the fact that DFID's Freetown office ramped up their Ebola activity in September as colleagues returned from leave and, as they told me at the time, received instructions from London to work exclusively on Ebola.

It was very welcome. The UK had told President Koroma in August that they would support an ETU in Freetown and they sent an experienced humanitarian consultant, Peter Rees-Gildea, who had a budget of 25 million pounds to help support the national response.

Some improvements in the national response kicked in around this time as well. The CDC was working to improve the data. The President appointed a new Ebola Operations Coordinator, Stephen Gaojia, to help lead the EOC. This was a surprising decision, as Stephen, while a politician, was not a member of the President's party. Having worked closely with Stephen in the past, though, I thought it was a smart move. He had been a government minister in the previous administration, and I saw him as competent and well-intentioned. After the small political party that he had been a part of had failed to win any seats in parliament in the 2012 elections, Stephen had returned to work in the US until President Koroma unexpectedly called him home. Whilst it was good news from my perspective to have Stephen on board for the fight against Ebola he told me his elderly mother in southern Sierra Leone saw things quite differently!

I helped Stephen get a handle on the response, introduced him to the key players on the international side, and even started sending him lunch daily once I found out he was in meetings until 10 p.m. every night and was starting to look a bit gaunt. I wouldn't have predicted that 'lunch provision' would have become one of my Ebola activities, but these were not normal times. For his part, Stephen gave me the inside track on developments within the EOC and did his best to address issues that I would raise with him.

Despite these positives, my memory of Freetown at this time is of running just to stay still. The epidemic was getting dramatically worse, while we were getting only marginally better at dealing with it. On a group email chain, one phrase used seemed apt, that we were "trying to bail out a leaky rowboat with teaspoons."[5]

A rock and a hard place

I wrote to other donors in early September suggesting we reallocate all our regular programme budgets to Ebola:

> The Monrovia scenario looms even larger with increased cases in Freetown and the North and no beds ready yet and not nearly enough isolation space. We are not at Monrovia level yet, but the window to avoid a catastrophe like that is a narrow one and we need to fight hard and resource quickly in the next 2–3 weeks.

I went on to say I thought we should focus on getting beds up and running in Freetown and the north of Sierra Leone. While Kailahun and Kenema made up about two-thirds of the total case numbers so far, the districts of Port Loko and Bombali had more new cases than Kenema in the first week of September. At that time, Irish Aid had $1 million we could use towards this effort to get more ETUs off the ground, but NGOs volunteering for clinical work were thin on the ground.

Sometimes, outside of our Ebola bubble, when we talked about 'beds' people would think we were talking about a shortage of wooden bedframes, and would wonder why this was such a problem. Some people even kindly got in touch offering to send over shipping crates full of beds. But the real barrier to having enough beds was actually sufficient staff willing and trained to treat Ebola patients, massive supplies of all of the associated necessities like PPE and chlorine, and an organisation willing to manage the Ebola unit.

I strategised with Peter, the DFID consultant, who was actively seeking organisations to open units. I was a bit baffled by the absence of organisations willing to engage in treatment, even given the significant risks involved. It was a humanitarian crisis and we had some of the world's most experienced organisations like Oxfam and World Vision in the country already, organisations that took risks to save lives in other settings. And yet the only organisations volunteering to open new Ebola units were King's, the small Italian NGO Emergency, and International Medical Corps (IMC), an American NGO that didn't even work in Sierra Leone at that time. These organisations didn't have any Ebola experience, but we didn't have any choice. Together with the US and the EU, we came to an agreement to fund IMC for an ETU in Port Loko district, but it would take weeks to build from scratch.

In the meantime, we were between a rock and a hard place. The Ministry was starting to set up isolation units around the country, but we worried the hurried way these were being done could make the situation worse. There were no good alternatives. In Sierra Leone alone, we already had three times as many cases as the worst prior outbreak of Ebola in history.[6] We were completely overwhelmed.

Distractions

Frustratingly, while the epidemic raged, September was also characterised by many distractions. Because the coordination of the response was still weak, both nationals and internationals wasted the EOC's valuable time with their new ideas for what should be done.

One example of this was the red herring, supported by UN Women and others, that women were more likely than men to contract and die from Ebola. This garnered a lot of attention at international level, including an article in *The Guardian*, and there was a flurry of meetings and time taken up in the EOC discussing the implications.[7] But it was simply not supported by the data.[8] I ended up in the odd position, given that Irish Aid was the lead donor on women and girls' rights, of arguing against this focus, which was distracting from the real fight.[9] Whether the motivations were genuine or whether people were just trying to create funding opportunities for their organisations, or a bit of both, we just didn't have time for these distractions.

Unfortunately for Oliver, around this time I created a distraction for him. We didn't know each other very well at that point but I had been working a bit with his colleagues to try and raise awareness of the situation and needs at Connaught. My colleague Emma suggested we offer King's a grant for some supplies. I was able to write a cheque for $4,000 from our micro-project fund on the same day we got the proposal. I felt quite virtuous about how speedy we were. One of our drivers brought it to the hospital to give to Oliver. Job done. Or so I thought.

Emma came into my office a couple of hours later to say that, having had to queue for an hour at the bank, Oliver had handed over the cheque only for it to be rejected. This was not because the Irish Embassy was bankrupt, I hasten to add, but because Sierra Leonean banks are incredibly strict about how cheques were written, presumably as a safeguard against fraud. Any tiny error or extra stroke in my signature and they rejected the cheque. Having terrible handwriting in general, I always struggled with this, but it was never as much of an issue as when a busy and exhausted Ebola doctor had to stand in line only to get a cheque rejected because of my incompetence! Not wanting to risk a repeat performance, we ended up sending the cash equivalent over to the hospital.

OLIVER

Going on the offensive

By the start of September, it was very clear to me that the status quo was untenable for King's. The Ebola unit at Connaught was full, there were very few other isolation beds in Freetown, and the number of cases was still rising. It didn't seem from the meetings I was attending that anybody else was stepping up to open many more beds quickly. If King's limited its support to just one hospital then it seemed like only a matter of time before Connaught, and the city, became overwhelmed by the sick and the dying.

We had started recruiting more international volunteers, and two doctors and a nurse had arrived to join the team so far. We were still desperately short-staffed but I made the call to stretch us even thinner and go on the offensive. We needed to replicate what we had done at Connaught at health facilities across the city, but we were going to have to do it faster and with less direct management support from King's.

First, I needed to understand what was there already, so I went to visit 34 Military Field Hospital, located on a military base next to the President's house up on the hills overlooking Freetown city centre. Following major reforms after the end of the civil war and with strong support from the UK, Sierra Leone's military had developed a good reputation in the country and I had previously worked with the doctor in charge of their medical unit, Col Dr Foday Sahr, as until recently he had also been Provost of the medical school. 34 Military was one of the few isolation units still open and accepting suspected cases in the city at that time, the only other facilities being Connaught and a two-bed unit at the trauma hospital run by the Italian NGO Emergency. Driving into the 34 Military grounds, I saw a cluster of neatly erected tents off the road to the right – their isolation unit.

To my surprise, on getting out of the car I was met by a friend, Lt Dr Mohamed Boie Jalloh, who up until a few months before had been a medical student based at Connaught. He had been the head of the student Muslim association, so I was more accustomed to seeing him dressed in a long *thawb* shirt and prayer cap than in military fatigues. After just a few months as a junior doctor, he had been tasked with setting up an Ebola isolation unit at the hospital, just as a contingency measure. Now he found himself in the same position as we did at Connaught, thrust into the middle of a humanitarian crisis.

Mohamed seemed delighted to see a familiar face and was eager to share notes with me about tackling the myriad logistical challenges involved in running an Ebola unit. He and I suited up so I could take a look around the fenced-off red zone of their unit. It was extremely well-organised, as you might expect from an army-run facility, with the buckets and beds arranged in crisp lines inside the tents.

They had also come up with a few innovations I immediately wanted to adopt at Connaught. My favourite was their simple solution to providing each patient with their own toilet, which was important because shared toilets could lead to Ebola spreading between suspected Ebola patients who actually did have the disease and those who didn't. Back at Connaught, we simply gave each patient three small black plastic buckets, sealed with lids and lined with watertight bags – one for urine, one for faeces and one for vomit. Whilst the buckets might have been practical from our perspective, they were an undignified solution for the patients, and those who were really sick were at risk of falling if they tried to squat. Mohamed's pragmatic solution was to buy a dozen cheap plastic garden chairs and cut a large round hole in the seat to make a crude commode, with a bucket underneath. Comparatively, this was a huge improvement.

The visit was a reminder to me of how much could be achieved within government systems using minimal resources and national staff, provided the right leadership was in place.

But one thing, above all else, stood out to me. Whilst Connaught had been turning away suspected cases that morning, due to a lack of beds, the 34 Military isolation unit was only half-full. Alongside opening new Ebola units to increase total bed capacity, coordination across the city also urgently needed to be improved so that we could make use of every bed that was already available.

Establishing more units and citywide coordination

It was also clear we needed more control of the system as a whole, because the isolation units were just one cog in a much bigger machine. Each unit had to coordinate with others at every step in the process: the government's Central Medical Stores sending PPE and supplies; ambulances bringing suspected cases from the community; labs collecting blood samples and giving test results; ETUs accepting referred patients who had tested positive; burial teams taking away the corpses. In fact, most of our senior clinicians' time was not actually spent looking after patients, but managing all this coordination and logistics. Freetown needed a local operational command centre to coordinate the clinical response.

My ideas about citywide coordination were not really new – I had been pressing the Ministry about them for weeks. But although they had agreed on how the command centre would operate, and had identified a senior Ministry official to lead it, there had been no actual progress on setting it up.

Meanwhile, an Australian friend of mine, Ali Readhead, was now working as an advisor in the EOC, and got in touch with me to ask for some help. Ali's day job was serving as an advisor to the President's Chief of Staff, as part of Tony Blair's Africa Governance Initiative (AGI). This was an NGO that embedded advisors into ministries in a number of African countries to help them to strengthen their management. She had been brought in by the former Minister of Health in July to set up the hotline for people to report Ebola cases, along with a dedicated Sierra

Leonean lab scientist called Reynold Senesi who had been supporting the Case Management Pillar. With the hotline set up, Ali started looking at what else she could help with.

There were two ETUs being planned for Freetown at that time, but both were facing significant delays. So Ali suggested to the EOC that she work up a plan for an interim solution involving setting up new units. She asked me for my input. She was preaching to the choir on this and the next day we set off with a Sierra Leonean epidemiologist to visit possible sites.

Top of my list were government hospitals, as they already had the infrastructure and health workers that would be needed to run an isolation unit, and we would not face the delays and politics of negotiating permission for new sites, as Red Cross had in Kenema. We visited about five that day, including a small one called Rokupa, which had previously housed a makeshift isolation unit. Without proper systems or expertise, eleven of their staff had become infected in August – of these, nine had died. When we arrived, we were alarmed to discover the unit had still not been decontaminated and was an infection hazard. The staff were clearly traumatised from their recent loss, but with a redesign and the right management we thought it could be made to work.

We regrouped in a hotel restaurant back in town and put together a plan for each of the sites. But when Ali presented at the EOC the next day, she received little support, despite all our efforts.

So, instead, she arranged to be deployed to the headquarters of the Freetown District Health Management Team (DHMT), where the local response was being organised, to try to push some tangible progress on the command centre idea that we had also discussed. There she found herself once again sitting in endless meetings with local Ministry officials and WHO staff, meetings that had no structure, no agenda and no sense of urgency. To say we felt frustrated by the lack of action in the face of such evident suffering across the city wouldn't do justice to how incredulous and distraught we were in those meetings. We were positively vibrating.

Despite this discouraging atmosphere, we pulled all the strings we could and managed to get approval for the Command Centre to go live the following Monday. The two of us, along with Amar and Ali's colleague Victoria Parkinson, headed down to find a room in the DHMT, settling on their conference room as the best option. Ali and I went to meet the Freetown District Medical Officer for his approval. Whilst professing, with a wry smile, that he always welcomed more help, he was clearly put out at these young foreigners turning up and telling him how to do his job. We got permission to use the room, but were told it was only temporary and could be revoked at any time.

The Command Centre had a couple of early successes. Amar and Victoria formed a team, and pretty soon they had made full use of the empty beds at 34 Military. But this was just a tiny first step towards what was needed. They set up whiteboards to keep track of the suspected cases in the community, and that list soon had about sixty names, with nowhere to isolate them. Each day a few more names would be added, whilst several would be crossed off after news came in they had died at home before they could be admitted. Only a small number of suspected cases could actually be taken to an isolation unit.

The focus of the response up until that point had been on increasing the total number of isolation beds, which needed more health workers and organisations willing to work clinically with Ebola. But we realised through the command centre that what really mattered was the throughput of suspected cases that we could isolate and diagnose each week. If we could identify and fix bottlenecks in the system, then the existing units could become more efficient.

So, if patients could be tested quickly, and then either discharged or referred to an ETU within two days rather than four, that doubled the number of patients we could isolate. Usually more than half the patients in an isolation unit were suspected cases that didn't actually have Ebola, so spending less time there was safer for them and better for overall capacity. Also, it did not require a single extra health worker or the construction of any new units.

For instance, at 34 Military, we found their main bottleneck was a rather grim one. They did not have a morgue inside the unit, so corpses had to stay on their beds until the burial teams could come to pick them up. When an extra tent was added as a morgue, the corpses could be moved straight away, allowing a new suspected case from the community to be brought in immediately.

Despite this progress, the workload and the politics at the Command Centre were almost unbearable for Victoria and Amar, who felt they were facing constant resistance and hostility. The officials at the DHMT were always frustrated with them, asking why all the suspected cases couldn't be transferred immediately. The officials would stare in disbelief at the whiteboard that listed the Ebola isolation facilities in the city and their available beds. Next to each was always the same number: zero.

Though the Command Centre was desperately understaffed, when Victoria and Amar tried to recruit medical students to help, the DHMT staff delayed the process. I didn't understand why the DHMT were so reluctant to recruit these eager medical students until a Sierra Leonean doctor explained that they were wanting to give these jobs to their relatives and friends who would give them kickbacks.

There was a clash of professional cultures at the heart of this tension. The King's and AGI teams were trying to create a rules-based system where a set of policies would be agreed upon for an operational team to then implement. However, this conflicted with the culture of the DHMT where, as in many other institutions in the country, decisions were often made from the top on a case-by-case basis. Unfortunately, we saw how personal relationships, financial interests and political pressures often influenced these decisions in unhelpful ways.

Whilst our relationship with the District Medical Officer became increasingly tense, what we perhaps didn't appreciate was how much pressure he was getting from cabinet ministers, business leaders and sometimes even foreign embassies, who would call him to demand immediate action on particular cases. He was loath to give up personal control, making this constant turf war with his office unavoidable. It was a sensitive situation, and we probably didn't help matters by being so assertive.

Regardless of the outcomes of these battles, however, there was only going to be so much efficiency the Command Centre would be able to squeeze out of the system, and no matter how quick we were with the turnaround, there was no way of getting round the immediate need for more beds.

Back at Connaught

I was still busy working in the Connaught isolation unit, and while it was gradually becoming better staffed and supplied, there were still constant challenges.

Maintaining a basic level of medical care across the hospital was difficult, as many doctors had stopped coming to work. Given the deaths of so many of their colleagues, their absence was understandable, with many of them facing intense pressure from their families to stay at home. A number of doctors had been quarantined when their colleagues had fallen sick, and one senior physician had even heard his own death announced on the public radio.

When our volunteer consultant physician Terry arrived back from London, he set about maintaining some level of care on the medical wards with seemingly inexhaustible energy. From the moment he had arrived a few months previously, he had insisted on living alone in the on-call apartment for junior doctors, next to the mortuary, so he could be closer to his patients. The nurses would often wake him in the middle of the night when a sick patient needed urgent review. Working largely alone on the medical wards, he would undertake epic twelve-hour rounds, alternating between the sixty male and sixty female patients each day. His work was heroic and also a reminder of the broader consequences of the outbreak on the health of the population as it vastly depleted the health workforce.

Meanwhile, the unit had challenges of its own. Ensuring we had a regular supply of PPE was still a daily struggle. I had a particular problem because we often only received the suits in one size, normally a medium or a small. For a six-foot-two tall person like me, this presented a considerable challenge, especially as the suits included a hood and the arms needed to reach as far as your wrists. A trick we were taught by a seasoned Ebola expert was to cut a hole in the sleeve to put our thumb through, between the first and second pair of gloves, so that the sleeves did not ride up and expose our skin. For me, however, this meant I became mummified inside the smaller-sized suits, unable to bend my head or stretch my arms fully. On more than one occasion I found myself ripping the arms off the suits at the shoulder when I leant forwards, breaching the PPE and requiring me to go through the tedious process of decontaminating and re-dressing.

We were delighted when a large supply of PPE was delivered to us, which we were told was a donation from the Chinese government, flown in as a demonstration of their friendship with Sierra Leone. Unfortunately, we discovered over the coming days that the quality of the supplies was abysmal, with the surgical gloves often peppered with small holes and tearing at the slightest insult. We had to scramble to find replacements.

There were also shortages of chlorine, which was essential for decontaminating the beds and also our own bodies when we removed PPE. The Ministry delivered large barrels of it to us, but the labels had often worn off, which would leave us concerned about what was inside. Was it concentrated enough? Was it expired? One Saturday, I came in for a shift and we had completely run out, so I had to send a security guard to local grocery stores to buy small packets of household chlorine tablets. By the time the guard returned, I had gone inside the unit to check on a distressed patient and he had to toss the packets to me through a window.

Despite all this, the standards of safety and patient care were actually getting better. Realising drastic action was required, we had demolished the wall at the end of the corridor so the unit could have separate entrances and exits, which made for a much safer design. We had also implemented much stricter oversight since we had taken over the unit after Dr Cole's death, and we had a clearer understanding by this stage about exactly what was required to stay safe. We only took risks when we felt it was unavoidable and when our patients desperately needed us to.

The human tragedies we were faced each day meant that this happened all too often however. When I was walking through the Emergency Department to the isolation unit one morning, I saw a motorbike pull into central arch where the ambulances usually parked. The rider was a young man in shorts and a t-shirt, and collapsed in his arms was another man of a similar age who I later found out was his brother.

The rider's face was splattered with drying blood that had sprayed from his brother's bleeding nose and mouth while they were riding. As they came to a stop they fell sideways, the bike's burning hot engine trapping them underneath. I knew already that this was most likely an Ebola patient, but I couldn't stand by while they cried out in pain. I called for our nurses to quickly dress in PPE while I grabbed an apron, gloves and a face shield for myself, and ran over to wrench the bike off them, doing my best to stay at arm's length from the blood until my colleagues came to take over. Actions like this were risks, but deliberate risks, and I would do them again.

After reporting the incident to my colleague Colin back in London, he decided I should start the first of many twenty-one-day countdowns, recording my temperature on a log sheet twice each day and hoping no symptoms would emerge. Even the slightest hint of a headache or sore throat would fill me with dread, and I would lie awake in bed at night planning out what would happen if I became sicker by the morning. How I would call Marta, who would arrive in PPE to take a blood sample. How I would hear the ambulance arrive to take me to the RAF Hercules plane that would be waiting at Lungi Airport. And in my darkest moments, I would envisage my death, imagining myself looking up at a single-strip light on the ceiling of a London hospital ward, through the plastic sheeting of a Drexler medical tent. It was a scenario I'm sure all frontline staff in the response feared and prepared themselves for. I was one of the lucky ones.

Death was everywhere

When I would arrive at the unit for the morning shift, the first question I would ask our nurses was how many of our patients had died during the night. Yusuf Koroma, an Ebola survivor who had been isolated at Connaught, later recounted what it felt like to be a patient at that time:

> We heard rumours that at Connaught they'll kill you. I was in Bed 1. There were five other beds. All five were dead in the morning. I couldn't run because they had security. I was afraid to walk. When I went to take my first bath, I had fear, people were lying in the corridors dying. I could not imagine to be there again. People were dying every day.

On one occasion, I walked into the room for high-risk patients at the start of the morning shift to find all six of the patients were dead. Their corpses were splayed over the beds and the floor, and I was alone. It was eerie. Our cramped unit had only one gurney for holding the bodies until the burial teams arrived, so I had little choice but to stack the body bags one on top of the other in order to make the beds available for new cases right away.

Whenever a bed opened up, we would report it to the Command Centre and ask them to send one new patient, but when the ambulance arrived we would sometimes open the doors to find six or seven people inside. The surveillance officer would have gone to the house of a known suspected case to collect them, only to find three generations of the same family now showing symptoms. We would then have to work out what to do with them all.

On one occasion, I left what I thought was a single patient waiting in the ambulance for about an hour while I moved a corpse and decontaminated the bed to make space. But when I opened the door of the ambulance, I found three teenagers inside, two brothers and a sister, and I was horrified to realise that two had already died, leaving the elder brother entangled in the limbs of his dead siblings. I tried to comfort him and lead him out, but he was catatonic, unable to move or speak, and it was almost an hour before he would let go of their bodies.

Despite the enormous challenges, we did try our best to give dignity to the dead. When a well-known local doctor passed away in our unit, my colleague Dr Ahmed Seedat and I found a Bible and a flask of holy water by her bedside. So, it fell to the two of us, a Muslim and an atheist, to observe her passing as best as we could. Unsure what she would have wanted us to do, we sprinkled the holy water over her body and held a moment of silent prayer out of respect for our fallen colleague.

Closing the gates of the hospital

We had managed to increase the number of beds in the unit to eighteen, squeezed into a space where there had previously been nine. But we were still having to turn away patients who probably did have Ebola, as there was nowhere for us to put them. Every few hours, someone would collapse in the entrance of the Emergency Department, creating a major safety risk to other staff and patients. Something had to change.

We met with the hospital management and agreed to move the screening point from inside the hospital to outside the main gate. We built two huts, one as a screening area and another as a waiting area for patients who were flagged as possible cases. Some of the Ministry officials and members of the public were vehemently against these huts, however, as they were thought to be scaring away general patients. It was a legitimate concern, but we felt we had no choice.

To his great credit, Dr TB Kamara stood up to the delegations that regularly came to Connaught demanding the huts be demolished, including groups from the Mayor's Office, the Ministry and even the Cabinet. He knew that this measure, whilst not ideal, was critical to everyone's safety. This issue also led to many calls for the isolation unit to be closed down. For months, the tickertape that ran along the bottom of the screen of the national news channel included a permanent item that read, "His Excellency the President has instructed Dr TB Kamara to close the Ebola Unit at Connaught Hospital", but the doctor's strong leadership ensured this never happened.

"We'll kill you if you come inside"

There were still ongoing tensions with patients. One night I got a call at about 3 a.m. from Joseph, the night nurse, who said the isolated patients were threatening him. A mother and daughter had been sharing a bed, and the child had died early in the night. The patients were understandably outraged that nobody had come sooner to remove the body and Joseph was afraid to enter on his own.

I called Marta and picked her up in my car, and we went together to Connaught. After trying for nearly an hour to negotiate with the furious patients through a window, we decided we had to enter the unit ourselves so we could console the mother, remove the corpse and restore order. But some of the patients inside were still threatening to attack us, so we decided to ask the soldiers who guarded the main gate to dress with us in PPE, so they could protect us if needed. Even though contact with Ebola patients was strictly against their orders, the soldiers and the officer in charge bravely agreed to help us out.

Our hope was that the mere presence of the soldiers would restore calm, and this proved correct. Patients were being pushed beyond their limits. Officials would often describe them as "incalcitrant and uncooperative" with no recognition that, at that point, we were expecting people to put up with conditions that were unthinkable and inhumane.

Separating families

When we received a positive lab result for a patient, we often struggled to convince them to get into the ambulance waiting to take them to an ETU. From our perspective, the urgency of this was very clear. We thought they would have a better chance of survival at an ETU. We also wanted to free up their bed for the suspected cases who were collapsed outside the hospital gates and desperately needed care.

For the patient, though, the decision to leave was not so simple. For starters, we would often isolate a whole family together, but find that only one family member would test positive, or test results would come back at different times. Understandably, the families did not want to be split up. And until mid-September, the only ETUs were far away in Kenema and Kailahun. These were both many hours' drive from Freetown, and the patients had most likely never been to these places. Their family would be unable to visit them, and their bodies would never be returned if they died. And who knew whether these foreigners in space suits were telling the truth about what would be done to them there? On top of everything else, by the time a positive result came back the patients were often very sick, leaving them exhausted and confused.

This set the stage for challenging negotiations, which, in the heat and stress of a busy day, I wasn't always very patient with. After an hour of listening, counselling, negotiating and begging, I would sometimes start to get desperate. I always resisted the temptation to lie to them, but I did sometimes exaggerate the benefits that going to an ETU would likely bring, and on more than one occasion I ended up frog marching a confused patient to the ambulance with the help of a nurse. I hated it, but as with so much of our work during that period, I believed difficult compromises had to be made.

Mutiny in the team

We also had the continuing threat of riots at the gates of the hospital. This came to a head one day when Marta and Andy Hall were inside the unit and an angry crowd appeared at the main gate, furious they were not allowed to conduct a proper burial for a relative who had died inside. The two had a heated exchange about whether to evacuate, but ultimately stayed and the situation calmed down.

Unbeknownst to me, however, the confrontation had a deep impact on the rest of the King's team, who were feeling exhausted, traumatised and increasingly isolated in Freetown. As the number of cases had grown, we had been stretching ourselves thinner and thinner. We now faced not only the threat of Ebola but also the possibility of physical violence. A couple of days after the incident, on a Sunday evening, I got a call from Amar to check that I knew the team meeting had been moved from 7 p.m. to 8 p.m. "What team meeting?" I asked. In the history of the King's programme in Sierra Leone, the only person to have ever called a team meeting was me.

Amar had to explain awkwardly that the team had organised their own meeting that night. Nobody had gotten round to informing me about it, although I didn't know if this was deliberate or an oversight. It felt like a coup. Sitting together on the balcony of one of the King's houses, looking out over the Atlantic, the team looked shell-shocked and despondent. As we went around the circle to air our views, one person after another said they felt exhausted and overwhelmed, that we were out of our depth, that it was time to evacuate.

Once again, our continued presence was on a knife-edge. After Marta gave a passionate speech about the importance of our work, I tried to address each of their concerns. "If anyone wants to leave, you know you'll have my full support," I promised. "I know this isn't what you signed up for and I can't tell you how it's going to end. But Marta and I believe we can make a real difference, so she and I are going to stay, and we could do with all the help we can get." By the end of the night everyone had agreed to remain for now, and though they looked weary as they left, they seemed to walk a little lighter.

Opening other isolation units

By this time, we had finally been able to get the permission we needed to reboot a couple of the isolation units at other local hospitals. An energetic director from the Ministry, Dr Alie Wurie, had been appointed to co-lead the Case Management Pillar alongside Dr Bash-Taqi, and it was now providing better coordination for the oversight and scale-up of isolation units. This enabled us to get approval to scale up. King's was approached by the DFID consultant Peter Rees-Gildea and secured funding from DFID for the infrastructure and supplies, and the Irish NGO Goal offered to undertake the construction required.

The first hospital we got approval for was a small one near Connaught called Macauley Street. The hospital had seen the city's first case on its general ward, following which it had largely closed down. As a result, their staff expressed some scepticism and anxiety, but were willing to give it another try. I assembled an A-Team from King's to go with me to set it up.

We knew it was a race against time, so we kept things simple and moved quickly. Whilst Andy and the Goal team were busy digging an incinerator pit and constructing a decontamination tent, our pharmacist calculated supply needs and one of our doctors trained the small staff. He also brought them to Connaught to work under Marta for a few days to get hands-on experience with Ebola patients, which was far more useful than showing Power-Points or doing endless dry runs in a classroom.

After about a week, the unit was complete. The skeleton staff we'd assembled were showing nerves, but with just six beds we thought they could handle it. I gave Amar a call and asked her to refer a single patient from the community by ambulance at midday. The Command Centre was critical here, as it gave us control of the stream of patients and allowed the new staff to start with a manageable caseload. The first admission was a success, with the King's team available but largely taking a back seat and observing. The Sierra Leonean staff handled it calmly and with great pride.

With a first new unit established, we were asked to turn our attention to Newton Community Health Centre, which was on the eastern outskirts of the city. We headed over with Dr Wurie and were met by a young community health officer called Fatmata Koroma, who ran the clinic. She was wearing a huge and improbable hat (think Dr Seuss) and was quite a quirky conversationalist. I learnt she had only recently graduated and that this was her first posting. Once again, the team set to work getting the unit open, with the staff getting training at 34 Military and, in just over a week, the first patients arrived.

Fatmata knew the place inside and out, and over the coming months she impressed us all with her thoughtful and steely leadership, coupled with her close links with the community. She proved you didn't need to be a doctor to be a leader in the fight against Ebola.

Shutdown

For weeks, there had been rumours of a three-day, government-enforced shutdown of the entire country in mid-September to allow surveillance teams to go house-to-house to identify suspected cases and isolate them.

It was a controversial plan, one that I argued against and considered to be a distraction. Ultimately the plan was modified to focus on awareness-raising rather than finding cases, but inevitably government workers going to every house in the country to talk about Ebola would come across suspected cases. One positive outcome of planning for this, though, was that it energised the Ministry to get more beds open.

It was becoming clear that small, scattered units like Macauley Street and Newton, whilst effective, could not absorb the huge numbers of cases we knew we might see if case numbers kept rising exponentially. In just a week, between 8 and 14 September, the total number of cases in Freetown had leapt from 71 to 109.[10] For months, the Ministry had been pressuring King's to open our own ETU but we had resisted, as it seemed beyond our capacity.

But Dr Wurie then announced that the Chinese hospital at Jui, a pristine facility that had only recently been constructed, was now available to be converted into an ETU. I was very tempted. Since coming to Sierra Leone, I'd had a dream of making a success of Jui Hospital, which was underused as it was too expensive for patients and most of the staff only spoke Mandarin.

To my surprise, the rest of the King's team was open to the idea as well. I did some back-of-an-envelope maths and came up with a proposal. King's would run an ETU at Jui with staff provided by the Ministry, logistics managed by IRC and funding from DFID. We could open thirty-two beds within two weeks, expanding it to sixty-four beds shortly after that. We would aim to achieve in days what others were struggling to deliver in months. It was wildly ambitious, but with our experience to date, it seemed feasible.

We rapidly got approval from our respective headquarters, and on Friday 12 September we went for a final visit, along with the Chief Medical Officer and a representative from the Chinese Embassy, who both confirmed there was a green light. But the following day I got a call from Dr Wurie. The plan was off – the

Chinese had vetoed it. I was gutted, as I believed our ETU could have had a decisive impact on the outbreak in Freetown and because we had all become so energised by planning the project over the previous few days.

Apparently, when Beijing heard that the British were going to be taking over a Chinese hospital, they found it unacceptable, and had decided to open it as an ETU themselves. That same day, on Saturday 13 September, the Chinese military medical team had received orders to embark on a "rescue mission".[11] They would be arriving in less than a week, although not in time to get the unit open for the shutdown as we had planned.

One major achievement that did come out of the pre-shutdown push was the opening of the ETU in Hastings, on the east side of Freetown. The Ministry had become increasingly frustrated with the escalating delays in constructing two internationally led ETUs in Freetown, especially the one at Kerry Town that the UK had committed to in early September, and had decided to build one on their own. The site was at the national police training school, an open, grassy and spacious complex with a cluster of separate single-storey buildings that used to serve as classrooms.

The Ministry, using entirely its own resources and expertise, had set to work converting it into an ETU and were determined to do whatever it took to get it open before the shutdown. It had become not only a key part of their plans to increase bed capacity, but also a symbol of what the Ministry, and Sierra Leone, could do on its own during a period of heavy criticism. My colleagues at the Ministry were hugely optimistic it would be finished on time and to a high standard, but many of us, including me, were deeply sceptical given the disasters we had seen at Kenema and Rokupa in previous months.

The Hastings ETU was due to open on the 20th, the second morning of the shutdown, and I decided to head down to see for myself what the situation was. It was a bright sunny morning, and the site was a flurry of activity when I arrived. There was a sense of excitement in the air, reminding me of a summer festival in England.

As I toured the site with Dr Bash-Taqi, who was dressed in jeans and baseball cap and spoke of the ETU like a proud father, I was deeply impressed with what they had achieved. The buildings had neat rows of beds on clean tiled floors and the whole site was carefully fenced off. A mountain of supplies was piled up in one of the offices. Whilst their planning for the buildings had gone relatively smoothly, they had struggled to find enough Ministry doctors to work there, and so a last-minute call had been made to Colonel Dr Foday Sahr at 34 Military, requesting the Sierra Leone military take the lead clinically. A small team from their staff, including my young friend Dr Mohamed Boie Jalloh, had been dispatched to the Hastings ETU and given just a few hours to familiarise themselves with the facility and get ready to receive patients. It seemed crazy, even by King's standards, but I was underestimating them. They immediately established themselves as a critical part of the clinical response in the country, admitting about fifty Ebola-positive patients in their first weekend alone.

It was far from perfect, like all ETUs. There were problems with the construction and allegations of corrupt contracts and political interference that would become increasingly problematic. Still, the opening of Hastings was a huge boost to the response at a critical time, and evidence of what the government system could achieve.

SINEAD

Controversy continues
The shutdown, later known as the 'house-to-house' campaign, was something I worked on a lot in September, mostly shuttling

between NGOs, UN and the government to communicate concerns and try to find ways of mitigating the risk of it all going horribly wrong.

I had first heard of it when I got a call from MSF. They told me the Ministry had raised plans for the campaign during an EOC meeting, but MSF were concerned it would result in the discovery of a large number of cases that could overwhelm the existing capacity for isolation, treatment and safe burial. However, the MSF representative admitted to me on the phone that they had perhaps not expressed themselves as constructively as they might have in the EOC meeting. As she described it to me, they were tired and frustrated, and had refused to be associated with the initiative. With their "reputation for being sanctimonious", it had not gone down so well. They were now not sure if they would be welcome back to the EOC. Would I mediate?

I was happy to help. As far as I was concerned, it was critical that MSF remain a presence in the EOC. The EOC folks were gracious when we met. "We need MSF on the team," they said. "And its good for them to challenge, as long as they stay and help."

When the President of MSF-Belgium visited, I reiterated this message and requested they be more flexible on helping with these kinds of 'least worst' options, because these were, realistically, all we had in the short-term. She got it and agreed. I also asked her to call up other NGOs' headquartersand encourage them to come and do treatment in Sierra Leone. We were trying, but it would make a big difference if they got the nod from MSF.

The controversy about the shutdown plan reduced when the campaign became focused on awareness-raising rather than 'rooting Ebola cases out of their houses', as many of us had initially feared. But even the new plan divided opinion. For instance, most Sierra Leoneans didn't have their own water supply at home and many in urban areas could only afford to buy food a day at a time. Would telling them they had to stay at home for three days under these conditions lead to hardship and civil unrest?

The government was firm however. Experience with teams going house-to-house for mass vaccination campaigns showed them that Sierra Leoneans responded well to this kind of initiative. Much of the population was still not cooperating with the Ebola response, and some still didn't even believe Ebola was real. Case numbers were going through the roof, and this kind of drastic measure was imperative.

My colleagues and I agreed and decided to look for some funding to support the campaign. This enabled us to be in discussions around mitigating some of the risks, like organising food provision in the slum areas of Freetown and ensuring teams were trained for what to do should they come across people suspected to have Ebola.

However, at the last minute, the debate blew up again. The Friday afternoon before the campaign was to start, the Minister for Information did a CNN interview and referred to the campaign as a nationwide "lockdown" and gave the impression that it was indeed about finding Ebola patients.[12] President Koroma later clarified the true purpose but not before this interview went viral, and international organisations in Freetown started getting calls from their headquarters saying, "What's going on and how can we stop it?"

When donors and the UN met the following Monday, four days before the campaign was to begin, some of the donors said, "We should try to get the government to cancel it." I had to remind them that the plans that we had all supported three days before hadn't actually changed! It was one of the many times during the Ebola crisis when perceptions appeared more important than reality.

The plans went ahead nevertheless and despite concerns about civil unrest, the three days were remarkably peaceful. I only heard of one incident, on the outskirts of Freetown, where a burial team was confronted with angry community members. Aside from that, the mood was eerily quiet. Many internationals had underestimated the resilience of Sierra Leoneans to cope with difficult times.

Opinions on the success or not of the house-to-house campaign and associated shutdown were, and still are, divided, including between myself and Oliver. The government and some internationals declared the campaign a success; 85% of households in the country were apparently reached with awareness of Ebola. Others felt it was a distraction from the day-to-day response work and questioned the quality of the awareness work. Personally, I feel that while some of the criticisms are valid, it was a significant psychological turning point in the response and galvanised important action, such as the new ETU at Hastings.

Announcements

A week after receiving President Johnson Sirleaf's letter, President Obama announced a response "so massive it stunned even his own advisors."[13] The US would send 3,000 troops to Liberia to build 1,700 beds and open a joint command operation in Monrovia to coordinate the international response.[14]

In Freetown, we awaited an announcement from Downing Street about what the UK would do. Sure enough, on 17 September the UK government announced they were going to support 700 beds in Sierra Leone (and six days later announced that they would commit £100 million [$163 million]).[15]

A participant in the critical meeting at Downing Street which made the decision later described it:

The general mood in the meeting was for the UK to do more. But one Minister in particular seized the moment. MSF had called for 1,000 beds by the end of the month, and he said, "Well let's do it." He set out the perfect rationale in five sentences. The humanitarian rationale and the political rationale. Sierra Leone was an old friend. The UK had intervened in the civil war, and Ebola was an awful war. Should UK intervene? Absolutely. The UK public would support this use of aid money. And that was that.

Interestingly, it seems that politicians were pushing DFID officials to do more, rather than the other way around. One senior UK official later noted: "The UK took too long to realise how big and bad things were. It was a shock to the system. Eyes were not wide open enough. In the end, there was strong political leadership telling officials, who were in denial, saying we'll manage it."

Many of us felt that there was also a self-protection rationale in the UK's decision, with the media still being alarmist about the possible spread of Ebola to the West. Either way, the politics worked in our favour. I was ecstatic when Peter West texted me with the news.

But there was more to come. The next day, I happened to be meeting with UN colleagues at the Radisson when we got news about an historic UN resolution on Ebola that called the epidemic "a threat to international peace and security."[16] The resolution also set up a new mission to be based in Ghana, called the UN Mission for Emergency Ebola Response (UNMEER).

There were a few reasons why this was historic. It was only the third time in the UN's history that the Security Council had convened to discuss public health (the first two times concerned HIV/AIDS). It was also the first time in its history the UN would launch a "system-wide organisational crisis response mechanism."[17] And finally, the resolution, which was passed unanimously, had the greatest ever number of co-sponsors

(234 countries). The UN Secretary-General called for a twenty-fold increase in assistance, expressing the UN's intention to raise $1 billion in the next six months.

Interestingly, despite the optimism, even euphoria, emanating from New York about this resolution, the mood of my UN colleagues in Freetown when we got the news was decidedly muted. They stressed that this 'Ebola Mission' was uncharted territory and there were therefore risks that would have to be managed carefully, especially that of losing precious time adjusting to a new structure like this. A few minutes later, I got an email from a UN staffer in New York who was working internationally on Ebola: "Honestly, don't expect too much", she wrote, "It's not promising."

When I left the Radisson that night, I had more questions than answers. Why was UNMEER to be based in Ghana rather than one of the three affected countries? Would this mean we would finally get a proper presence of the Office for Coordination of Humanitarian Affairs? How would this fit in with the ramped-up role of the UK in Sierra Leone? And, most of all, what would UNMEER actually do? Unfortunately, these were questions I would continue to ask for some time.

Private sector energy

While things were starting to look hopeful on the response side, it seemed to me that the secondary impacts of the crisis on the general population were still not getting enough attention.

On 24 September, State House put out a press release quarantining Port Loko and Bombali in the north, and Moyamba in the south.[18,19] In the previous two weeks, case numbers in Port Loko and Bombali had doubled and in Moyamba they had tripled. These three districts joined Kailahun and Kenema, which had been quarantined since the end of July. Almost half of the districts in the country were now under quarantine, with their population of over one million unable to leave. This meant a loss of livelihoods for many people, such as those who brought their agriculture goods to sell in Freetown's markets or those who migrated to other districts for temporary work.

It also didn't seem to make a great deal of sense to quarantine so many people within these large districts, where they could still move around and potentially infect one another. It made sense to my Sierra Leonean friends, though – they saw it as being all about the government protecting Freetown, the historical divide with the rest of the country rearing its head yet again.

This district quarantine came on top of a host of other measures that affected peoples' lives and livelihoods, even if Ebola had not affected their community directly. Most significantly, schools had not reopened in September, leaving 1.8 million children at home. Other educational institutions such as universities were also closed, as part of the ban on public gatherings. In addition, at different points in the response, many markets around the country were closed, restaurants and shops had to close at 6 p.m., nightclubs and video clubs were closed entirely, and motorbike taxis, a key mode of public transport, could not operate after 7 p.m. The Minister of Finance announced that same week that Ebola had already put 24,000 jobs at risk, and there were likely to be many more.[20]

Much of my understanding on these issues did not actually come from my work day but from my social life. Most of my Sierra Leonean friends worked in the private sector and, by September, they were anxiously trying to keep their businesses afloat and their staff employed. The economy was collapsing, partly because of Ebola and partly because the price of iron ore had plummeted, and the economy had become very dependent on this export income.

It is surprisingly easy for internationals in the aid sector to lose touch with the perspective of the general population at the best of times, and this became even more likely during Ebola when we were dashing from pillar to post. To counter this, I tried to stop by the local restaurant Balmaya once or twice a week, provided whatever meeting or reception I had hadn't finished too late.

Balmaya was one of Sierra Leone's oldest restaurants and a Freetown institution, presided over by its indomitable seventy-something proprietor Aunty Joy Samake. My friends and I would converge around her as she held court at the corner table of the restaurant's breezy open-air terrace, slightly elevated above the busy main road. While we couldn't escape the incessant traffic noise, Aunty Joy had surrounded the terrace with large leafy plants, so at least we could imagine we were somewhere less congested. In those days, I would generally not make it into a seat before my friends would start interrogating me on the Ebola situation since, ironically, despite being Sierra Leonean citizens, they had much less access to information on the crisis than I had. "Is it true that there are now cases originating in Freetown, not just coming from Kenema?" "Is the government finally getting a grip on it?" "Is there any news on a vaccine?"

In turn, I would grill them on how people and companies were coping. I would then use the information I would get from them to feed into the lobbying we were doing on the State of Emergency measures. Although quarantine was our biggest concern, we felt the whole suite of emergency measures should be reviewed. We were convinced that, apart from being damaging to people's livelihoods, they were probably also not doing much to stop Ebola. But the government's policy on these measures was firm: by deliberately causing the population inconvenience in their daily lives, the measures showed the population that Ebola was real and had to be taken seriously.

So while we continued to lobby, we were not terribly optimistic. Over the course of those evenings in Balmaya, another possibility to mitigate the increasingly dire situation of the private sector started to emerge. It started off back in July when some of my Sierra Leonean friends, or friends of friends, wanted to make donations of money or goods to the response. They didn't trust the government, however, so would ask me how to donate and I in turn would link them up with whichever NGO I thought could most use their soap, mattresses or cash at the time. People then started approaching me offering to volunteer their time. They were deeply worried about their country, had skills, knew the terrain and how to get things done. Most people couldn't afford to volunteer for very long, or make too many donations, though. They needed their companies to survive.

There was work available for companies, but it was related to the Ebola response and tended to be cornered by government, UN and NGOs. This gave my friend Memuna Forna and me an idea. Always glamorous in her tailored black dresses, Memuna was a communications specialist and did a lot of work promoting Sierra Leone as a location for international investment. She and I decided one evening that what was needed was a 'matchmaking' initiative. Rather than importing everything, we needed the international responders to know what goods and services they could get on the domestic market, and we needed the local companies to know where to look for contracts.

Memuna got to work on the supply side, putting together an Excel spreadsheet in which companies detailed the goods and services they could provide. Ultimately there were over seventy companies in the database with goods and services, such as buckets and bed clothes for ETUs, and trucks to transport food for quarantined homes around the country. I worked on the demand side, lobbying the international agencies like DFID or World

Food Programme to look at what was available domestically before flying in goods or consultants.

We brought both sides together at a launch in late September. There was great energy at the event. Private sector folks were keen to get involved and some responders saw this as a way to solve some of their supply problems. In addition, the more progressive responders saw the benefit of helping the struggling domestic private sector survive and recognised that domestic know-how would often be superior to anything brought in from overseas. For instance, instead of flying in communications people from abroad to help with social mobilisation, we encouraged them to hire a Sierra Leonean communications company who already knew their way around.

There were limitations to the initiative however. The domestic private sector didn't produce some of the things the response needed, such as PPE or chlorine, while some international agencies were too set in their ways in terms of importing their supplies from established systems abroad, which was disappointing. Still, it was something.

The first ministerial visit

The day after the launch event for the matchmaking initiative, we got word from our headquarters that the Minister of State for International Development, who oversaw Irish Aid, was interested in coming to Freetown. This was a surprise. At this time, international hysteria about Ebola was still strong and, apart from public health specialists, most travellers were heading away from Sierra Leone, not coming in. We couldn't think of a single politician from any other country that had visited Sierra Leone since the virus took hold – Minister Seán Sherlock would be the first. He had been recently appointed to the job and when he had a discussion with Irish Aid officials about his first country visit, they agreed that Sierra Leone would be the best place at that moment in time. He would be able to learn a lot about our aid programme and hopefully have a bit of an impact too.

We were delighted with this prospect for a couple of reasons. High-level visits were always a useful way to pass messages to the powers-that-be in that country, and, God knows, we had a lot of messages to pass to the Sierra Leonean government at this time. Secondly, we thought a ministerial visit might help to clarify that the region was not as dangerous as it was commonly misunderstood to be. Surely a minister wouldn't visit if he thought he was at risk of infection?

Every diplomat will tell you that a big downside of any high-level visit is the preparatory work: organising the visits the VIP will go on; doing pre-visits to check journey times and make sure that everything will work well on the day; putting together detailed briefing documents on every aspect of the visit. In this case, though, we just didn't have time for all the usual bells and whistles, so we did the bare minimum of preparation, hoping that it would be enough.

Given this, I was a bit apprehensive when I took the boat over to the airport to meet the Minister when he arrived. My concerns were soon allayed when he got off the plane wearing a pair of long khaki shorts and sporting a broad smile. He was about forty years old, full of energy and with little interest in formalities or protocol. We would get on just fine.

As we filled him in on the situation and took him on visits, the Minister became increasingly incredulous at the state of the response and particularly the vast gap between the needs of the situation and the paltry resources that were being put into it. When, on his visit to the Freetown Command Centre, he saw that the data on cases was being recorded with markers on whiteboards, he was appalled. We had to point out that, basic as it was, it was actually huge progress that data was being recorded transparently at all.

Next stop was our meeting with President Koroma. The Sierra Leonean government was happy to see the first foreign ministerial visit since the start of Ebola, as they were keen to retain some sense of normality in the country so the President had gladly assented to meet.

En route to the meeting, the Minister and I stopped off to meet with colleagues from the UK to prioritise which concerns we would emphasise in the meeting. At the time, there were enormous problems with health workers not receiving their hazard pay, and sometimes their salary, from the Ministry of Health. We had also heard many rumours of corruption. So we proposed the Ebola payment system be moved outside the Ministry. We were not sure the President would be open to this, but when asked in the meeting, he responded that he would indeed be open to a different way of doing things. He knew about the strikes, and could see the current system wasn't working. I called Peter on the way to our next visit and told him the prospects for a shift were looking promising.

The next day, as I drove to a meeting with diplomats and donors at the Radisson with the Minister, we came across an unexpected traffic jam. People living in shanty housing opposite the hotel were protesting because there had been a death in the community and despite calling the hotline as they were supposed to, the body had still not been picked up after three days. It had now, as they told us, become bloated and had an overpowering stench.

To highlight the issue, the community members had blocked the road close to the Radisson. Fortunately, when our driver spoke to the protestors, they agreed to let us pass. When we got to the Radisson, my colleague Emma called the Command Centre to alert them, and they collected the body soon afterwards. So, it was a pretty effective form of protest. I felt a bit uneasy about this, though, as I was aware there were many other uncollected bodies around town, some for days longer. The resources simply were not there at the time to keep up.

The day after the Minister left, a Sunday, I was back at the Radisson again. My first meeting brought a rare moment of light relief. I was meeting the President of the Sierra Leone Football Association, who was a friend. The football team was supposed to go to Cameroon for a match, but the hosts were so nervous that the Sierra Leonean team had been asked to bring a doctor with specialist knowledge of Ebola along with them. Could I help?

At first, I had to suppress a laugh. We barely had any doctors with specialist knowledge of Ebola to actually work on Ebola, let alone travel to football matches. But, at the same time, the conversation did bring up a serious point. Even though Ebola was a huge problem for Sierra Leone and some of the population were directly affected, most Sierra Leoneans were just trying to get by and earn a living in whatever way they could.

My next meeting that Sunday evening was with Oliver, actually the first time we had worked together substantively, apart from that small grant we had given King's earlier for supplies. He wanted to talk about an untenable situation affecting efforts to scale up isolation beds in the city.

OLIVER

Troubled waters

Despite the opening of new isolation units at Macauley Street and Newton, troubled waters lay ahead. There was growing recognition at all levels that the outbreak in Freetown was spiralling out of control and becoming a real threat to the country. The

President appeared increasingly desperate about what to do, and put immense pressure on his officials to get the situation under control. This pressure put our plans at risk, since our approach required caution so as not to overwhelm these small new facilities. At the heart of this lay the question of who, in this partnership between King's and the Ministry, was in control of the isolation units.

The first skirmish was at Connaught Hospital late one afternoon, when I happened to be in a meeting with the Chief Medical Officer in the Ministry. I got a call from Marta that a senior politician from the Ministry had arrived at the hospital accompanied by a convoy of ambulances filled with suspected Ebola patients she had arranged to have rounded up from the community. Of course, all this had been done outside of the Command Centre system, which was supposed to be managing these referrals in a planned and coordinated way. On learning the Ebola unit was full, the politician demanded that alternative beds be found. "Just relocate patients from one of the general wards at the back of the hospital," she instructed the Ebola unit staff, "and turn that into a second Ebola ward so that we can move these patients up immediately."

At King's, we fully agreed there was an urgent need to isolate all suspected cases in the community, which is why we had been working tirelessly to set up the new units. But to suddenly fill a ward with Ebola patients spelt disaster for the hospital and patients alike, and would likely result in multiple staff infections and a total collapse of the hospital.

So I sat with the Chief Medical Officer in his office, both of us on speakerphone with Marta and the politician, to negotiate a solution. I acknowledged that we at King's were just external partners and that the government, of course, had the right to ignore our advice about how to manage their own hospital. However, I pointed out that the government did not have the right to put my team at risk. I explained that if the door to a single one of those ambulances was opened, then I would have to consider Connaught an unsafe working environment for my team. If that were to happen, I would instruct Marta to immediately evacuate the King's team from the hospital, until the facility was once again safe.

Knowing that Connaught could not run the isolation unit without King's, the Chief Medical Officer overruled the politician, and it was agreed that Connaught should not at any time isolate more Ebola patients than its designated bed capacity. This seemed like a victory, but it came at a cost. I was later informed there had been nowhere else to put the patients, so they were left in the back of the ambulances overnight, with a number of them most likely dying as a result.

Round two came not long afterwards when I got a call on a Monday morning from Amar. She was worried that something was not right at Macauley Street. We had taken our eye off this unit while we concentrated on Newton, and I had, wrongly, figured that one of the staff would call me if they encountered a problem. It turned out the Freetown DHMT had decided, without informing us, to significantly expand the Ebola unit at Macauley Street over the weekend and fill it with more patients.

The expansion had been very poorly thought through, to say the least. The original isolation unit had been carefully designed to ensure safety. Now the DHMT, with the support of WHO, had simply converted a room in the main hospital building into an Ebola ward, thereby compromising the entire facility.

It wasn't until we arrived at the hospital that we discovered quite how catastrophic this act had been. The nursing staff we had been nurturing had fled, feeling understandably overwhelmed.

We were told that three corpses were scattered across the site, including one that was slouched against the door of the medical superintendent's office. Faeces and blood were smeared on the walls, including in the PPE dressing room and the decontamination area. The patients who were still alive were wandering listlessly around the compound. Normally, when people compare a situation to a horror film or zombie movie, they are exaggerating. This was no exaggeration.

As usual, there was nobody we could call for help. As far as everyone else was concerned, we were the help. We didn't have time to ask how this had been allowed to happen or to let our frustration get the better of us. My newly arrived colleague, Dr Dan Youkee, and I had to get to work.

There were two jobs that needed to be done. One of us needed to coordinate with the Command Centre to arrange ambulances to relocate the remaining patients and for burial teams to come for the corpses. The second person had to go alone into the devastation to find the patients and help the burial teams, when they arrived, with the bodies. Since I was the only person who knew how to manage the coordination, it fell to Dan on his second day in Sierra Leone to get suited up in the emergency PPE I kept in the back of my car, and go inside. It's a job he took on without hesitation.

After a few stressful and strenuous hours, the site was made safe, but it was still a huge loss. The unit had collapsed, and its staff members were reluctant to return. It was just one of several similar setbacks we experienced around that time.

So, I picked up the phone and started firing off emails to my most senior contacts in the national response and international community, including Sinead, asking for action to be taken to prevent this from happening again. In an email to Daniel Kertesz at WHO and the health lead at DFID, I said,

I have grave concerns about the way in which the response
in Freetown is being managed. There is no clear plan, the
new units and the Command Centre have been pushed to
the point of collapse. The situation has become absolutely
untenable. These are not problems of strategy, technical skills,
human resource capacity or funding – it is exclusively an
issue of political leadership and support at both the macro
and micro level.

I had also spoken with senior colleagues at the Ministry, who had
set up a meeting with the Freetown District Medical Officer to
discuss it, but after two hours of talking, nothing was resolved.

Sinead heard my alarm bells, however, and quickly engaged
her counterparts from WHO and the US and UK governments.
A group of us met in the Radisson hotel restaurant one evening.
There, I explained my frustration at how King's finally had the
staff, resources and know-how to significantly increase the number of isolation beds, but were being obstructed at every turn by
individuals at the Ministry, who were more focused on using the
response as a way to score brownie points with the President, or
to avoid blame.

I explained that we needed new leadership, in the form of a
senior Sierra Leonean who could oversee the response in Freetown outside of the DHMT, and clear protocols to prevent the
meddling in the Command Centre and isolation units. These
problems would obviously be more difficult to resolve, but the
team promised to take it up with urgency and at the highest levels.
At that time, I did not know Sinead well, but she had an impressive reputation and I was hopeful she and the other major players
would find a solution.

But as September drew to a close, more bad news came in. Dr
Ian Crozier at Kenema had become sick a couple of weeks previously, and we now heard our friend and colleague Dr Michael

Mwanda at Emergency was infected as well. To Marta and me, it felt only a matter of time before it would be our turn.

At the same time, the CDC published a new model predicting that unless the response improved, then, in the worst-case scenario, there could be 1.4 million cases of Ebola in Sierra Leone and Liberia by 20 January.[21] As I drove home in the rain after hearing the news, I passed people walking, bicycling, driving, and I could not shake the image of one in ten of them being dead in just a few months' time.

SINEAD

Devastation in the north

The announcements about the new UN and UK missions in the second half of September had given us hope. There was also promising news from the first-hit districts in the east. The combination of an improving response, strong local leadership and changes in community behaviour had resulted in progress quashing the local outbreaks in those districts. In the first week of October, the district of Kenema reported just five cases and Kailahun only three.[1] I later asked Yoti Zabulon from WHO what had made the difference in Kailahun. "We worked with the chiefs and the religious leaders," he told me. "There were chief-led efforts at mobilising communities as well as talks in mosques and churches. It was a community-led effort to break transmission." Leaders had worked with their communities to come up with local rules about how to deal with the epidemic and had then enforced them, such as having a rule that any visitors ("strangers") had to be announced to the chief.

Community engagement varied considerably around the country but another bright spot at that time was Koinadugu district which had, thus far, managed to avoid a single Ebola case, the only district to do so. Granted, geography was helpful as Koinadugu was relatively remote. Critically, though, since Ebola had first hit Sierra Leone, community leaders in Koinadugu had undertaken vigorous mobilisation and, with voluntary input from local residents, set up a network of checkpoints all over the district to monitor and restrict movement. One community leader later said: "For that time, coming to Koinadugu was more difficult than going to the USA!"

At the same time, leaders in Koinadugu put systems in place to support the population to continue with trade and agriculture despite the movement restrictions. A fleet of communal trucks was made available to the district's food growers for the export of their produce and goods to neighbouring markets.[2]

I had heard about these initiatives from a friend of mine who happened to be from Koinadugu and who was involved in their District Taskforce, and we had been happy to give them a small grant from the Embassy, as this was the best example I knew of where communities had taken action themselves which made a real difference. We kept our fingers crossed for them.

But this good news was overshadowed by the dire situation in the country as a whole. There were 290 new cases that first week of October, almost double the 157 cases from the first week of September.[3,4] Of these 290 new cases, 233 were in Freetown and its surrounding rural areas, and in two northern districts: Port Loko and Bombali.

By early October, horror stories abounded in the north. The *New York Times'* Adam Nossiter, one of the journalists who won a Pulitzer Prize for his long-term coverage of Ebola, wrote about 'A Hospital from Hell' that he visited in Bombali, the President's home district, about a three-hour drive from Freetown. Adam's article showed that all of Oliver's worst fears about hospital preparedness had been realised:

> A 4-year-old girl lay on the floor in urine, motionless, bleeding from her mouth, her eyes open. A corpse lay in the corner – a young woman, legs akimbo, who had died overnight. A small child

stood on a cot watching as the team took the body away, stepping around a little boy lying immobile next to black buckets of vomit.

The hospital director described the training they had received on Ebola as "just PowerPoint".[5]

The government had been setting up Ebola isolation units (sometimes called 'holding' units) in these northern districts, but these didn't have anything like the standards the King's team were using.

In Port Loko district, which sits between Bombali and Freetown, there were so many cases that people were being taken to local clinics that didn't even have an isolation unit. A CDC staff member visited one of these facilities and wrote in internal emails:

5 Oct – 18 patients lying around the outside of the facility. We don't know if they walked there or if transported by community members . . . The patients were in various stages of illness, delirium, and starvation. Those that were able were crawling in a field of cassava leaves trying to eat the raw leaves. There was nothing there for them . . . [Port Loko] is in urgent need of assistance.

6 Oct – 18 people suspected to have Ebola are sleeping outside a [clinic] that is not a holding facility. They have no food, no shelter, no water. They are sleeping outside and are receiving no care. IS ANYONE OUT THERE? We need help and we need it now. There is nowhere to transport these people.

7 Oct – The two nurses at this health facility are also symptomatic . . . Essentially, [the patients] were dropped off to die on the front steps and that is exactly what is happening.

It was catastrophic. On 7 October, Sierra Leone surpassed 2,500 confirmed cases of Ebola.[6] This was the context that the new UK mission entered into.

OLIVER

The UK gets to work

At Connaught, the tent outside the main gates was now overflowing with desperately sick patients with nowhere else to go, so we had all breathed a huge sigh of relief when the UK had announced their major response effort in Sierra Leone. This was to be underpinned by the British Army, with 750 military personnel committed for deployment. It felt like the cavalry was finally coming.

The UK response, known as the Joint Inter-Agency Taskforce (JIATF), rapidly contributed to a fundamental shift in the urgency and professionalism of the response. After months of inaction and infighting, I found myself transported into a world of terse discussion and swift decision making.

JIATF was set up at a former UK military base nestled on the hill next to the US Embassy. In recent years, the base had become more of a residential complex for UK officials, and it had somehow managed to re-create the feel of a sleepy English village, which of course meant that there was a pub at the centre. With the arrival of hundreds of military personnel, though, the base had reverted to a much more hurried atmosphere. A training facility was converted into an Ebola operations centre, with a hive of British soldiers in military fatigues busying themselves around long rows of trestle tables equipped with secure telephone lines and military laptops.

Retooling this military machine to support a civilian health emergency would require some work, however. Soon after the UK team arrived, I was invited to one of their evening meetings, the Commander's Update Brief (but referred to universally as the CUB), where the various UK teams would provide updates. Nobody was allowed to sit or get too comfortable, which might explain why these meetings were so efficient!

I had been asked to stay behind at the end to give input on the UK's plan for isolation in Freetown. I dusted off the proposal for quick new isolation units that Ali and I had drawn up a month previously only to have it largely ignored by the EOC, bar the couple of units we'd eventually gotten approval for. Whilst the plan was the same, the audience couldn't have been more different. We stood in the centre of the hall around a high table, upon which enormous maps of the city were laid out. Donal Brown, the senior DFID official who had been appointed head of JIATF, led the meeting and was joined by the senior UK military officer, Brigadier Steve McMahon, and Peter West, the British High Commissioner, as well as a cluster of other senior military and humanitarian staff. As I spoke about possible sites, soldiers scrambled in the background to work out their GPS coordinates and update the maps.

At the end of my presentation, a team of military planners then discussed plans for a kind of isolation that was very different from the one I had been thinking of. They talked in heavy military jargon about plans to lock the city down in the event the government collapsed, including how to secure power grids, water supply systems and key transport routes. I did my best to convince them that such contingency planning might be somewhat premature.

It was a sign of how seriously they saw the Ebola threat, but also of how the UK's thinking was being led by a military rather than a public health approach. Ebola had become the "enemy", decisions were made as orders rather than through consensus, and constant parallels were drawn between this outbreak and the "insurgency" these soldiers had cut their teeth on in Afghanistan and Iraq.

I left the meeting encouraged at the level of professionalism and urgency the UK had brought, as well as the sheer scale of people and resources now at our disposal. The JIATF model was impressive: it integrated teams from a range of different government departments into a single team and chain of command, creating what the military guys described as a 'uniformity of effort'. Internally, there was talk of a 'trinity'; Donal was the overall lead and managed the money, Brigadier Steve managed the military side, and Peter managed the politics. In what would soon become a pattern, however, I was alarmed that nobody from the Sierra Leone Ministry, WHO or CDC had been invited to the meeting, with the UK appearing more than comfortable going it alone.

I also had to come to terms with my disappointment that this UK military intervention was not the one that MSF, and indeed King's, had been calling for back in September, when we had imagined field hospitals and soldiers in hazmat suits. I was told that, apart from a small Ebola unit under construction at the Kerry Town ETU to care for internationals and some national health workers, the soldiers were explicitly barred from direct contact with Ebola patients and would not actually be staffing or running the UK's 700 beds. Instead, the UK government had decided that they would outsource that task to somebody else, without specifying who. The role of the UK personnel would be restricted solely to engineering, coordination, training and logistics.

The UK prioritised the safety of its own staff from the start. This was true of many international organisations at the time, including the CDC and UN agencies, but nobody took this to a greater extreme than the UK military, who had been instructed to ensure a 'zero casualty rate' and placed enormous emphasis on 'force protection'. Thus, while they were often out and about during the day at various field sites, under no circumstances could the soldiers get too close to the clinical Ebola frontline, which included visiting me at Connaught for much of the outbreak. In the evenings, they were largely confined to base.

At the time, I was pretty incredulous about this approach, since an ability to handle risk was one of the main reasons we had called on the military's help in the first place. At the time I assumed it was purely a political decision, which it likely was in part. The word on the grapevine was that the Prime Minister didn't have the stomach for the public fallout that would occur if one of their soldiers or civil servants became infected. It was only later that a senior army officer explained another dimension to me, which was how much the deaths of young British soldiers in Afghanistan and Iraq, from such threats as roadside bombs, had affected the psyche of the army. Though this was understandable, it limited the usefulness of the UK military in the Ebola response.

The constant concern about staff safety also applied to DFID staff, and a few days later I was back at the UK headquarters to meet their new health advisor, Susan Elden, who suggested we meet at the pub there. Susan was American, a former nurse by background, with bright red hair and a mischievous grin, and she insisted on buying the beers. "Honey," she said, "this is the least I can do given everything we'll be asking of you over the next few months."

The massive surge in DFID staff included several other health advisors who were redeployed from other offices around the world, as well as programme managers and logisticians. The DFID health advisors had an informal style that emphasised relationships, and understandably they tended to focus on the technical health aspects of a problem. They embraced complexity and were usually quick to ask questions and challenge their seniors. Whilst the DFID team's more nuanced approach was vital in some instances, the military team tended to be laser-focused on delivering on their orders. This made them great at getting things done, although they could oversimplify things and treat every challenge as a logistical problem.

Donal was a good choice, as head of the UK mission, to span the culture gap that existed between these two very different

communities. Wiry and athletic, in his mid-fifties, he carried a
military bearing and could only really be distinguished from the
soldiers by the fact he wore wide-checked shirts rather than military fatigues. He would often delight in reminding colleagues that
his background was as a large-animal vet. He had a dominant and
assertive disposition, which I appreciated since it enabled him to
push through some of the political obstacles that had been holding us back. Some people complained this went too far and that
Donal was brusque and uncollaborative, but this was never something that caused me any problems personally.

Instead, Donal took on an almost paternal role towards me and
went to great efforts to seek my advice and to make sure I was supported. On one occasion, when the clutch on my car broke as I
pulled into the UK headquarters (the British High Commissioner
had to tow me through the gates), he arranged personally to get
it fixed by mechanics and even gave me use of his own official
Toyota Land Cruiser to get to key meetings in the meantime.

One group that had a surprisingly limited role on the large
UK team were public health and disease outbreak specialists,
who you might reasonably have expected to be at the forefront.
Although Public Health England had many qualified experts with
extensive international experience, the agency had no mandate
to work abroad, and claimed they were too short-staffed to do
so whilst also managing the UK's domestic public health issues.
The small number of Public Health England epidemiology staff
that did deploy to Sierra Leone generally did not stay long, and
many of us on the ground were gobsmacked as we watched them
get recalled to London, often against their will, to resume their
day jobs tackling far less hazardous threats such as salmonella.
With the shortage of epidemiologists within the UK mission, I
was often called upon to fill the gap and give advice to Donal and
his team. I would routinely make frantic calls to Colin Brown in

London to check my maths with him as I made my way to a meeting with the UK, to which he once replied: "What you've sent me does look correct, but how on earth are you, with no formal training in epidemiology, the person giving advice on this?" It was an excellent point.

The main brains behind the UK response was DFID's London-based Chief Scientific Advisor, Professor Chris Whitty, who, as luck would have it, was an infectious diseases specialist. It was Chris who had geared the response to focus on transmission and the concept of 'R', which is a technical way for epidemiologists to describe how many new people, on average, one person with Ebola is infecting. If R is 1 then it means each person infected by Ebola is infecting 1 other person. As Chris and his colleagues explained in a published article at the time, "According to our analyses, R in Sierra Leone is currently between 1.2 and 1.5. In some areas, R is considerably higher. If R remains above 1, any public-health intervention (except a vaccine) will eventually be overwhelmed by the number of new infections. Getting R below 1 is the single strategic aim of the UK effort at this stage of the outbreak."[7]

Whilst this relentless drive to reduce transmission made sense from a public health perspective, especially given how quickly the outbreak was spiralling out of control, over time I began to realise that this sometimes came at the expense of improving the survival rates for individual patients and that it did not address the wider secondary impacts of the outbreak.

SINEAD

The British gel
I was thrilled when the new UK Ebola mission arrived. The fact that Donal, their head, had strong Irish roots was obviously even more reassuring!

JIATF hit the ground running on various fronts. The military component included a huge incoming contingent, as well as the International Security Advisory Team (ISAT) that had already been in Freetown before Ebola. ISAT was the latest incarnation of the large UK military mission that had done such a great job training the Sierra Leone military since the end of the war. While they were just eight advisors by then, ISAT laid the groundwork for the UK's first big impact on Ebola: burial logistics.

We knew that transmission from dead bodies was a key driver of the epidemic. This was difficult to quantify, since some of the people involved in burial ceremonies were also involved in caring for the same individual at the late stages of the disease, so it was often impossible to tell when transmission occurred. But burials were definitely a significant avenue of transmission, with estimates ranging from 10% to 60% of Ebola infections being related to burials.[8,9,10] However, while the government had mandated that all deaths should have a safe burial countrywide, they completely lacked the capacity and the organisation to conduct such burials.

It was the risk of community anger about burials escalating into widespread civil unrest that made some officers from ISAT decide to look into the issue. One day in late September, having heard there had been an unburied body in one busy urban area for six days, they visited the DHMT for Freetown to try to understand what was happening with burials. There, they found King's, AGI and the Irish NGO Concern Worldwide running the Command Centre with great difficulty, and found that the system to organise burials was barely functioning. There was just one person mainly responsible for organising burials, no clear system had been established, and in addition to this there weren't enough vehicles and the quality of the few that had been allocated was very questionable. All this meant that very few bodies were being buried on a daily basis and hence they were piling up in communities.

Over the following three weeks, ISAT, AGI and Concern, with the help of some government officials, leadership and funding from DFID, advice, logistics and manpower support from the Sierra Leonean military and technical advice from the CDC, designed a new system for burials. It was piloted on 18 October. Fiona McLysaght from Concern described the first morning:

The ISAT guys slept in the PPE store on the Saturday night before we took on responsibility for burials the next morning. I came in at 6 a.m. and met them, they were wrecked. They helped us to set up the system for the first 10 burial teams, which became more or less the system we would maintain over the next twelve months. We got the role on a Friday and it was to be sorted by Sunday a.m. Late on Saturday night, we were fuelling vehicles and seriously wondering what we had had agreed to take on. It was crazy.

Crazy as it was, it worked. Within three days, the backlog of bodies in Freetown was cleared and the UK asked the President to authorise this as the national system, which he did. The UK then led the same process in Port Loko district, where there had been no safe burials at all up until that point. According to one UK staffer, within four days of the start of the programme, all bodies were being buried safely within twenty-four hours.

Several of those who were involved in that pilot burial initiative told me about the unique partnership which made it work, the combination of individuals and organisations with flexibility and sufficient knowledge of the context to try something new in the face of the desperate situation. As Fiona said: "There was a feeling of all being in this together as a leap of faith, there was sadness, but humour and a sense of collective achievement towards a common goal." All agreed with the sentiment that, as Victoria from AGI put it, "the British provided the gel to bring burials together." Their creation of the platform through which others could act was central to the effectiveness of the UK Ebola response.

This concept of the platform is illustrated by the fact that the main players in the pilot burials initiative were not actually the new UK arrivals – they were people who had been in Sierra Leone for some time. Even key UK figures such as Edward Davis (later known as 'Dead Ed' due to his central role in the burials process) had been in the country before Ebola as DFID's Education Advisor. But, with President Koroma's blessing, the UK took on a mandate to sort things out, finding ways to work around the problems of capacity and politics that had hampered the response up until then. They brought in a ton of resources and they took others along with them, such as NGOs.

Admittedly, sometimes 'working around' problems looked a little like bulldozing, and the approach was far from perfect. But, in the case of the logistics around burials, the UK provided the leadership that had been missing for all those months, pulling people together for urgent action. As John Raine, a UK staffer who worked on burials in Port Loko said:

> Early UK scale-up was remarkable, the most impactful thing I have ever done. When we went to Port Loko, no bodies were being buried, within 96 hours we had 100% buried . . . we were given what we needed, it was liberating to work for Donal and Steve, we got in and sorted it out.

However, reflecting back on it later, John raised one very large caveat to this achievement which was not new but which would continue to haunt the burials process: lack of community buy-in. This was still the 'biomedical' model of burials that clashed profoundly with communities' spiritual and practical needs. As John says:

> Whilst we got the logistical issues resolved we were always
> playing catch up on the cultural issues. I feel we never really
> won over the rural communities in the matter of burials. We
> failed to secure the highest level of trust. Setting up the logistics
> infrastructure was, with hindsight, easy. Winning community
> trust and confidence was far harder.

At the time, though, I was not thinking about this. On the contrary, I and others around me felt an enormous sense of relief and a stirring of hope. It wasn't just the UK's first success, it was the first significant countrywide achievement of the response. As such, it had an important psychological impact, giving confidence to the President and to many of us international partners at a time when we were despairing: something could be done.

Trying to square the circle: re-vamping the national response

When the new UK team first arrived, my main concern was that they would focus on managing their funding and getting 'their' promised 700 beds up and running, but wouldn't focus on the gaping holes in the national response as a whole. Donal laid this concern to rest in our first meeting. The UK was determined to get Sierra Leone to zero cases of Ebola, with anything less considered mission failure. With particular assistance from Kate Airey, the Deputy British High Commissioner, they brainstormed from early on ways to improve overall coordination of the response.

By mid-October, coordination at a national level was still being led by the EOC, which was co-chaired by the Ministry and WHO. This was still proving ineffective, despite the improved WHO leadership. The situation was worsening fast. I was gutted when Koinadugu finally fell victim to the disease with two cases reported there on 15 October.[11] The next day, the EOC reported that Sierra Leone had surpassed 3,000 confirmed cases, 37% of these in the previous three weeks.[12] Worse than that, we had no idea how many cases were outside the system – CDC estimated that for every two Ebola patients we knew about, there were five others that went unreported.[13]

In the face of this worsening situation there were huge holes in the EOC's response. A group of us had been engaged in discussions for weeks about how coordination could be improved. Within the donor and UN group, we had a spectrum of views on what a new leadership structure could look like. I hosted a working dinner in my apartment in mid-October to thrash this point out. Donal from the UK was keen to have a coordination structure that was distinct from the Ministry, given their failure to deal with the crisis so far. Daniel from WHO, on the other hand, could not conceive of a structure to defeat an epidemic that didn't substantially include the Ministry. After all, at the district and local level the only people who had the skills we needed were Ministry employees, people like district surveillance officers and nurses. If you took their bosses out of the leadership of the response, how would that work? Personally, I identified very much with Donal's view that there were huge problems with the Ministry, but I also tended to agree with Daniel that they needed to be engaged nonetheless. It was difficult to know how this circle could be squared.

On 17 October, the President appointed Palo Conteh, then Minister for Defence, to be the new National Ebola Coordinator. Palo, a tall and dashing lawyer and ex-army Major, was someone I knew well as we had been in the same running group since I'd arrived in Sierra Leone. Palo had held the 400-metre sprint record in Sierra Leone since 1982 and was still in good shape; he enjoyed when new arrivals in the group would try to guess his age and generally understate it by 15 to 20 years.

I thought Palo was a good choice for that job. Though he didn't have any health qualifications, the army had been doing some solid work on Ebola, in addition to which, we all felt by then that our main problem in the response was not technical knowledge of Ebola, but 'command and control', putting in place systems and procedures and ensuring accountability. Importantly, Palo had a background living and working in the UK, and the assumption that he would work well with the British in their role as lead donor was probably a key factor in his appointment. Indeed, this turned out to be the case.

Who's in charge?

The President also announced the creation of the National Ebola Response Centre (NERC) to take over from the EOC as the main coordinating body of the response. It would have a staff of Sierra Leonean government officials, led by Palo, with a strong representation of the Sierra Leone military, and it would provide a platform for international organisations to contribute to the response. The UK had proposed a structure for the NERC to the President and they worked with Palo over two and a half weeks to set it up. The NERC ultimately became an important force in coordinating Ebola efforts and resolving problems.

Unfortunately, however, some aspects of the way the NERC was established would haunt it, particularly in terms of its relationship with the Ministry. It had not been made clear how the transition between the EOC and the NERC should happen, and so the EOC, which consisted mostly of senior Ministry staff and UN agencies, continued to meet after Palo's appointment, awaiting some kind of notification. Meanwhile, the NERC also started to meet and so the two bodies met in parallel for at least a week, both ostensibly making decisions as the leadership of the national response. One of the international EOC members later told me:

> For weeks Donal and Palo etc. would be having meetings in one room . . . while Stephen Gaojia, the Chief Medical Officer,

myself and others were having meetings separately and they
didn't tell us. And they didn't have the epidemiological data.

When senior Ministry officials from the EOC were eventually invited to attend the NERC, one apparently refused to attend for a month in protest at the disrespect he felt they had been shown with this transition. Others, however, said this was just an excuse and that the Ministry officials would never have cooperated with the NERC anyway, as they resented that people with non-health backgrounds were now in charge of this huge health crisis.[14] These tensions over power and control including, of course, control of resources, continued and became a major fault line in the response.

The pendulum swings to command and control

The NERC set up shop at the complex that used to house the Special Court for Sierra Leone, which undertook prosecutions after the war. When I went to the former Special Court building to attend my first NERC briefing, I was amazed to see soldiers at the door turning people away. Fortunately, I had happened to mention to someone in advance that I would be attending so I was on the list. I was further surprised when I was directed to a seat with 'Irish Embassy' written on it. These people were organised.

As I sat down on the plastic swivel chair, I realised I had been in this room before. It was not an actual courtroom, but a large semi-circular side room with curved rows of grey desks and a big screen at the front of the room that could be used for watching court cases as they happened. A group of us had gathered here in 2012 to watch the result of the court case against Liberian warlord and former president, Charles Taylor, which had concluded its proceedings in The Hague. Charles Taylor was imprisoned for fifty years for his role in starting the war in Sierra Leone.

The room had been transformed into the NERC 'Situation Room'. It was a far cry from the EOC meeting room, crammed into a corner of a building at WHO. Most of the others in the Situation Room that day were military, either from Sierra Leone or newly arrived from the UK. It was incredibly odd, six months into the crisis, to be discussing Ebola in a room where I didn't recognise most of the faces. Another oddity was the hushed silence, not something one experiences often in Sierra Leone. I eventually realised that everybody was waiting for Palo's arrival. And indeed, bang on the hour, he swept in with Donal and a contingent of military, and the meeting started right away.

The briefing was managed by OB Sisay, an energetic Sierra Leonean based in the UK who had come back to work on the response and became the Situation Room Coordinator. OB would work through the agenda point-by-point and call on presenters, mostly Sierra Leone military, to present updates to Palo, referred to throughout as "Sir". Palo sat with Stephen Gaojia, who had become his deputy by then, and Donal, at the hub of the room.

Opposite Palo, presenters would show the data they were discussing on the big screen and, at the end of each presentation, OB used the screen to show an Excel spreadsheet of colour-coded action points. Sometimes, when action points were marked as 'not done', Palo would bark at the presenter, "Why was that not done? Who is responsible for that?" and there would be a brief conversation about following up. At the end of the meeting, Palo, after some whispered discussion with Donal and Stephen, gave a series of instructions. It was another world compared with the EOC. This felt like an emergency response.

But a few things about the meeting made me a bit uneasy. I was struck that none of the epidemiology experts from WHO or CDC had spoken during the meeting, although Daniel and the

CDC head were present. The focus was mostly on operational issues and logistics, rather than public health or epidemiology. I felt this might have been related to the fact that neither the UK nor the Sierra Leone military working in the NERC had strong public health or epidemiological expertise on the ground. As one donor official said after their first NERC meeting, "If you have lots of hammers, you tend to see a lot of nails."

This public health gap was part of a broader concern I had about the meeting, which was the lack of opportunity for discussion or questions. The briefings were given, instructions relayed, and that was that. Alternate views were not requested and absolutely did not feel like they would be welcomed in the militarised atmosphere. Even knowing Palo well, I didn't feel comfortable raising my hand that day, despite there being a couple of points I thought were questionable. For instance, I knew some NGOs were providing supplies to quarantine homes to supplement what the government system was doing, but when the situation of quarantined homes was discussed, there didn't seem to be much knowledge of this.

This related to my other concern, which was that there were no NGOs in the room. This was extraordinary given they were managing much of the frontline work, such as treatment and social mobilisation. Without NGO input, how would the NERC discussions be based on the reality on the ground? I raised this after the briefing and I was told they were going to be engaged in a separate forum, which they were. These meetings, though, were absurdly infrequent: the NGOs asked for weekly meetings with the NERC, but the second meeting was scheduled for over three weeks after the first. Three weeks in the middle of an Ebola epidemic when strategy changed on a daily basis was a very long time.

So, the command and control we had begged for was there, but in those early days of the NERC the pendulum had swung rather too far in that direction. I raised these concerns with the other donors and the UN, who had had similar observations, and over the weeks that followed, we supported the NERC as they made adjustments to fill some of these gaps. However, quite a few of the international responders had considerable experience in other emergencies and couldn't understand why we were having to reinvent the wheel in this response, when the humanitarian sector had decades of experience setting up coordination mechanisms that ensured the inclusion of different voices.

While trying to strengthen coordination and raising the issues of frontline players was still a big part of my role in the response, I found other aspects gradually started shifting in the second half of October. There was less need for 'alarm-raising' about the crisis at national and international levels – we had most of the resources now and, on the international side, the UK were showing real leadership. As a result, I focused more on giving feedback to the UK to try to influence their response as the dominant player.

This evolved naturally, rather than being a plan on my part. Most of the UN and NGO actors were receiving funds from the UK, and some of them felt uncomfortable with criticising the hand that fed them. So, they would tell me about issues, and then I would tell the UK. In a way, I was well-placed for this role, because even though Irish Aid was deeply engaged in the response, we were not one of the big financial players and thus were not 'in competition' with the UK. Peter and I developed a routine of drinking a Coke on my apartment balcony in the gap between the end of the work day and the start of the evening meetings, and I would give him my latest 'key issues' list as well as, of course, my unsolicited performance review of how the UK were doing!

UNMEER arrives with a whimper

Apart from the UK team, the other new player in October was the much-hyped UN Ebola mission, UNMEER. If the UK had arrived with a bang through their work on burials, then UNMEER started off with a whimper. UNMEER was to bring in a new set of staff while also bringing together the UN agencies already in the country, such as WHO and UNICEF, under one umbrella. In theory, it should have become the third leg of the response leadership, along with the NERC and the UK. In practice, it didn't.

There were a few reasons for this. A big one was that this was a UN mission without any precedent. The UN, like most big bureaucracies, is not known for its agility even at the best of times.

In mid-October, the UNMEER coordinator for Sierra Leone, Amadu Kamara, arrived and I went to meet him for a cup of tea at one of the local hotels. I found Amadu to be pleasant and collaborative, although not particularly assertive, and my first thought was, "I wonder how he will get along with Donal!" Amadu was a peacekeeping specialist, so he didn't have particular experience with health emergencies, and with few resources at his disposal in those early days, he was left a bit toothless.

That day, Amadu told me about the difficulties he was having in recruiting staff for the Sierra Leone office, even though these were not medical roles. It was a common problem. One international NGO even said, "We had people lining up to get shot at in Syria, but we couldn't get anyone to come to West Africa."[15] This reluctance was probably a combination of fear encouraged by media hype and justifiable concerns about visa restrictions – a number of countries had, by then, instituted rules that imposed various kinds of quarantine on people returning from Ebola-affected countries.

Despite the anticlimactic beginnings, I tried really hard to help UNMEER get off the ground, as they had the mandate to lead the coordination of the international community on Ebola and to play a key role in the national response. At that time, I was very focused – in hindsight probably too focused – on mandates. I helped Amadu and his small team to get the lay of the land, set up coordination meetings with donors and NGOs, and try to define their role. But their progress was painfully slow.

Dying alone

The epidemic was not waiting around for us to get our houses in order, and every day brought more horrendous stories. These stories came from all over the place, field visits, coordination meetings, phone calls from an NGO, WhatsApp groups. I had stopped watching television, having previously been in the habit of switching on the news late at night when I got home from meetings and was getting ready for bed. After Ebola started, though, some of the stories were so disturbing I wouldn't be able to sleep for hours. I would lie there feeling guilty about the huge cleavage between what we were trying to do and the suffering that people were going through. I had the same feeling after I got a call in the car one day about a situation that shook me to my core.

The parents of a family in Freetown got sick with Ebola and died, leaving five children in the house. The house was quarantined and the children were left alone there for a week. The fifteen-year-old girl who was, in effect, the head of the household, started having symptoms. To protect her siblings, she quarantined herself on the small balcony of the house and eventually died there alone.

I couldn't get the image of this girl out of my head. The loneliness she must have felt. Five months into the epidemic in Sierra Leone, and this is where we were? This is all we could manage to do for these children?

There was so much wrong with this story, so much that we were not even close to fixing. But one issue I felt we could make some progress on was the situation of quarantined homes. Around this time, Paula told me she thought we needed to get involved in this issue. Her nutrition contacts were telling her about households being left without any food for several days, or getting a bag of rice but not any water or cooking oil to do anything with it. Sometimes people in quarantine did not have access to soap or cleaning supplies, while at the same time being locked up with others who might have Ebola. We had raised these concerns before, and we knew NGOs were trying to help here and there, but clearly whatever was happening was not nearly enough. We decided to get involved.

The only problem was we were one of the most vocal opponents of quarantine. We were continuously lobbying the government and international agencies on it. Paula had produced a policy paper presenting the evidence that it was not working, which we had sent around to our contacts and presented on at meetings. We were thus faced with a real dilemma. By engaging in making quarantine better, would we undermine our own lobbying that quarantine was harmful to the response as a whole?

In the end, we had to acknowledge that our lobbying seemed to be going nowhere, as the government felt very strongly about quarantine and we didn't have enough powerful allies on our side. For instance, it was not a significant priority for the UK. So, we put the humanitarian priority first and got involved.

Paula got a working group going on nutrition issues related to Ebola, along with the other key players in that area such as the Ministry and UNICEF, and this group came up with procedures for supplies to quarantined homes. We then funded a programme to deliver food, disinfectant, and other practical needs like mobile phone credit. Paula coordinated the programme, with strong funding support from the UK and with the NGO Plan International as the lead implementer.

In districts that the Plan couldn't reach directly, Paula and the working group tried to ensure that other organisations supporting quarantined homes followed the procedures. This was surprisingly difficult. Paula used to come back to the office from meetings fuming that some organisations wanted to cherry-pick what they would provide rather than delivering the agreed upon package: "It was as good as doing nothing because if you provided food, but not drinking water, people wouldn't be able to survive without breaking the quarantine to get water."

What shocked us most was the failure of a lot of organisations to give any consideration to the gender and protection issues that were emerging. Unlike the earlier myths that women were more likely to be infected by Ebola, we were getting reports of violations that were really happening to women. As Paula said:

> Organisations threw away their guiding principles with Ebola. Like there were organisations saying they took gender perspectives in their long-term programming. Then you would be in a meeting about quarantined households and no one mentions women and children. The failure of a lot of partners to give any consideration to things like the supply of feminine hygiene products, or the increased risk of domestic abuse and sexual violence in quarantined households, was particularly disappointing and a bone of contention.

This was not to be the only time that we felt that consideration of basic human rights and dignity seemed to be 'on hold' during the Ebola crisis.

OLIVER

'Moving': establishing the Freetown DERC

The establishment of the NERC at national level shifted the leadership of the response away from the Ministry, and the same process happened, to varying degrees, at the district level. For us in Freetown, this was a positive development as it meant that the Freetown Command Centre could finally be lifted out of the DHMT and given more independence.

It had taken a few weeks, but the changes that Sinead and I had talked about in our meeting at the Radisson, regarding removing the political obstacles in Freetown, were finally happening. Using the pretext of a lack of office space at the DHMT, the UK had set up the burials operations in the huge British Council auditorium in the centre of town, and the Command Centre that Amar and Victoria had been running was soon relocated there too.

The UK military seemed much less encumbered by bureaucracy or the need for political tiptoeing than other agencies had been and were quickly able to sort out the logistics of laptops, Wi-Fi and other office equipment. Amar, Victoria and their dynamic group of medical students no longer had the DHMT officials looking over their shoulders all day, and instead could look to this new structure and the NERC to provide them with political cover. A large banner with the new name of the Freetown District Emergency Response Centre (DERC) and crested with the logo of the government of Sierra Leone was hoisted to hang from the rafters. Amar's team became known as 'Live Case Management' and, section-by-section, the hall became filled as additional teams were established to work on specific issues, including surveillance, quarantine and social mobilisation.

The new structure was about more than just moving operations out of the politics of the DHMT. It was also about creating order out of chaos. Organograms, decision trees and process flows were collectively developed and dictated how the response should be managed operationally, with teams being held accountable to deliver results.

At the same time as the UK team had scaled up, we had seen a surge in the number of public health, epidemiology and infection control staff deployed by WHO and CDC, who gradually took on different support roles in the Freetown DERC. They brought useful skills and capacity, but the downside with both organisations was that these staff tended to be on short-term deployments of four to eight weeks. The CDC was bound by US government restrictions on their staff staying for longer than twenty-eight days without having received comprehensive Ebola training, and the WHO experts were on temporary secondment from their day jobs, which they had to return to. One UK representative commended the consistently high quality of the CDC staff's work but described their turnover as "a killer". He explained, "They would want to give presentations at 8 a.m. with their new ideas but they wouldn't have done a handover and we had usually already tried what they were suggesting. It was exhausting."

At Connaught, and at the other isolation units King's was supporting, we immediately felt the difference of the DERC, as we now knew who to go to when we had a problem and had confidence it would quickly be resolved. For example, daily delays in transporting lab samples from the isolation units to the newly established South African lab on the outskirts of the city were resolved by handing over this task to a team of soldiers in Jeeps.

On another occasion, I arrived at Connaught to discover the main downtown water supply had been shut off and the hospital had completely run out of water. This was critical for us, because without water we couldn't decontaminate safely when leaving the unit and ran the risk of repeating the mistakes that had led to Dr Modupeh Cole's tragic death. So I rang Kate Airey, the Deputy British High Commissioner who was by then a UK liaison officer with the NERC, and she immediately sprang into action. "I'll sort it," she promised me. "Just give me twenty minutes." After failing to resolve the situation through the relevant ministry, she co-opted a general from the Sierra Leone military who was based at the NERC, who threatened the local water company that if they didn't send a water tanker to Connaught immediately, he would send his soldiers down to commandeer one. A water truck soon arrived, but the hospital's water tank wasn't ready to receive the water, so the truck tried to leave. I ran in front of the moving truck to block its escape while I called Kate again for help. It was at times like these that the impact of the NERC and DERCs was truly felt on the ground.

I also approached Kate to ask how we could get the NERC to appoint a senior Sierra Leonean to lead on case management in Freetown, so that Amar and I could play more of a support role to a local leader. Despite suggesting various names, we had struggled to get anyone approved to take this on, so Kate suggested that I present at a NERC Situation Room briefing the next day. I hurriedly prepared some slides and when I raised the issue, Palo Conteh stunned all of us, most of all me, by what he said next: "This is clearly a problem that needs fixing. Oliver, I'm appointing you as the case management lead for Freetown going forward. Okay, what's next?" This was the exact opposite of the plan! Me taking on this role would make the Ministry officials feel completely disrespected and likely make the situation considerably worse.

Kate could see the horror on my face, so she grabbed me at the end of the meeting to have a one-on-one with Palo Conteh, where I was able to convince him to reverse the decision. A crisis was averted, but it had given me a real insight into how fast, but non-consultative, the NERC decision-making structure was and how the Ministry seemed to be side-lined.

Meanwhile, the Freetown DERC soon became the flagship site for the response and over the following months experienced a constant stream of visiting dignitaries, including UN Secretary-General Ban Ki-moon, WHO Director-General Margaret Chan, Tony Blair, the UK Foreign Secretary and even the Archbishop of Canterbury.

'Red-eye': visit by Justine Greening

An early visitor to the Freetown DERC was the UK Secretary of State for International Development, Justine Greening. I was actually back in the UK for a fleeting visit home when I got a call requesting I cut my visit even shorter so I could fly to Freetown that night with her, in order to brief her about the on-the-ground situation as we flew. With just a few hours' notice, I rushed to get the last train to RAF Brize Norton, a UK military airfield near Oxford, where a commercial plane had been chartered and was scheduled to take off at around 2 a.m. I was seated next to her in the small first-class section at the front of the plane, with over a hundred British soldiers sitting in the economy section behind us.

She listened politely as I launched into a rapid-fire exposition of everything that was going on with the response. I could see her attention gradually drifting (it was about 4 a.m. by this point) but I couldn't stop myself and carried on talking at her even as she closed her eyes and reclined her seat to horizontal. It was only when she put her eye mask on that I finally ground to a halt and let her get some rest.

Also in the front with us was BBC journalist Tulip Mazumdar, who had been providing valuable and balanced coverage of the outbreak. We arrived mid-morning, and after being shuttled to the city in the President's speedboat, I didn't get a chance to go home or return to the office. Instead, I had to rush straight to our Macauley Street clinic to make sure it was ready for the Secretary of State's imminent visit. With both a military and a BBC film crew present, things had to go right. Firstly, the community health officer running the unit led Justine Greening around to the central area of the facility and introduced her to staff.

She was also reintroduced to Will Pooley, the nurse from Kenema who had been med-evaced home after becoming infected in August. Will had experienced a quick recovery at the Royal Free Hospital and had been discharged in early September. He was determined to return to Sierra Leone and had chosen to join the King's team, which we were delighted about. He had become a minor celebrity following the media coverage and had met Justine Greening previously at a photo op with the actor Idris Elba, so the media teams were eager to include him in her Freetown visit.

The Macauley Street staff then insisted, to everyone's surprise, on leading the Secretary of State around to the back of the isolation unit, a journey that required her to climb over a small rubbish dump. She then found herself face-to-face with a group of confirmed-positive Ebola patients who stood just a metre or so from her, separated only by a wire fence. This was an awful lot closer to the disease than any of us had intended to let her get, and to the Secretary of State's credit, she kept her nerve and wished them good luck with their recovery, before hurrying back to her car, where an aide was ready with a generous dose of hand sanitiser.

'Firsts': opening more Ebola isolation units

Macauley Street and the other Freetown isolation units were faring better now that their influx of patients was being carefully managed by the Freetown DERC, although the constant problems with hazard pay meant staff were always stressed out and were regularly going on strike.

We were receiving strong encouragement to open more beds from both the UK and Dr Wurie at the Case Management Pillar. A priority for King's was to open a unit at Kissy Psychiatric Hospital for mental health patients, since we were concerned about how we would safely care for an Ebola-infected mental health patient in one of the general units.

The staff at Kissy Psychiatric explained to us that often relatives or 'friends' of their regular inpatients would take them home on Sundays, but some patients, rather than being cared for, would be mistreated and forced to do horrendous and dangerous manual labour such as digging out sewage drains. These days out might also expose them to infection, so the staff wanted to make sure there was an isolation unit available in case any of the patients contracted Ebola.

As a result, we helped them set up the world's first psychiatric Ebola unit. The mental health nurse on the King's team drilled us on how to physically restrain somebody in a way that was safe for them but also did not breach our PPE, since knocking off our goggles or scratching our skin could prove fatal. Two people would hold either arm of the patient and secure it close to each of their bodies, allowing you to frog march them around. That's easier said than done in full PPE, believe me, but fortunately I never had to put these new skills to the test, although my colleagues did when they had to isolate a number of suspected Ebola cases with psychosis.

By this stage, more international medical teams were finally starting to arrive and a number of these were interested in learning from our experience with isolation units and clinical care. Amongst these was the US NGO Partners in Health (PIH), whose co-founder was Paul Farmer. They had decided to largely emulate our approach to supporting government-run Ebola units. It had taken time, but in October PIH arrived, ready to work.

A thorny issue at the time was how to support pregnant women who were suspected or confirmed to have Ebola, since symptoms of Ebola could mimic or be suppressed by pregnancy. Ebola infection could also cause a woman to go into labour early. So, if a woman was rushed to hospital already in labour, confused, bleeding and perhaps feverish, it was very hard to assess whether she was a suspected case or not. The clinical outcomes for pregnant women with Ebola were reported to be terrible, and we had heard of only one case, from Kenema, of a baby surviving after being delivered from an infected mother – the rest had all died. The process of delivering a baby also exposed the midwife or doctor to enormous amounts of infectious body fluids. Indeed, many Ebola units refused to accept pregnant women due to the risk, leaving them to fend for themselves.

Never a man lacking ambition or commitment, Paul Farmer gamely volunteered PIH to support Freetown's maternity hospital and run their obstetrics Ebola unit, the world's first. He also offered to take on the toughest hotspot in the country, Port Loko, from which stories were coming in every day about overwhelmed facilities and widespread infections. Although some people later criticised Partners in Health for their levels of staff safety and for not delivering on some of their loftier promises, I remain grateful to them for taking on some real challenges at a time when nobody else wanted to go near them.[16]

Jumping over the fence

Medical teams from Cuba and China also arrived in October. The Cuban team of 165 health workers was being managed by WHO, who were trying to identify a safe facility where these health workers could be placed. Meanwhile, the Chinese team had arrived at Jui Hospital to open up an ETU and lab. Their deployment to Sierra Leone was pioneering for them but, like the Cubans, they faced the practical challenge of having very few English speakers on their team. This language barrier became a huge issue for both groups, although surprisingly the Chinese fared better since there were quite a few Sierra Leonean health workers who spoke Mandarin, having received scholarships to study in China over the previous decades.

However, since the ETU at Jui had opened, there had been a steady trickle of alarming stories about what was going on inside. Ambulances and lab vehicles reported being forced to wait outside for hours before being allowed through the gates to deliver their sick patients or urgent samples. People arriving at the facility with symptoms and asking to be isolated were left standing on the road. A Sierra Leonean staff member based at the hospital told us the Chinese staff mostly remained inside their office watching the patients on CCTV, afraid to go near them. One report from the Freetown DERC read:

> Yesterday, two positive patients [from Jui] escaped by jumping over the fence of the compound, and made their way to Connaught. They both reported not being fed, not getting their results, and not receiving treatment. One was a nurse from Rokupa.

The DERC decided to suspend referrals to Jui until the problems could be sorted out, even though the overall shortage of beds in Freetown was severe.

The King's team ultimately built strong relationships with the teams from both countries. Marta's Spanish came in very handy, as she was able to provide rapid on-site training to many of the Cuban doctors at Connaught. Meanwhile, one of the leaders of the Chinese team, an oncologist who spoke good English, reached out to us for help. She acknowledged it was the Chinese military's first independent humanitarian mission overseas and they were keen to learn. My team spent time in Jui giving them advice on how to improve their systems, and they turned out to be a gregarious bunch that delighted in having visitors, always insisting on treating us to an excellent Chinese lunch in their canteen afterwards. We became such good friends we even got invited to their Chinese New Year dance celebration.

The most useful thing we did was probably to plug the Chinese ETU into the DERC so they could better integrate their systems around referrals and lab transportation. The Chinese team later described how, prior to this, "communication [with] health administrative officers was poor because of language and cultural differences."[17] We had started holding a meeting each week for all of the Ebola units in Freetown to share best practices and give feedback to the DERC team. These meetings became so productive that even MSF, who were described by one WHO colleague as normally being "allergic to coordination meetings", started to attend regularly.

In an effort to encourage units to maximise their throughput of patients, we also developed a league table, based on the data the DERC was collecting, to keep track of the efficiency with which each unit was moving their suspected cases through the system. In their first meeting, the Chinese Jui team was at the bottom of the league, with a slow average turnaround time, and scored a bright red classification. They later told me they were hugely embarrassed by this public shaming and organised an urgent meeting when they got back to Jui to discuss how to turn things around. Within weeks, they became one of the top-performing units in Freetown and had been upgraded from red to green in the table.

It was easy to forget sometimes, when staring at spreadsheets or calling out patient ID numbers over the phone, that there were real human consequences when our coordination was poor. This was brought home to me when a Sierra Leonean businessman found me in my office at Connaught just when I was heading to the Freetown DERC for a meeting. His five-year-old daughter had tested positive at Connaught, but he couldn't find out where she had been moved to. I checked our records, which clearly stated she had been taken to the Hastings ETU. But when I called colleagues there, I was told she had never arrived and that her ambulance must have been redirected while en route. I gave him the contact numbers for the other ETUs, and he set off in search of her. I felt deeply ashamed. I could only imagine what he was going through, and was appalled at how we had failed to keep track of his daughter.

'No-touch care': the Ebola Training Academy

As more international medical teams started arriving to open new Ebola units, there was a growing need to recruit large numbers of Sierra Leonean nurses and cleaners onto their teams.

The Ministry and WHO had therefore set up an Ebola Training Academy at the national stadium, where they were running an introductory course on the disease and teaching people how to dress and undress in PPE. The creation of a centralised site to run this was useful, as it allowed people to be trained rapidly and at scale. After a few weeks, the UK team took over the Training Academy from WHO, as they were considered better placed to sort out all the logistics. This did create some problems, however.

The first issue was that the teaching was delivered by UK and Sierra Leonean soldiers, most of whom had never set foot in a real Ebola unit or managed an Ebola patient. This was a broader issue of internationals in the response providing Ebola training without any experience. With some exceptions, such as the WHO doctors in Kenema, this was even the case for WHO and CDC staff. As one international doctor who had worked at Kenema put it,

> CDC wouldn't allow their staff to go into the hot zone. And then WHO said the same thing soon after that. It was impossible for them to do training if they couldn't go into the red zone; they didn't have the credibility. But it was also a psychological thing for the national staff that these internationals wouldn't go in.

Moreover, the curriculum for the Ebola Training Academy was flawed, it focused on how to protect yourself from Ebola, instead of how to care for Ebola patients or manage an Ebola facility. A central tenet of the training, which the UK said they had inherited from the previous WHO curriculum, was that of 'no-touch care': staff in PPE should try to avoid touching patients at all cost. Many Sierra Leonean healthcare workers who attended the training told me they found this deeply offensive, seeing it as the UK dehumanising Sierra Leoneans and having no interest in trying to save lives.

It didn't seem the UK military was getting this message, though, as their 'force protection' rules helped keep them in a bubble. Curfew and other restrictions prevented them from interacting after-hours with frontline Sierra Leonean or international health workers, meaning there were no informal opportunities for the military to get feedback on the training they were conducting.

The problems were not due to any one individual, but were structural. In fact, the soldiers involved worked tirelessly and were deeply committed to the project. Despite all these shortcomings, however, the academy still managed to provide some useful PPE training to many people, even if it could have been done much better.

Bureaucracy slows us down

The UK's promise to build six new ETUs to get to their promise of 700 beds was at the forefront of everybody's minds, since the number of new cases each week was continuing to outstrip the number of available beds. Donal had approached me about King's running one of the UK ETUs, in collaboration with the Sierra Leone military, at Hastings Airfield, which was close to the existing Hastings ETU near Freetown. We had agreed, thinking we could get it open quickly, and that this would relieve the pressure on our isolation units. We also hoped that collaborating with the Sierra Leone military would allow them to further strengthen their capacity to respond to any future outbreaks independently. I was worried we might be taking on more than we could handle, but thought we had to take every chance we could to get beds open fast.

It was in these discussions about the Hastings Airfield ETU that I realised I had another misconception about the UK military. I had assumed they would be able to set up field hospitals at lightning speed and that we could have the ETU open in one or two weeks, especially since we were building on an airfield, unlike the Red Cross, who'd had to build their Kenema ETU in the wet jungle. But the plans the UK proposed to us, whilst impressive, were also totally over-designed and we were being told it would take over a month to get the facility ready.

As Marta, Dr Mohamed Boie Jalloh and I pored over the designs, we found all sorts of things we didn't need, such as piped chlorine water – we were happy with just a couple of taps in the facility so we could prepare the chlorine in buckets by hand.

Despite the experience of the Sierra Leone military and King's in managing Ebola, we were not allowed to make most of the changes we wanted in order to simplify the design and speed up construction. The UK were later heavily criticised for how long it was taking them to open the promised ETUs, especially since MSF and the Ministry had shown it could be done far more quickly. The UK claimed it was the NGO partners, who were slated to manage the ETUs, who had insisted on the elaborate designs that had made the process so slow.

While I can't speak for others, I can categorically state this was not true when it came to ours at Hastings Airfield. When we challenged the plans at the time, it was explained that the UK military engineers were under orders to ensure anything they built met British health and safety standards. The sentiment that the UK should only provide what they themselves would use was a nice thought, but when there was a severe shortage of beds it was a luxury the response simply did not have time to wait for and was not an effective approach in delivering desperately needed care to the Sierra Leonean population. Unfortunately, the bureaucratic approach of the UK government, including the UK military, was undermining their ability to be effective in the response.

When I met with Donal, I did my best to explain to him that whilst 700 beds might be enough to stop the outbreak if they opened right away, they might not be enough in a couple of months, as every day the number of cases was increasing exponentially. This meant that having fifty beds next week was far more useful than a hundred beds in a month. Donal understood the issue, but said it was difficult to shift the UK plans which had been agreed in London. Whether Donal's hands were really tied by his headquarters in London, or whether he was just trying to shift my ire in their direction, I didn't know, but either way I was hugely frustrated by the unnecessary delays.

I also raised these concerns in the international media, in the hope it might pressure them into speeding up. This would usually lead to some icy comments at the next evening briefing along the lines of: "Some people present have been on the media again today, criticising the hard work you've been doing. I hope they're enjoying the attention." I got the sense that bad press about the UK response must be avoided at all costs, lest it embarrass the British Prime Minister. This exposed the dual mission of the UK response: they wanted to support the Sierra Leonean government to bring the outbreak to a close, whilst also delivering for the UK's domestic politics. Whilst these two missions were often aligned, they could also be at odds.

It was not just me making this criticism, however, and the UK started to come under heavy pressure from officials at the Ministry, who were smarting because they felt the UK had encouraged the President to take leadership of the response away from them, and they now seemed to delight in being able to criticise the UK back. So Donal proposed a compromise: whilst the construction of the six ETUs would continue as planned, the UK would support other options to open beds more quickly.

SINEAD

Bed shortages

The discussions I was part of in October were also largely about beds, specifically three questions: how to fill the gap until the UK beds came online, whether they would be enough, and if not, what in God's name would we do then? The question of how many beds we needed was a surprisingly contentious topic that month.

On 8 October, WHO had said we had 304 beds out of the 1,148 we needed at the time in Sierra Leone, just 26% of what was necessary.[18] However, the same day, Daniel from WHO sent me an email with some projections for the coming weeks that made the gap look even more concerning. One of their epidemiologists had just run the numbers, based on the case numbers and various factors such as the average number of days the beds were being used for, and found that "In 5 weeks we will need 1,400–2,800 holding beds and 2,400–4,800 treatment beds." This was a shock. It meant that, even if all 700 UK treatment beds were opened by mid-November, added to the 304 already open, they still wouldn't be anywhere close to enough. I brought up these figures in numerous meetings, hoping that someone, maybe the CDC, maybe the UK, would be able to dispute them by pointing out a mistake in the projections, but nobody did.

It got even worse when WHO took a closer look at the quality of some of the existing beds. In mid-October, they did a survey that found that only 213 beds had adequate supervision and were "quality assured", while others had no direct supervision and were "highly variable". We knew by then what that meant – beds being provided without proper supervision could actually spread Ebola rather than contain it.

Hopes seemed pinned on the UK's beds, but these numbers suggested we needed to look far beyond these. I raised this issue every chance I got, as by then VIPs had started visiting thick and fast, and some of them were offering to scale up what their institutions were doing. When I heard Samantha Power, the US Ambassador to the UN, was to visit on 27 October, I thought it might be an opportunity to ask the US for help on this. By this time, we had had 3,760 confirmed cases of Ebola and 1,057 deaths in Sierra Leone that we knew of.[19]

Samantha Power

One point that doesn't seem to get much recognition in discussions on the Ebola outbreak is the role of the US, particularly President Barack Obama and Ambassador Samantha Power, in lobbying the rest of the international community to do more. They were chairing the UN Security Council at the time and Samantha Power regularly called meetings on Ebola, which my colleagues in the Irish mission at the UN in New York attended, while President Obama made phone calls to other heads of state to request they increase their contributions. In one meeting in October, Samantha Power was critical of the still-slow international response, noting that "We are asking too much of frontline workers and should be asking more of ourselves." This certainly rang a bell in Freetown.

Generally, the understanding was that the US 'had Liberia' while the UK 'had Sierra Leone', but the US lobbied for other countries to do more in all three of the most affected countries, and their own funding and engagement was definitely strong in Sierra Leone as well as Liberia. The CDC presence in Sierra Leone was actually greater than it was in Liberia, and the US Embassy and the Office for Foreign Disaster Assistance were very active on the ground.

The US engagement had pros and cons. I had been frustrated early in the outbreak when the CDC experts didn't seem to be able to significantly influence the Ministry or the EOC. When I had discussed this with Director of CDC, Tom Frieden, and his team on his first visit to Sierra Leone, they had made the point that these were technical staff who did not have experience in advocacy to governments, so the dysfunction of the response was beyond them. It was a fair point, but did make me wonder whether they should be better trained to deal with politics.

I had a very good collaboration with the US Embassy and with their aid programme. Two women in particular stood out. Kathleen Fitzgibbon, the Deputy US Ambassador, was a fiery redhead who spoke her mind and was a key voice trying to raise the alarm in the early days. She would also do things like bake brownies for NERC meetings or send care packages to nurses in Kenema which meant a lot to people. Sonia Walia, a soft-spoken, determined and experienced health specialist, was the head of the US Office for Foreign Disaster Assistance in Sierra Leone for six months during the crisis. Perhaps, in part, because neither Ireland nor the US were in the lead position like the UK, we worked very closely together, along with our Dutch colleague Esmee de Jong, who worked for the European Union, to see how we could fill some of the gaps in the response the UK hadn't managed to cover.

It was in this vein that I saw the visit of Samantha Power as an opportunity to lobby the US to help us get more beds up and running. We were starting to see a slow-down in the rate of infection in Liberia after the horrendous highs of 300 to 400 new cases per week in August and September, but the US had committed to building eleven ETUs there that weren't even close to being finished.[20] Surely, they could instead transfer some of those resources to Sierra Leone, where the epidemic only seemed to be getting worse?

The day of the visit, we were at the Radisson for the fourth time that week. I was excited to see Samantha Power, in part because of what I saw as the potential for the US to help us get out of the hole we were in, and also because she was a bit of an idol of mine. When I had been a college student at Harvard in the late 1990s, interested in human rights and development, Samantha came there to be the founding director of a human rights centre. I took her seminars and she was kind enough to offer me career advice as I headed off to India to volunteer after graduation. It obviously also helped that Samantha was born of Irish parents and had spent her early years in Dublin.

We were scheduled to have two interactions with Samantha Power that evening. First, a reception with a broader group of stakeholders, and then a smaller meeting with a group of diplomats. But she was running late. I tried to make good use of the time by cornering the global head of the Office for Foreign Disaster Assistance and trying to persuade him the US needed to come in on beds. He, though, was having none of it. It seemed they'd had their fingers burnt in Liberia, where it looked like they would end up with a vast excess of beds far too late, and this coloured how they viewed the situation in Sierra Leone. I tried to make the point that how many beds we needed depended on how quickly we could produce them. It was clear the UK beds were going to take more time, so if the US could help us with some beds quickly since they already had resources in the region, it could avert many Ebola cases later on.

Samantha Power arrived at the reception and gave a strong speech about the need for a greater sense of urgency at the international level. It was now after 10 p.m. Since the US Embassy folk had told us she had been up since 5 a.m., we expected our smaller meeting with her to get cancelled. But no. We kicked off at 10:30, Donal and Peter from the UK, me, the Chinese Ambassador and Samantha Power and her team.

She made some interesting points in her introduction. At this time in the US there was a huge controversy over mandatory quarantines that some states wanted to impose on returning health workers from Ebola-affected countries. Given our desperate shortages of health workers, this was the last thing we needed, as it would discourage people from volunteering. Samantha Power talked about the need for us to change the narrative – rather than talking about how many international health workers were being infected, and possibly bringing the virus back to the West, we needed to talk about how many were *not* getting infected.

Then it was the Freetown group's turn to speak. I went first, as was the local custom, since I had been in-country the longest. I recapped the dismal numbers comparing cases with available beds and reiterated my plea that the Americans help us to get more ETUs up and running quickly. I noted that part of the problem was our failure to provide quality care and focus enough on the survival of patients, which was further discouraging people from reporting suspected cases. The UK had made quick progress on burials, meaning if someone in Freetown called the Ebola hotline about a death, a burial team would be prompt to pick up the body. But if they called to say someone was sick, there was a good chance the response couldn't do anything for them as there were no beds. This had led one local man to comment, "The government cares more about us dead than alive." I wasn't sure exactly how the US could help, but I was sure they could.

Samantha Power responded quite positively, to my delight. She was interested, even after a seventeen-hour day. I felt like I had gotten somewhere. However, Donal Brown spoke next and what he said essentially translated to, 'No thanks, we've got it covered'. I couldn't believe my ears! How could he say that when there was such a huge gap between the beds we needed and the beds we would actually have anytime soon? Our bipolar views didn't escape Samantha Power, who asked us to "Go at it" so she could better understand our divergent views. We did this for a while, but our poles didn't come any closer together.

I knew that there was very little chance that my voice would overrule Donal's, as the UK was the lead donor. I was very frustrated as I had never heard him or anyone from the UK dispute the WHO projections, so I'd thought we were all on the same page that we should do anything possible to get more beds. I didn't understand why that should exclude asking the US for help. Of course, I couldn't guarantee they could help, but I figured it was worth a try.

Fairly or unfairly, I felt that the UK had excluded this possibility because they wanted to take the credit for sorting out Sierra Leone. In a similar vein, a UN official later told me that, in December 2014, he had been involved in an effort to transfer bed capacity from Liberia to Sierra Leone, "but the UK kept giving green lights on their bed capacity and it was simply not true on the ground. They did not want a role for others, they were under pressure." Along the same lines an MSF interviewee said, "The UK kept saying 'we have enough', when all beds are online, but week by week there weren't enough beds, especially because ETUs open slowly."

However, the notion that the UK did not want a role for others does not entirely make sense because, at the same time, the UK were building an incredible platform which enabled about ten other countries, such as Norway, Denmark, Australia and Holland, to contribute to the response. They had also hosted an international conference in London on 2 October which mobilised millions of pounds for the response in Sierra Leone. Was it perhaps that the US was too big and had the potential to threaten the UK's profile in the Sierra Leone response? Later, it occurred to me that maybe Donal genuinely thought assistance from the US would do more harm than good as it would bring more bureaucracy into play and wouldn't produce results any quicker. I certainly learnt a lot about US aid bureaucracy during this response, and may have been naïve in thinking more American resources would have helped at that point. However, that night I was baffled and annoyed.

Anyway, it was time for bed. But not before I got a selfie with Samantha Power, who kindly claimed to remember me, and then another one with her and Kathleen from the US Embassy, who quite rightly pointed out that "We redheads need to stick together . . ." I sent the pictures to my mother on the drive home. We still claim Samantha as Irish after all.

OLIVER

'Designed by committee': Kerry Town gets off to a troubled start

At the start of November, the existing Ebola units were still unable to cope with the number of patients, with about 400 new confirmed cases per week in Sierra Leone. At the same time, the UK kept telling us that we would have to wait until early December for most of their new ETUs to open.

The one bright spot came when the flagship UK ETU in Kerry Town opened on 5 November. The ETU was split into two parts, with eighty beds managed by Save the Children for general patients, alongside a specialist twenty-bed unit run by the UK military for foreign nationals and certain Sierra Leonean health workers. Unfortunately, a series of mishaps quickly turned this achievement into a liability.

A few days after the President opened the facility to great fanfare, only four beds had been made operational and one health worker – a doctor from the Cuban Medical Brigade – had already been infected.

The ETU had been under enormous scrutiny because of the delays in getting it open in the first place. We had been hearing about an ETU at Kerry Town since August and, although the UK was credited by some with constructing it in "just eight weeks",

this seemed a very long time compared with what other organisations had achieved.[1]

The UK now came in for intense criticism. Palo Conteh, the
head of the NERC, held a news conference where he said that,
"Save the Children do not have the expertise . . .That is something we must all accept, and say the Brits got it wrong with Kerry
Town, handing over the facility to Save the Children who have
never run an Ebola facility."[2] The criticism was widely reported
in the local and international press. Donal called an urgent meeting with Save the Children to discuss how to rectify the situation,
asking the King's team to attend and give independent advice.

The Save the Children team and the UK military engineers
put most of the blame on fundamental problems with the design.[3]
"It's the Ministry's fault," the lead engineer insisted, "they
had already started construction before we took over and their
original design is unworkable." But while I agreed the layout was
not ideal, I wasn't terribly impressed by this as an excuse, given
the success the Sierra Leone military and King's had had opening
units in various awkward locations.

It became clear to me that a much more significant problem
was the leadership and management of the site, which consisted
of a cumbersome and chaotic consortium that included the
Ministry, DFID, the UK military, Save the Children, Public
Health England, WHO and the Cuban Medical Brigade. Also
involved were UK-Med, a group managing the recruitment of
health workers from the UK.

The saying goes that a camel is a horse designed by committee.
The various organisations involved in designing the ETU were
prone to micromanaging, often insisting on their own standards
and requirements. Some of these decisions appeared to have
been made around conference tables in London rather than on
the ground in Freetown, like insisting on exactly what face mask

had to be worn, overruling the objections of the health workers on the ground who found them claustrophobic and unsafe. Kerry Town was the flagship ETU for both the UK and the President of Sierra Leone, so everyone had an opinion. Save the Children were clearly struggling to get a grip on all the different organisations and agendas.

I proposed the King's team go to Kerry Town to undertake an assessment of the ETU ourselves. My boss Andy was visiting, so he joined Marta and me at the facility. We were met by a British nurse who, though an effective and experienced health advisor for Save the Children, was clearly very stressed. She welcomed us cautiously, perhaps a little threatened by our presence there, before leading us down gravel paths between the warehouses and Portakabins that had been constructed in the green zone, to the entrance of the ETU itself.

As we stepped into their PPE dressing room, we realised they were operating on an industrial scale compared to what we were used to at Connaught, with enormous racks of PPE and rows of mirrors to dress in front of. A Canadian nurse impatiently checked whether we had dressed appropriately in their complex MSF-style PPE, which included head drapes, two masks and a heavy reusable apron. By the time I eventually got the PPE on, I was already sweaty and exhausted – and I hadn't even entered the unit yet! It was far hotter and more claustrophobic than the WHO-standard PPE we wore at Connaught, and whilst you certainly felt well-protected inside it, I could imagine staff getting overheated in it quickly and making mistakes as a result.

The ETU had scaled up to a couple of dozen patients by this point, and as we walked into the ward, I was impressed by the level of care being provided. Their drug cabinets were far better stocked than ours at Connaught, with almost every patient receiving IV fluids and an array of strong painkillers. This was a long way from the 'no-touch care' so many people on the outside thought that the UK ETUs would be providing.

At the same time, basic tasks seemed to have been overcomplicated, which we thought presented risks for both safety and patient care. For example, the corpse of a small child who we were told had died during the night had been left on one of the beds. At Connaught, the corpse would have been removed and the bed cleaned within minutes. I asked why this hadn't happened yet, especially as there were nurses standing around in the ward who didn't look terribly busy. The doctor explained that everything at Kerry Town had to be done according to a specific protocol. Only burial teams could collect the corpses, which had to include at least six people to move a single body. The nurses had apparently called the office to report the death, but it was taking time to assemble a team to do this one task.

Marta, Andy and I all agreed on the problem – Kerry Town was overstaffed and had too many protocols, some of which apparently required sign-off from London to change. In short, it was an orchestra with no conductor. We believed what they needed was a clinical coordinator in charge of each shift that could use a bit more common sense to get the job done, something that Save the Children acknowledged and worked hard to fix.

Overall, I left feeling impressed by the quality of care the clinical team was providing, but frustrated they were opening beds so slowly. A Sierra Leonean doctor later shared similar sentiments:

> They wanted to get everything perfect before they started
> receiving patients. It was very frustrating. Can you imagine? We
> were turning away Ebola patients. They met the case definition
> but we would send them home and say come back tomorrow.
> Maybe somebody would have died by then and we would give
> them a bed. That's how bad the situation was.

A week after the government-run Hastings ETU had opened, they had 120 beds open compared to the four they had managed at Kerry Town.

Kicking and screaming: why the UK struggled to respond to a health emergency

A couple of Save the Children staff mentioned surreptitiously during our visit that they didn't think it was a great idea for the NGO to be running an ETU in the first place. We'd heard the UK government had put pressure on them to run it, or, in the words of one UK official, "dragged them kicking and screaming." This was in part, I suspect, because they wanted their signature ETU to be run by a British NGO. Since Save the Children had taken over the UK NGO Merlin in 2013, which specialised in running medical programmes in humanitarian emergencies, there was a widespread expectation that they ought to have the capacity to take it on. But a senior Save the Children official acknowledged that "when we were asked to take on the centre, we made it absolutely clear that this was new business for us. We have never run frontline health services at this scale."[4]

The UK, one of the world's biggest aid donors, is also home to the National Health Service, which, with its nearly two million staff, is the fifth-largest employer in the world.[5] You might therefore expect the UK to be a leader in the medical response to international health emergencies. In fact, the country has very few agencies with this capacity. Neither the British Red Cross nor MSF UK deploy internationally, unlike their counterparts in several other countries. The other big humanitarian NGOs in the UK, such as Oxfam, ActionAid and Christian Aid, focus largely on issues like food, water and sanitation. This meant that the other five ETUs supported by the UK in Sierra Leone were all to be run by foreign NGOs such as Goal (Ireland), Emergency

(Italy), Aspen (Australia), Médecins du Monde (France) and International Medical Corps (US).

In the globalised world of humanitarian relief, you might wonder why it matters which country an NGO is based in: I would argue that it matters quite a lot when it comes to a medical emergency. The biggest challenge with organising a medical response is being able to recruit experienced clinical staff and getting them released from their day jobs quickly. Building this network of potential volunteers and having arrangements with hospitals in place for the staff to be released when needed requires constant and active engagement with the national health system.

Additionally, there are often profoundly different cultures of practice amongst health workers in different countries. Sometimes this is as simple as language barriers, such as Spanish-speaking Cuban doctors struggling to communicate with their British colleagues at Kerry Town. Often, though, it goes beyond language to what clinical protocols are followed, what skills health workers have, and how hierarchies and power dynamics play out within clinical teams.

A clash of medical cultures later became apparent at the UK-funded ETU run by the NGO Emergency, whose mostly Italian medical team was supplemented with British staff deployed through UK-Med. Some of these UK health workers quickly rebelled, citing "grave concerns" at how "complex and controversial therapies took priority over basic patient care . . . to the detriment of patients." They also complained of an "overall management culture of Emergency [that] discourages staff from raising patient safety concerns, and questioning the decisions of the leadership".[6] Their complaints grew so loud that there were calls for DFID to pull their support to Emergency entirely, and ultimately the UK-Med team were withdrawn from the ETU. There are lots of lessons here, but one of them is that, in the midst of a fraught emergency, it's much wiser to deploy teams of health workers with a shared medical culture and practice, avoiding the need to negotiate compromise whilst also trying to navigate an ongoing crisis.

SINEAD

The world outside

Though we had been fully occupied with the Ebola outbreak for all these months, this had not, of course, meant that other aspects of our lives had stood still.

My mother had been diagnosed with cancer. Fortunately, it was a treatable form that was caught early, but nevertheless it seemed a good time to go home to Ireland and finally take the leave I had been postponing since 1 August. I booked flights for the first week of November.

A few days later, however, while I was in a meeting at DFID, I got a call from my mother's doctor at one of the main hospitals in Dublin. She was very apologetic, but told me the hospital's new protocols on Ebola meant that if my mother's temperature changed within twenty-one days of meeting me, then she would have to be taken to Ireland's national isolation unit. My mother was having chemotherapy, meaning there wasn't much doubt her temperature was going to fluctuate. So, I cancelled my trip. There was no way I could put my mother under that kind of stress, but there was also no way I was going to Ireland without seeing my mother.

I had to go somewhere, though, as my headquarters was becoming insistent that I take a break. Plus, like others who had been involved in the response since the beginning, I hadn't taken a full day off since June and I was beginning to feel a strange kind of weariness. I tried to ignore it. It felt ridiculous given that so many others in the response were under so much more pressure than office workers like me. But it persisted. During the workday I would be fine, running from meeting to meeting or scrambling to get through my emails or make calls. During breaks in activity, however, I would often feel submerged beneath a wave of exhaustion. Even climbing the single flight of stairs to my apartment would suddenly seem like a challenge, and I would find myself clinging on to the bannister. I was thirty-six-years-old and supposedly fit. I needed a break.

As it happened, I had been invited to the wedding of a close college friend in Mississippi in the US, which normally I wouldn't have missed. But I was worried. On 8 October, a Liberian man, Thomas Duncan, had flown to the US and died of Ebola in Texas.[7] Two nurses had been infected while caring for him. Fortunately, both survived, but hysteria had broken out in the US. Texas is not a million miles from Mississippi – what if just one person at this wedding was freaked out by my being there? Then my presence would become a source of stress for the bride and groom. I told my friend that, regretfully, I had decided not to go. A few days later, my friend called. "To be honest, I thought you were overreacting a bit," she said. "But when I said you weren't coming, several people told me they were so relieved. I was shocked." Welcome to our world!

In the end, I decided to go to a yoga retreat in Morocco for five days, as it was one of the only direct flights we still had from Freetown. But, as so often happens when you take a holiday after a tough period of work, as my departure date arrived, I could feel that I was getting sick, just when I was about to finally experience the airport's endless temperature checks and form filling about my health status that everyone had been telling me about for months. My flight was late at night and as I rushed around finishing up meetings before I left, I brought my own thermometer and checked my temperature every hour or so; I had no interest in going through the boat trip and airport ordeal if they weren't going to let me on the plane. Fortunately, I didn't have a fever so the whole process went ok, although it was exhausting.

In Casablanca, as I stepped off the plane onto a creaky walkway, I was greeted by four men in PPE, who directed me to an elaborate walk-through infrared thermometer and another round of form filling in relation to my health and plans for my time in Morocco.

From the airport, with my cold getting worse by the minute, I took a five-hour bus ride to Essaouira, a small seafront town where the retreat was. I had been in my hotel room for about ten minutes and was getting ready to crash when I got a call from reception. The local health authorities had come to enquire about my health. "You've got to be kidding me," I said to the receptionist. It was a bit of a pain as my health was in fact, not so great and I was dying to go to sleep, but at the same time, I couldn't help but be impressed by their efficiency. On my last day in town, the same two men even came to wave me off to the airport, just to make sure I really was getting out of their hair.

The Moroccan government deserves a lot of credit for allowing Royal Air Maroc to continue flying to Sierra Leone and Liberia during the crisis. As a middle-income country heavily dependent on tourism, it would have been hugely damaging for them if they had imported even a single case of Ebola. But they and Brussels Airlines continued to be a lifeline for the two countries after everybody else had pulled out.

Though the retreat was marred by my being sick for the whole week, in an odd way this contributed to making it more of a break. Given it took almost all my energy just to get to the yoga classes, beyond checking in once a day with Freetown and sending a few urgent emails, I didn't work and was largely out of the 'Ebola headspace' for the first time in six months. I felt refreshed on my arrival back in Freetown, even though I went straight from the overnight flight to our 8:30 donor meeting at DFID. This was helped by the fact that I was by then, predictably enough, fully healthy again.

As far as my mum was concerned, one consolation for my cancelled visit was all the media interviews I was doing at the time, which provided a great distraction for her. There would first be a couple of hours of calling and texting around to friends and family, telling them, "Sinead's going to be on the radio." And then I would be on the radio. And then there would be a couple more hours of fielding calls of, "I just heard Sinead on the radio." It helped to pass the time on her sickbed.

Managing fleets

The day I got back from Morocco, I had a discussion with Paula and Emma at the Embassy about how to adapt our approach to the new scenario in the country. There were now many more resources and the UK was taking a leading role with the NERC. The acute shortage of beds was still preoccupying me and I kept raising it, broken record-like, every chance I got. But it was just not looking like anybody was about to step in to build any new centres before the bulk of the UK beds opened, so there didn't seem to be a whole lot we could do about that. Meanwhile there were other problems and gaps all over the response so we discussed where we might add the most value.

The process of figuring this out would have been easier if UNMEER had taken a strong role in coordinating international partners, as had been the plan. However, that hadn't happened, so, as usual, we worked things out informally. Emma found out through the grapevine from the UK that there were now a lot of vehicles being used for the response, but that management of these vehicles was chaotic, particularly outside of Freetown. I could testify to that. On one trip I had made to Bombali district that month, the DERC had pleaded with me for two more motorbikes so that surveillance officers could do their jobs at community level. This despite the fact that for weeks I had been seeing about fifty brand new motorbikes in the carpark of the NERC awaiting distribution. In this instance, I was able to pass the information on and two motorbikes were sent to Bombali. Clearly, though, there needed to be a better system.

Apart from ensuring vehicles were not misused or stolen, and were properly maintained, it was crucial that ambulances were decontaminated between patients. On one trip to Port Loko, I had heard about a stand-off where community members had, quite understandably, refused to get into an ambulance with vomit in it, and the driver, also understandably, had refused to clean the ambulance for fear of getting infected himself.

The UK could see the management of about 1000 vehicles being used for the response outside Freetown was a big problem, and they had money to address it, but lacked the manpower to sort it out themselves. We, though, were happy to take it on. There was only one problem: we had no idea about fleet management. We had never engaged in any programming related to transport and had only three cars and two motorbikes at the Embassy! Despite this, we had a trump card – we had just found out we were being sent Irish Defence Forces personnel to help with the response. So, we made a pitch for fleet management experience on that team and agreed with DFID that Emma would manage the programme, with army colleagues monitoring the technical side. We would put in whatever budget we could, and DFID and the US would cover the rest between them.

Enter the Irish army

We were a bit apprehensive in mid-November when the first team of four Irish army officers was due to arrive at the Embassy. None of us had ever worked directly with the military before.

We had lobbied for Irish health workers to support the response, many of whom did deploy independently through WHO, but it had never occurred to us to ask for the Irish army. When the idea was suggested by our headquarters, we were initially sceptical. The original proposal was that they could help with Embassy security, but we still felt very safe in Freetown. Remarkably, despite all of the hardships the population had suffered, there was very little unrest outside of isolated incidents, such as the riots that took place at Connaught and Kenema hospitals. We had given that feedback to our headquarters, but were still worried, as arrival day approached, that we would end up with camouflage-clad army officers patrolling the Embassy all day long for no particular reason while we scrambled around trying to do our Ebola work.

Fortunately, our trepidations were quickly allayed. After explaining the situation to the first team of four clean-cut, straight-backed officers on their arrival, they immediately offered to help with whatever we thought the pressing needs were. "Headquarters discussions are headquarters discussions," they said. "We've been sent here to work for you." I liked the sound of that! There were, however, some institutional cultural challenges we had to resolve. As I gave them a tour of the Embassy on the first day, they kept calling me 'Ambassador', which nobody else at the Embassy did, and I thought, "This is going to get a bit old." So I told them the story of how, on my first day in 2011, one of our drivers Desmond had nervously called me "Madam" all morning. I had said to him at the time, "Desmond, that's no problem. You can call me 'Madam' if you like. But just so you know, I'll have to call you 'Sir'." And that was the end of 'Madam'. They laughed politely and assented to call me Sinead. But Paula later told me that they reverted to 'Ambassador' the moment I was out of earshot. I wasn't totally opposed to the culture they brought, though, and frequently mentioned to my staff how refreshing it was that the army officers did everything I asked them to do. Sadly, all my staff did was laugh at this evidently strange quirk.

Emma wasted no time on their first day, drafting one of the officers to work with her on the fleet management programme. By then, she had worked with DFID to contract a consortium of NGOs, led by World Vision, to set up fleet management systems in each district alongside the DERC. Ably armed with her masters in human rights law, twenty-seven-year-old Emma spent her evenings googling decontamination techniques and run-off systems.

As she recalled to me later:

> It was so surreal. For the first couple of months it was like we were all coming up with it ourselves, how to decontaminate ambulances, how to set up fleets. As if it had never been done before. We couldn't figure out where the experts were. We chased WHO and eventually they came through with guidance but it took time.

The main issue with the programme was the potential for the theft of fuel and vehicle parts, and heavy resistance to the attempts of the NGOs to enforce a system of control. In one instance, a brand new vehicle left Freetown and, by the time it arrived in Port Loko two and a half hours later, the gearbox had mysteriously aged ten years. Another time, a driver was caught emptying the fuel tank fifteen minutes after leaving his base. The NGOs tried to retroactively create an inventory of the vehicles, as none had been kept initially at central or district level. The programme was, as Emma described it, "a nightmare". Nevertheless, there was strong support from the NERC and the other donors, the implementing NGOs did a good job under very trying circumstances and the army guys helped strengthen the technical aspect of the programme. Slowly, things got better.

Apart from their fleet management role, over the months that followed we lent the army officers out to Irish NGOs to assist with specific jobs, such as helping Goal set up their UK-funded ETU. They were a huge hit: highly skilled in engineering and logistics and extremely motivated to boot. Soon after that, the Irish Defence Forces deployed five other medical army personnel to work with the UK, which also worked out well. These weren't big numbers, but they were high-quality people. And as we saw time and time again, strong individuals could have a disproportionately large impact on the response.

Down your tools

The day after I got back from Morocco I got a call from Hussein Ibrahim, a British-Sierra Leonean who was the country director for International Medical Corps (IMC). We were funding them to build an ETU which was due to open soon and would be Port Loko's first (and desperately needed) ETU. He and his colleagues were working around the clock to get the ETU opened as soon as possible. Hussein was clearly stressed when he called and he told me why: "The chief told all the workers on the site to down their tools and threatened the contractor that they better not pick them up again."

This was a shock. After much to-ing and fro-ing by the government on different sites, IMC had finally been loaned this piece of land to build the ETU, with the personal involvement of the President and the senior chief in the district. And now a local chief shows up at the site and demands payment? Clearly seething, Hussein went on "He said his family owned this land and they could no longer farm and needed compensation. But the reason the land was chosen in the first place was because it was a land not used!" When I got off the phone to Hussein, I then called Palo, the head of NERC, who promised to sort it out.

I decided to visit Port Loko a couple of days later to check in with Hussein and also to see how the general situation in the district was developing. Emma and two of the army team were due to go there to do some work on the fleet management programme, so we headed up early one morning and they dropped me off at the IMC site. There I found Hussein chain-smoking and sleep-deprived. He updated me that the issue with the chief had been sorted the day before, but not without the direct engagement of President Koroma, who had had to personally send a delegation to meet with the chief. In the end, it seemed like just another example of politics getting in the way and people trying to profit from the response, making hay while the sun shone.

Despite the obstacles, however, progress had been made. When I walked around the site in the wellington boots they had me put on at the entrance, most of the construction of the white-tented ETU was finished, the beds were in place, and they were in the process of stocking up on PPE and training their staff.

Speaking truth to power: showdown in Port Loko

Next, I went to the DERC, which was housed at the site of the slightly ramshackle district health offices, now crammed with military officers and epidemiologists. I ran into a UK staffer that I knew in the car park and he gave me an update as we walked in. The situation they were dealing with in the district was still terrible. The previous day alone, thirteen of the country's thirty-nine new confirmed cases were in Port Loko.[8] Since the beginning of the outbreak, Port Loko had had 792 cases, making it the country's second worst hotspot after Freetown, with only a fraction of the population.[9] What's more, cases in the district were still rising week-on-week.

But the beds for people were just not there yet. The IMC and Goal ETUs were still under construction, while Partners in

Health were trying to improve the previously dire-conditions in the Ebola unit at Maforki, close to the town of Port Loko. Four smaller units had also opened, but given the case numbers, these were a drop in the ocean.

Nevertheless, I felt a palpable energy as I walked through the building on my way to the WHO office, passing desks of Sierra Leone and UK military officers coordinating the logistics of beds and burials, and WHO and CDC staff huddled in corners discussing particular villages, or tapping new data into the system.

The larger-than-life WHO lead for Port Loko, Sierra Leonean Kande-Bure O'Bai Kamara, was on the phone when I arrived in their makeshift office, talking in Krio and gesticulating wildly. KB, as he was known, was an epidemiologist normally based with WHO in Geneva, and was one of the few people in the response who combined high levels of epidemiological expertise with cultural knowledge. He was also practical, energetic, and angry at what was happening to his people, making him one of the key forces behind the effectiveness of the Port Loko DERC.

I was keen to congratulate KB for his role speaking truth to power on a visit President Koroma had undertaken to Port Loko shortly before.

In October, President Koroma had started to undertake tours of the country, mostly during the weekends, pushing local leaders to support the Ebola response and mobilise their communities. This was, in part, a response to complaints from the DERCs and others that some politicians, government officials and chiefs were routinely interfering in the functioning of the response in order to advance their own agendas or make money. This sometimes took the form of soliciting bribes from international organisations – one friend of mine had been asked for $5,000 by a Ministry official for 'permission to work' – or allowing secret burials to take place. In addition to his team of senior officials, the President was usually accompanied by representatives from the UK, such as Peter and Donal, and by UNMEER.

When the President started these tours, some politicians were keen to tell him what they thought he wanted to hear, others what they thought would make them look good. So on the President's first visit to Port Loko, a prominent national politician originally from the area reassured the President that things were fine, that he and his supporters were taking care of matters. Alarmed, KB, who was sitting at the back of the room, pulled aside one of the UK representatives and told him that things were not at all fine. This was passed on to the President who stopped the meeting, dismissed the attendees and asked for a technical briefing by the WHO team.

KB briefed him on the real situation, that cases were skyrocketing and yet the response was weak with considerable political interference. Quarantine was doing more harm than good. Burial teams and surveillance workers were not receiving their hazard pay. There were so many rumours circulating that communities did not know what to believe. Chiefs should have been the key entry-point to the local population, but had not been engaged by the response and so were not cooperating.

As one participant on the visit later told me:

> Visibly angry, the President then went to the town hall meeting and spoke forcefully to the chiefs and other political leaders, telling them that they better stop hiding information and start cooperating properly with the district response. Particularly impactful was his threat to the chiefs present that he would take away their staffs of authority, you know the stick that symbolises their chieftaincy, if they didn't sort out their chiefdoms before his next visit.

Incentives were used, as well as threats. As KB had suggested, chiefs were given funding to lead social mobilisation in their areas, which often proved to be effective. It was fascinating to me that chiefs were central both to the problems and the solutions in the response, harking back to what I had read about in Sierra Leone history books about the contested history of chieftaincies since colonial times as forces both for and against democracy.

While these kinds of political issues did not go away, the President's frequent trips to the districts made a big impact on the engagement of local leaders and were seen by many as a game-changer in the response.

Just jingles

After KB had updated me on the somewhat improving situation with the chiefs, I asked him what he saw as the big issues at that time, aside from the chronic bed shortage. He answered without hesitation: "Community engagement." He went on, "You should spend hours every day with communities. You should meet in the morning and again in the afternoon. Communities should know that you're concerned, that you live with their problems. But a lot of what we have seen is just jingles."

There were still huge issues of communities not cooperating with the response, sometimes for very understandable reasons, such as there being no beds or burial practices that were unacceptable to them. As KB explained, what was needed was a dialogue with communities to find ways together to mitigate the dire situation, not the the top-down instructions that we had started with in the response. We discussed how, at times, our efforts at community engagement actually made it harder for communities to protect themselves. As one NGO worker specialising in social mobilisation had told me:

> Not only were community members not listened to, respected, supported with resources etc, but at times, they were actually held back from protecting themselves with their own resources. Early meetings were literally zoo-like. Everyone rushed to

'hotspots' and all the different agencies held their own meetings, questioning the same community members over and over again about the same things. Communities were expected to give up hours of their days to various agencies all working in siloes.

On a more positive note, I updated KB on some community action I was hearing good things about in the rural areas of the Freetown peninsula that one of our partners was involved in. Communities had set up their own taskforces, some of which were now being supported by NGOs. The taskforces came up with their own ideas for Ebola prevention in their community. One innovation was the 'Community Census book' where the Taskforce carried out a survey of the population and then paid daily visits to each household, checking temperatures and health status of each member. Taskforces in some communities helped the DERC with contact tracing, in other communities provided psychosocial and practical support to people suffering in quarantined homes. These taskforces seemed to be leading to more alerts coming to the DERC and overall better collaboration. KB was interested in this because WHO were trying to get this kind of deep community engagement started in Port Loko, despite the enormous challenges.

Leaving him to his constantly pinging mobile phone and conscious that everybody else at the DERC was also swamped, I set off to do a quick run around the desks to ask if people had issues that needed to be raised at higher levels.

The human rights void

As I was leaving the WHO office, I met Martin Cormican, a calm and experienced microbiology professor from Ireland, on his way in. A volunteer with WHO, he had been assessing government isolation units in Port Loko district that day, some of which were ill-equipped and poorly staffed. As we stood in the corridor he told me some of the horrifying things he had seen. His description of one holding unit in particular really disturbed me:

> The barrier between the red and green zone was a piece of tape.
> One patient asked about her lab result – it turned out she and
> her relatives had no symptoms but were described as 'strong
> contacts' – the Chief wanted them there. They were standing five
> feet from a very sick Ebola patient . . . Sometimes staff only went
> inside three times per day – early, lunch and late. That meant
> there was no staff maybe twenty out of twenty-four hours.

Two aspects of this were especially alarming. First, there was a high risk of infection of people who might not have Ebola – we knew that poorly managed Ebola facilities could spread the disease far more than they prevented it. What really struck me, though, was the violation of the patients' human rights. The woman and her relatives were being forced to go to the centre without meeting the admission criteria as suspect cases, solely on the order of the chief. They were then confined in a small space with people who actually did have Ebola.

Where were the human rights organisations to stand up for these people? Then another thought came to me: who was I to talk? I hadn't been framing the response in human rights terms either. Sure, I had been advocating for better services to communities, better care for patients, lobbying against quarantine. But I had not been framing these issues as questions of human rights. Did this matter? Or was it just semantics?

Actually, it mattered a lot. If we don't start off with a clear acknowledgement of what people are entitled to, simply by virtue of being human, we run the risk of dehumanising them. In the response, this presented itself when we talked about Ebola patients as statistics or even as 'vectors' of the disease, the danger of this dehumanisation being that we wouldn't fight hard enough to give Sierra Leonean Ebola patients the same conditions we would expect for ourselves or our families. We got caught up in the resources we had available, rather than what people were entitled to.

What to do while you're waiting? The controversy of home care

The human rights theme came up again in the last conversation I had at the DERC that day with John Raine. John, tall and fifty-ish with closely cropped hair, was a former British police officer whom I had known before Ebola when he was providing support to the Sierra Leone police. He was now the UK lead at the Port Loko DERC. He told me about the progress on the burial system, and generally about how the DERC was getting things organised. But he was also disturbed: "Sinead, there are still 200 to 300 people in this district in their homes, suspected to have Ebola. Beds will take a few weeks to complete. In the meantime, what are we doing for these people?"

John was absolutely right. It was preposterous what we were telling people and their families to do if they suspected they had Ebola. The standard line was: don't touch sick relatives and call the national 117 hotline. However, at the time, there was a very good chance that 117 would not be able to help the caller. Given the shortage of beds in Port Loko, they would likely be told to wait until a bed became available. But as one nurse from an ETU had said to me, "What to do while you're waiting? We didn't want to say anything about this, but it was inhuman. You wouldn't leave your child lying in vomit." Sierra Leoneans were going to continue to care for their loved ones whether the response told them to or not.

Since early October, we had been talking about this at the national level – surely, there was something we could do for people stuck in their homes? WHO even wrote a manual on how to do home care. But the issue was hugely controversial.

I told John how I had received a call a few weeks previously, from Adam Nossiter of *The New York Times*. He had asked me to comment on an article he was about to publish on how the EOC had passed a policy on 'interim home protection and care' against the objections of the head CDC official at the time.[10]

Personally, I was supportive of the policy. While working to get ETUs up and running, there should be provisions for people who were left waiting. The policy clearly stated that ETUs were still the preferred option, stating:

> Taking care of the patient suspected to have EVD [Ebola virus disease] at home is NOT recommended; all efforts should be made to safely transport patients to an appropriate Ebola care facility. While waiting for the ambulance to pick up the patient, it is important to maintain safety of family members.[11]

But the CDC official was quoted in Adam's article as saying: "It's basically admitting defeat . . . You push some Tylenol to [patients], and back away." This quote annoyed me; it wasn't fair. The new home care policy simply acknowledged reality: there weren't enough beds and there wouldn't be in the foreseeable future. But on that phone call, when Adam asked me to comment on this evident division in the response, I decided I had better not say anything. If I objected to the CDC's objections, it would just fan the flames of something that I didn't think should be a controversy at all and might lead to CDC hardening their position. Adam wasn't thrilled with me because he could sense, as a good journalist, that I was holding something back, but I had learnt during Ebola that trying to have the media work in ways that were good for the response was sometimes as much about what we didn't say. I hung up the phone to Adam, all sweetness and light, and promptly called Sonia from the US team to vent my frustration at the CDC quote.

Despite the passing of this policy, which even listed items for a 'home care kit', support for home care had not become a priority in the response. Hundreds of thousands of kits had been distributed in Liberia, but in Sierra Leone it seemed to be blocked, despite the US agreeing to fund it. I told John that day in Port Loko that I thought this partly came down to confusion over the objective of home care kits. They could potentially help with two things. The first was reducing transmission in the home by giving people tools to protect themselves, such as gloves, disinfectant, and hand sanitiser. The second benefit could be an increased chance of survival by providing oral rehydration salts to people suspected of having Ebola.

The transmission point was deeply controversial: there was a valid concern that providing some protective equipment might put people at more risk by giving them a false sense of security.

There was no controversy, however, about providing oral rehydration salts. It would not have done any harm, even if a person did not end up having Ebola, and if they did, once in a while, it might have made the difference between life and death. Unfortunately, partly because these two objectives of home care kits got entangled, even the straightforward and cheap idea of giving out oral rehydration salts never happened on any significant scale.

Clearly, time and competing priorities were also an issue here, but I think some people agreed with the CDC official – that home care would be tantamount to admitting defeat. The crazy thing was, as far as those households in Port Loko were concerned, in failing to get treatment ready for them in time we *had* been defeated. Rather than acknowledging this and giving them a bit of support, we gave them nothing at all.

I didn't have any answers for John that day beyond fully agreeing with him that home care should be a priority and saying I would keep trying to push it.

As I left the DERC, despite the horrendous situation, I felt oddly encouraged. I got the sense the response was on the right track in Port Loko and that the different organisations were working well together with a strong sense of urgency.

OLIVER

Reinventing the wheel: Community Care Centres

We were facing challenges at Connaught similar to the ones experienced by our colleagues in Port Loko, with a tent full of suspected cases outside the main gate. Out of desperation, we had started to make our own home care kits from spare supplies, after being unable to get any through UNICEF or DFID. These consisted of oral rehydration salts and medical gloves to give to the patients we were sending home. It wasn't much, but it was better than nothing.

The opening of a handful of beds at Kerry Town had not put much of a dent in the challenge we were facing. By this stage, I was in almost daily meetings with the UK on the beds situation, and they were grasping at almost any opportunity for new beds that presented itself. Their team clearly felt immense pressure to get on top of things. It was a chaotic environment, and the signs of exhaustion and strain were showing all around. One UK official described constant nosebleeds from the stress.

In early November, the UK had asked for my input into plans for increasing bed capacity through units called Community Care Centres (CCCs). For those of us who had been on the Case Management Pillar from the beginning, proposals from recently arrived colleagues for new models of care were frustrating. With isolation units, we already had a model that we knew could be effective; we simply lacked the resources and organisations to implement the strategy more widely.

I had first heard WHO talk about CCCs in a Pillar meeting back in September.[12] In their presentation, CCCs were described as tented structures built in villages where there would be limited testing and little treatment. Family members – without full PPE – would help care for the patients. All of us in the room voiced fierce opposition to the idea. Marta led the criticism, pointing out: "These units sounds like death traps, you can't have relatives in no PPE, they will be like factories for Ebola and will spread the disease everywhere." I noted that we had been working hard to encourage the public to seek out Ebola facilities voluntarily if they were sick, convincing them that these facilities were places where they would receive safe care and effective treatment. Even though we had more patients coming forward than we had available beds, we did not want to lose the trust of the public, and worried that CCCs, in the way they had first been described to us, could undo all our progress.

All this being said, the proponents of CCCs had some good arguments in their favour. They hoped the units could be built very quickly, as an interim measure while we waited for the ETUs to come online. Surely some care was better than no care? CCCs would also be closer to communities than ETUs, and in theory more acceptable to them as a result. The idea of CCCs became popular at the headquarters level in Geneva, London and New York, and the UK made a high-level decision to build 200 of them.

The exact definition of a CCC was open to debate, however. Susan Elden from DFID, with whom I'd developed a close bond since we'd first met over that drink at UK headquarters, reached out to people on the front line like me to get suggestions for "red lines", to ensure the CCCs were not unsafe or inhumane. After some fierce advocacy on her part, and weeks of negotiations, the final proposal for the CCCs looked very different from what had initially been proposed. Instead, they looked much more like the isolation unit model we were already using, with full PPE, trained health workers and supervision by international NGOs. But, of course, this landed us back at square one, since they would take weeks to build and there were very few NGOs willing to provide clinical supervision in the Ebola red zones.

The one red line that wasn't – but should have been – included in the final plan was that CCCs should, wherever possible, be co-located with existing local government clinics, just as our isolation units were co-located with local hospitals. When a person got sick, they didn't know whether it was Ebola or something else. So by locating CCCs separately from local clinics, you would have some Ebola patients presenting to the clinic thinking they had malaria, and some malaria patients presenting to the CCCs thinking they had Ebola. Both groups would then be stuck miles away from where they needed to be, with the staff at the clinics having to look after Ebola patients while they waited for an ambulance to come and transfer them.

Given the country's severe shortage of healthcare workers, CCCs inevitably ended up recruiting staff away from the clinics, where they were also desperately needed. If the clinics and CCCs had been co-located, then they could have shared the same staff and easily transferred patients between them. Furthermore, the massive investment in building CCCs could have been used to upgrade the clinics and strengthen the health system, leaving a lasting capacity to isolate Ebola patients in future outbreaks.

Despite my efforts to convince WHO and DFID to focus on government facilities, the plan for CCCs as primarily separate entities went ahead and UNICEF were given the funding to manage the project.[13] I then received a call from UNICEF asking if they could sub-contract King's to supervise the CCCs in Freetown! I declined, since we had our hands full already setting up isolation units.

Snubs, wounds and grudges: politics gets in the way again
Alongside all the talk about CCCs, we were continuing discussions about more isolation units in Freetown.

As much as I admired the can-do attitude of the UK, it came with an unhealthy tendency towards unilateralism that could create problems. Although the UK had pushed for the creation of the NERC, so that a Sierra Leone-led command structure could integrate all international partners, the UK then never seemed willing to truly submit to it.

Instead, it sometimes felt like the UK and the NERC were duelling leadership structures. The UK would seize on a new idea for an Ebola unit and quickly organise their own meeting, where decisions would be made without any Sierra Leoneans from the NERC present. As a result, multiple uncoordinated efforts for Ebola units started to spring up. I found myself constantly pushing the UK to invite Sierra Leonean colleagues to the meetings, such as the case management lead, Dr Wurie, and to look to them for leadership.

Over the previous few weeks, the Sierra Leonean military and King's had been busy preparing to run the new ETU at Hastings Airfield, going back and forth with the UK engineers trying to speed things up. But during this time, the Australian government had offered to run a UK-funded ETU through a private healthcare provider and I was abruptly told that a decision had been made to give the unit to them to manage instead. It was like Jui with the Chinese all over again! Although I was a bit disappointed, I knew it was the right decision and was happy to see a new organistion step up to run an ETU, as we still needed all the help we could get.

We decided to put the planning to good use regardless, and to jointly open up a second ETU nearby. But the Ministry blocked King's from collaborating there. A few days later, King's offered to help open an Adventist hospital as a smaller ETU, and the same thing happened.

The Ministry's intransigence on King's not running our own ETU probably comes down to a couple of factors. Firstly, the tussles that we had had with the Ministry in August and September over the isolation units and Command Centre meant we weren't universally popular, something I might have handled better if I'd been more experienced and less sleep-deprived. Now we were reaping the consequences.

Secondly, I think these blockages were partly due to resentment of the Ministry towards the UK. Although the creation of the NERC had taken the Ministry out of a lot of the decision making in the response, they could never be taken out completely, since the response had to be delivered using Ministry health workers and facilities. The tension between the two was probably impossible to fully resolve. But the bullish way in which the NERC and the UK managed the transition had been seen as disrespectful by the Ministry and had unnecessarily alienated some allies there who were essential to the response. Key people in the Ministry were now outmanoeuvring the UK and King's politically, finding opportunities to reassert themselves in the response and obstructing us both when it suited them.

Dr Salia

These dynamics were also evident in a tragic situation involving Dr Martin Salia, the young consultant surgeon who ran the Emergency Department at Connaught. Short and energetic, with a trimmed moustache and boyish grin, he had always been a supportive colleague with an impatient determination to get things done. I had considered Dr Salia a fantastic role model and a future leader. Then, in early November, he started showing symptoms of Ebola.

Realising he was sick, he drove himself to the Kerry Town ETU, only to find himself turned away by the security guards at the front gate. In Kerry Town's defence, they had an established protocol for only accepting patients by referral and not walk-in cases, and the security guards were simply following procedure. I doubt any of the doctors inside knew a Sierra Leonean doctor was at the gate asking to be tested.

Dr Salia then drove himself to the nearby Hastings ETU to be tested by his Sierra Leonean colleagues. When the rumour spread that one of Sierra Leone's most popular doctors had been rejected by the British, at the very unit the UK had promised would treat Sierra Leonean health workers, there was outrage. People talked about it on the radio and around town, and it contributed to a spike in anti-British sentiment in Freetown. For the first time in our two years in Sierra Leone, my team and I started to get heckled on the streets for our nationality.

That same day, as soon as I heard Dr Salia was sick, I called the medical lead of the UK military unit at Kerry Town. Though a bed was immediately made available, after his initial experience at the gate, Dr Salia declined the offer and chose to stay at Hastings. There was widespread relief when his blood test came back negative, and Dr Salia headed home.

His symptoms continued to worsen, however, so he came to Connaught. He was seen by Marta and Terry, amongst others, and was tested for a second time. The hours crawled by whilst we waited for the lab result, hoping desperately not to hear another close colleague was infected. The moment the appointed time for the lab results came, I pulled my car over by the side of the road and made a call directly to the lab. The result was positive.

I had experienced so much death by this stage, and was so accustomed to bad news, that I felt pretty numb about it when I heard. I also knew, though, that if anyone had a chance at beating the disease then it was Dr Salia, given how young and healthy he was, provided he could get the best care.

A fierce debate then raged between his relatives, medical colleagues and the King's team about which ETU he should be referred to. I was desperate for him to go to the UK military unit at Kerry Town, since I believed the level of medical care they would be able to provide would be by far the best in the country. But his family and friends were adamantly opposed. They were still furious at how he had been turned away at the gate the first time and believed that at Kerry Town he would experience the 'no-touch care' they had heard so much about from the UK-led training.

Marta and I did everything we could to try and convince him to go to Kerry Town. I rushed over to Dr TB Kamara's office to enlist his help. "Right now his life hangs in the balance," I said, "and I really believe that whether he lives or dies is going to come down to the next five minutes and whether we can convince him to go." But nothing worked. He was adamant that he go to Hastings, and was so suspicious we would try to trick him that his family escorted his ambulance all the way to the gates of the Hastings ETU.

After a few days there, his family in the US were able to arrange a med-evac to a specialised hospital in Nebraska. But it was too late, and the long transatlantic journey was too arduous for him. On 17 November, Dr Salia went into renal failure and died soon after arrival. He was forty-four.

I was desperately sad but also angry that he had been allowed to die. Angry at myself, at the UK, at him, at just about everybody. His death, in particular, seemed completely avoidable.

The same day, Sierra Leone surpassed 5,000 cases of Ebola.

Yokie, Sorie and Sewa

Whilst the UK military's specialised Ebola unit at Kerry Town didn't end up treating Dr Salia, it did provide life-saving care to some of our national staff at Connaught who became infected.

The facility had primarily been established to treat foreign nationals because, as the UK military explained, "In the early stages of planning, the UK government medical advice was to retain Ebola cases in [Sierra Leone] in order to reduce the risk of transmission in the UK."[14] Ultimately, however, all the foreign nationals were med-evaced to Western healthcare facilities soon after they were diagnosed. The specialist unit still had an important psychological impact, however, as it was very reassuring to international NGOs, including the King's team, to know that a safe and high-quality ETU existed nearby.

The UK government had publicly described the unit as being "specifically for health care workers and international staff responding to the Ebola crisis," but, in reality, the inclusion criteria for Sierra Leonean health workers came with a lot of fine print.[15] They had to be a health worker, not a cleaner or other support staff, even though these team members were critical to the operation of ETUs. Additionally, only those working at a UK-funded ETU were eligible. Each admission would also be at the "discretion" of the commander in charge.[16] A UK colleague told me, much to my irritation, that the UK military did not want their staff exposed to any more patients than was strictly necessary, nor did they want to risk running out of beds for UK citizens.

Fortunately for me, I had a good relationship with the commander, who was generally keen to help King's and wanted his clinical staff to get more experience treating Ebola. He knew they couldn't get this if the unit was always empty. I feel indebted to the UK military team for saving the lives of three of our young male nurses at Connaught, named Yokie, Sorie, and Sewa, all of whom were nursing students who had volunteered to work in the Ebola unit back in August when we were desperately short-staffed. They had quickly proved themselves to be invaluable.

When their families had heard that they were working in an Ebola unit, they had given each of the young men the same ultimatum: quit the unit or leave home. The three men chose to put their commitment to their country above their own interests and stayed at their posts. I hadn't been aware of this at the time, but the matron had found a small room at the hospital for the three of them to live in together.

The infections started when Sorie broke off the top of a glass vial to prepare some injectable medications. He had cut himself, but kept it a secret. A few days later he tested positive, but unfortunately, had already spread the infection to his colleague Yokie. With a sense of despondency, I called up the UK military medical commander and was able to convince him to admit both patients.

After Yokie and Sorie had been transferred to Kerry Town, I invited Sewa to stay with me for a few weeks since he no longer had a place to stay. Things seemed fine until about day nineteen of his twenty-one-day incubation period. By this late stage, it is exceptionally rare for someone who has been exposed to become sick. Yokie and Sorie had already recovered and been discharged back home, looking weak but in good spirits.

Sewa, who had moved to more permanent lodgings the day before, had started experiencing terrible headaches. He tested positive the next day and was quickly accepted to Kerry Town as well. Since Sewa had been living with me, my housemate and I became contacts ourselves. I wasn't too worried about myself, but I did feel extremely guilty for putting my housemate at risk, who had shared a bathroom with Sewa, when I should have known better. Sewa was desperately sick at Kerry Town for weeks but received exceptional care from the UK military staff there.

Unfortunately, not everyone we referred to Kerry Town survived, including Abdulai Sesay, our elderly but tireless cleaner, who died following a separate exposure at Connaught. But I'm still very grateful to the UK military for saving the lives of these three, who went on to return to work and later went back to nursing school. Overall, it is a tragedy that more Sierra Leonean health workers could not have accessed the specialist Kerry Town unit, which never saw more than ten of its twenty beds occupied at any one time and treated just forty-three Ebola patients over a period of about six months.[17]

Tipping point

After months of waiting, the five other UK ETUs finally started opening in December. An ETU run by MSF-Switzerland also opened in Freetown at around the same time, but unlike the UK, they had managed to complete construction in just twelve days.

The opening of so many ETUs and CCCs at once led to a massive increase in bed capacity across the country. It was a sudden and extraordinary shift, like someone had flicked a switch in the response. For the first time since the outbreak began, just like that, we had more beds in Sierra Leone than we had patients.

Alongside this was an enormous increase in the number of labs. Inadequate capacity in the previous months had led to significant backlogs getting samples tested, and become a major bottleneck in the response. Patients were often left waiting days for a lab result, meaning surveillance teams were unable to respond quickly when new cases emerged. As we approached the end of 2014, teams of lab scientists had flown in from around the world, including a large contingent from Public Health England, and a helicopter was made available to collect blood samples from remote areas. It suddenly became feasible to get a lab result back on the same day. Furthermore, we now had much stronger coordination of alerts and ambulances at the district level by the DERCs. Every known suspected case was able to access a bed quickly.

The tipping point had been reached. At Connaught, just before Christmas, we found ourselves with empty beds for the first time since early August. It was almost bewildering for me and the rest of the King's team. For so many months we had been at ground zero, desperately trying to keep Connaught open and feeling constantly overwhelmed and at the very edge of our capacities. And then, over the course of just a few days, we found out we weren't needed anymore. The situation was under control.

You might have expected me to feel relieved or overjoyed, and in many ways, the NERC, the UK, and everybody else involved should be congratulated for their achievement of getting the ETUs open.

However, while many people viewed this turning point as a success, for me it felt like it came too late. I knew we could have opened these beds much earlier, and that this would have saved countless lives.

NINE | Getting to zero

SINEAD

Hopeful signs

As 2014 drew to a close, things were looking up, helped by the end of the six-month rainy season. We started to see a reduction in cases as the various parts of the response, such as community behaviour change, safe burials and the availability of beds, finally came together.

There are different theories on what led to this rapid reduction in case numbers. One global health specialist who volunteered with WHO shared his view with me: "The outbreak stopped because of what happened in little villages. I suspect chiefs and imams and priests ending the body rinse funerals, and people becoming more hygienic and careful."

There is no question that communities changing behaviour was critical; no amount of beds and burial teams would have made any difference if communities hadn't fought the disease themselves. But in reality, it is impossible to say for certain how significant each of the different elements was in bringing the outbreak under control – what's certain is that, collectively, they helped reduce transmission dramatically.

After so many months of waiting for the response to improve while the situation got worse, it was amazing to me how quickly the improvements took hold. The last week of November had seen 711 new cases in Sierra Leone but, just four weeks later, the figure was down to 337.[1] There was similarly encouraging news from neighbouring Liberia where cases had been declining every week since mid-November. Guinea's epidemic had never reached the same catastrophic levels as Liberia and Sierra Leone, and tended to fluctuate with no discernible upward or downward trend. It was still persisting and reached 114 cases in the last week of December, although this was a drop from the week before.[2]

So, the picture was largely improving in December. Unfortunately, there was a snag.

Preparing for a bumpy landing

The snag was pointed out to us by Mike Ryan, a renowned epidemiologist from the West of Ireland who had worked with WHO in twelve previous Ebola outbreaks and who, with his down-to-earth and jovial nature, could communicate as effectively with President Koroma as he could with a district surveillance officer in Kambia. Mike no longer worked for WHO but, when he arrived in December, he made me realise this was exactly the kind of senior but operational leadership that we had been lacking from WHO Geneva.

In one coordination meeting at the NERC, I asked Mike to talk about the period after we would have enough beds, known as the 'getting to zero' phase. "Ah yes," he said, with a knowing smile and a shake of his head. "I hope you're all ready for a bumpy landing." He went on, "Lads, you shouldn't think that Ebola case numbers will go straight down the way they went straight up. They will get to a low level alright, but they might stay at that level for months, waxing and waning. It will take a ton more work to get to zero." There was a moment of depressed silence – we had all assumed when we started to see case numbers dropping that we were nearly at the end of the outbreak. It had seemed logical at the time. Then Sonia from the US bit the bullet and asked Mike to go into detail on what this bumpy landing concept would mean for the response. Mike told us that certain elements, like contact tracing and surveillance, would need to come to the fore and become absolutely top class. "If you want to get to zero, you can't miss a single contact. Not one."

Sonia and I exchanged an uneasy glance. We were very aware that contact tracing had been one of the weakest links in the response so far, and it was widely believed there was still a lot of transmission occurring under the radar. The response was routinely taking swabs from corpses, and 20% of these in Freetown and its surrounding rural areas were testing positive for Ebola. These were people who were not reaching ETUs, and if surveillance had been working well, we would have already known about them.

Back at the beginning of the response, when resources were completely stretched, the UN Population Fund (UNFPA) had gamely volunteered to lead on contact tracing along with the Ministry. But they didn't have any experience in doing this, as they were an organisation that focused mostly on reproductive and maternal health. Unlike some organisations who managed to take on new roles effectively, UNFPA never managed to get on top of this critical new responsibility. They carried out a lot of activities, like hiring contact tracers and equipping them with mobile phones, but the supervision needed to ensure that the complex work was done properly was often lacking. I remember raising a concern about UNFPA's ability to lead on contact tracing in a meeting back in July 2014, where I was told by WHO that they should really have been the ones doing it as it was a technical role, but they didn't have the capacity. So, it stayed with UNFPA, remaining a weak link throughout the response.

As the epidemic got worse, the numbers of cases got so overwhelming that contact tracing became next to impossible anyway. It could take as many as ten staff to monitor the contacts of one Ebola case.[3] Given that, for instance, we had sixty-seven new cases in Port Loko district in the second week of December, that would require up to 670 contact tracers in that district alone. But, as Mike pointed out, there was no way to get to zero without excellent contact tracing. WHO were going to need to step up.

In a similar vein, my recent trips to the north of the country and the conversations I'd been having with WHO colleagues in Freetown had made me realise that international WHO technical staff were now the most urgent need. So I decided to try to help this process along by suggesting to the donor group that we could write a joint letter to the heads of WHO and UNMEER, stressing the need for these additional technical staff to be deployed as soon as possible. The UK and the US both thought it was a good plan, so I drafted the letter with their input and sent it off to the head of UNMEER and the Director-General of WHO on Christmas Eve. I knew that WHO were already moving in the right direction on this, but hoped that this letter might give them an extra push.

It seems it did. One senior UN staffer was not too happy with me though, and cornered me shortly after that at the Radisson: "Oi!" he said. "I hear I have you to blame for the fact that I got a call from Margaret Chan on 26 December. As if what I need when I'm trying to have a nice Christmas with my family is the DG saying, 'How soon can you go to Sierra Leone?'" "Well you're here aren't you?" I replied. "Fait accompli!" All of the various efforts to push this meant that, by the end of January, we finally had the full complement of WHO technical staff that we needed to get us through the bumpy landing.

OLIVER

'Too many beds'

As more beds opened and fewer cases were identified, facilities that had been at breaking point just a few weeks before now started to look a bit empty. It was a stunning reversal. In October, the total number of beds had been just 304.[4] By January, the country had 1,046 treatment beds as well as a further 998 beds in isolation units.[5] After months of having to turn patients away at the gates, and of pressuring ETUs to open more quickly, those same ETUs were now suddenly fighting over the patients that remained. Clinical managers would call up the Freetown DERC to complain they were not being sent enough patients. A colleague even told me, much to my annoyance, that one ETU had entered into a secret arrangement with national staff at one of the King's isolation units, convincing them to refer any new positive patients directly to them rather than going through the DERC.

A total of forty-six community care centres (CCCs) had opened by the end of January, and in the three months since November had seen over 700 suspected cases, although only 17% of these had tested positive.[6] That was fewer than three Ebola patients per CCC.[7] After all the hype about them, this was a modest contribution to the response, with CCCs being most helpful in remote areas far from ETUs. However, some CCCs were now competing for patients with ETUs, where better care was likely available.

Part of the reason for the unseemly fight for patients was that these Ebola units were all extremely expensive to operate, and it quickly became obvious that a rationalisation process would soon start to close down redundant ETUs. After working for months to get the units ready, organisations wanted to see them put to good use caring for patients and allow staff to gain valuable experience treating Ebola. Some may also not have wanted to lose the significant donor funding they were receiving for their ETU.

The NERC and the UK were reluctant to move too quickly on downsizing though, since nobody wanted to close ETUs too early and end up with a shortage of beds in the event of a flare-up. Nevertheless, planning for the wind-down process started in January, and once it became clear the reduction in cases was being sustained, these closures began. In theory, this process was done objectively, led by the NERC and WHO and based on factors such as geography and clinical capacity. In practice, the process was extremely political, with behind-the-scenes horse-trading to ensure that the high-profile units such as Kerry Town remained open.

From the outside, it may seem like poor planning to have invested so much money in building these ETUs, only to start closing them when they had only treated a relatively small number of patients. But we were dealing with the unknown, and there were a lot of scenarios where these excess beds could have proven vital. So, whilst the UK can be legitimately criticised for being so slow to get the ETUs open, I wouldn't criticise them for opening too many.

The upside of the smaller number of patients was that the response was finally able to focus on providing better quality care. ETUs had enough staff to ensure patients received intravenous fluids and tailored clinical management. For the first six months of the outbreak the fatality rate for Ebola patients in Sierra Leone was about 70%.[8] Although it's difficult to prove this definitively, survival rates appear to have improved significantly in 2015.[9] Additionally, there was now the capacity to keep relatives regularly updated and provide psychosocial care to survivors and families. I was encouraged to see patients finally getting a decent standard of care, although, at the same time, the visible contrast with the degrading conditions from earlier in the response added to my feelings of guilt.

A new wave of international responders had started to arrive and my team and I were battle-weary and more than happy to let the fresh recruits lead the next charge. So we kept a watchful eye on the response and shared our lessons and experience where we felt it was useful, but increasingly took a back seat.

With the end seemingly within reach, I redoubled my focus on staff safety and became more cautious. During those months when we'd been overwhelmed, I'd accepted that I or someone on the international King's team was probably going to get infected. But it now looked like there was a real chance we would all get out alive and, having made it this far and with the situation finally under control, I felt that a slip-up would be inexcusable. I had developed a personal mantra of 'no more infections at Connaught' and it was constantly repeating in my mind. I was running down the clock on the outbreak, but it was anyone's guess when it would finally end.

SINEAD

Ebola persistence in the north

From February 2015 onwards, we had all the resources we needed to get to zero, and cases were dropping steadily in most of the country. But despite the much improved national picture, Ebola persisted, particularly in the two northern districts of Port Loko and Kambia.[10] The case numbers were lower than the catastrophic highs of 2014, but were not dropping as fast as other districts had. In the first week of February there were thirty cases in the two districts, and a month later that number was still twenty-five.[11] Enormous resources were poured into the districts. We even had the WHO's Assistant Director-General Bruce Aylward, an enormously experienced outbreak specialist, make repeated visits to the two districts to advise on strengthening surveillance.

I made quite a few trips to these two districts in 2015 and tried to figure out why they were so problematic. After all, even before the main surge of resources in the country, the eastern districts of Kailahun and Kenema had ended their local outbreaks, with a significant drop in numbers from September. There were a lot of theories. Some said that historically Northerners, many of whom were independent traders, had always been less inclined to listen to their leaders or work in groups – my Sierra Leonean friends called them "stubborn". Others said that these districts were more superstitious and had a stronger presence of traditional religions and healers. Others still pointed to problems with particular local leaders trying to profit from the response.

What I took from all of this was that, even when we thought we had figured out the beds and burials and surveillance, getting to zero was still going to be a grind because it could only be achieved when Ebola was eradicated in every single community and that would require lots of specific strategies village-by-village, and critically, community buy-in. Whatever confidence we had started to feel that we were nearly at the end when we reached the 'holy grail' of enough beds, was dissipated as the months wore on in these northern districts.

More carrots, fewer sticks

'Groundhog days' were common for me in 2015. I started to feel my most important function in meetings was giving introductions on the context to the perpetual stream of new people. In response to the continuous proposals of 'new' ideas, I also acted as a historian of the response, which generally involved me putting up my hand a lot and usually saying something along the lines of, "Actually, we already tried that and . . ."

Having said that, while it was far from perfect, the response did improve tangibly in many ways, and the positive developments got us much closer to the kind of response we should have had from the start. Early in 2015, however, the response as a whole retained its blanket punitive bent. Many responders from government, and some international partners, thought that this approach was all the more necessary given the "stubborn" populations in the north, but it backfired as people continued trying to escape the response, particularly quarantine.

So, in late February, I decided to renew my lobbying on quarantine at a meeting at the NERC. Fortunately, the Director of the Situation Room, OB Sisay, was a receptive audience: "Sinead, we are 100% on the same page, 100%. We spend so much of our time at the NERC dealing with complaints on quarantine you would not believe it. We urgently need to make it better or the response as a whole just won't improve." I knew from informal conversations with colleagues at State House that the political will still didn't exist to change the overall policy, but in collaboration with various NGOs and the UN, OB led a programme to improve the conditions of people in quarantine. It was still a hardship for the affected population, but better dialogue with them often found compromises that were more acceptable. For example, arrangements were made for other community members to tend the fields of farmers who were in quarantine. Small compensations like these were the very least the response should have provided to people, who were essentially being locked up against their will in the name of public health. But it had taken us an extraordinarily long time to get to them.

Sierra Leonean innovations
Improvements like this were a sign of the response maturing and becoming more empathetic, helped by strong leadership from the

NERC, including from its group of returned diaspora. In early 2015, they started holding regular 'command meetings', which comprised only the Sierra Leonean leadership of the NERC, to discuss issues before international partners were asked to give their input.[12] There would soon be a need for this Sierra Leonean leadership to come to the fore.

Mike Ryan's bumpy landing warning was coming to pass. Apart from persistence in the north, February saw new cases in Crab Town, a shanty town within Freetown, near the Radisson hotel. A highly regarded traditional healer had contracted Ebola, likely from trying to heal Ebola patients nearby. The healer's body was prepared for burial by friends, family and local leaders before the response got involved, meaning there was now a group of high-risk contacts.

KB of WHO had moved by then from Port Loko to support the Crab Town response. He looked at the high infection risk of the crowded living quarters and quickly saw the destruction that could be wreaked in Crab Town if rapid action was not taken. "I worried that whole generations would be wiped out in the community." He called Yvonne Aki-Sawyerr, the dynamic and inexhaustible Director of Planning at the NERC and said, "We've got to get the high-risk contacts away from their families."

Now this was not something the response usually did. We quarantined households on an involuntary basis but some of the highest-risk contacts of an Ebola patient, for example a girlfriend or boyfriend, might not live in the same household, and so wouldn't be quarantined. CDC had come up with the idea in Liberia that you could ask high-risk contacts to wait out the 21-day incubation period in a separate supervised facility. That way if someone did start to show a fever or other symptoms, it would be detected immediately, enabling rapid testing and treatment, while reducing exposure to friends and family.

KB came to the idea of voluntary quarantine when he was having discussions with community members in slum areas of Freetown, "I asked the community what they would do if they were WHO, in order to stop the outbreak." They responded that they would scrap quarantine, because many low-risk contacts were being isolated, whereas high-risk were not. This made KB think about voluntary quarantine of high-risk contacts:

> I immediately rang Yvonne and thankfully she listened to me. She immediately went to Crab Town and managed to take the nine contacts to a voluntary quarantine facility which she set up with UNMEER. She was there for five hours. They thought she wanted to kidnap them but she convinced them in the end.

Efforts were made to ensure the nine contacts had decent conditions, including televisions to while away the time. The fact the quarantine was voluntary reduced the potential for tensions that could have otherwise arisen with the community.[13]

All nine contacts tested positive for Ebola and were moved to an ETU, where five of them died. While this was a tragic situation, it is possible more of the contacts would have died had they not been in the facility as they would not have been diagnosed and treated as quickly as they were. In addition, the voluntary quarantine averted the possibility of their friends and families becoming infected, ensuring these cases did not lead to a major spike in Freetown.[14]

The implementation of this voluntary quarantine was not perfect and mistakes were made along the way. It will always be questionable how 'voluntary' such an initiative is, as contacts may be put under a lot of pressure by the government or other community members. Nevertheless, it was a step in the right direction, with voluntary quarantine facilities used for the rest of the outbreak in Sierra Leone to positive effect.[15]

"One day this land shall be ours"

Around the same time, while there was broad agreement on the quarantine improvements, one issue was deeply controversial: non-Ebola health care. This was a huge problem throughout the response, and one we failed to deal with. We often had it on the bottom of the agenda for meetings, but usually when we got to it, the response was a lot of hand-wringing. Nobody really took leadership on it. The sad fact was that the response was only focused on treating you for Ebola, but not if you turned out to have typhoid, meningitis or anything else. And you might not be able to get anybody else to treat you either, as often your local clinic didn't have any staff anymore. Maybe the staff had died of Ebola or maybe they had gone to work for an NGO-run health facility where they would get a better salary. What's more, from early on in the outbreak, people feared the health system as a place where you could contract Ebola. This was not irrational, considering the poor infection control measures in the early days. As a result, attendance at regular health clinics had plummeted.

In March, the NERC started planning a 'surge' of surveillance and awareness activities to drive down cases in the Freetown area.[16] At one particular meeting, several people from the government expressed their view that it would be very difficult to get better collaboration with communities in Freetown if the issue of non-Ebola health care was not addressed. However, a UK representative then stood up and made a statement to the effect of, "My government will not allow our funding to go to non-Ebola health care." He was presumably trying to make the point that the UK's top priority was getting to zero, and that it was important the response didn't get distracted from this. But his declaration did not go down well in the meeting. As one UN participant described it, there was "almost a riot". An impassioned senior

Ministry official stood up and said, apparently without any sense of irony, "One day, this land shall be ours."

The UK were not the only ones to have reservations about focusing on non-Ebola health care. While more efforts were made in this area from March 2015 onwards, including providing care to quarantined households, it never got nearly enough attention or resources and this failure was a collective one. I regret, looking back, that I didn't champion that issue from the very beginning. Like others I had it on my list but it was never near the top. I was caught up in the 'main event' of the Ebola response, but then again, so was everybody else. Later we would learn just how disastrous the lack of non-Ebola health care had been for the population.

Throw the office in the sea

Despite this 'near riot' over non-Ebola health care, overall the UK became a more collaborative partner in 2015, continuing to play a very central role at all levels of the response. Although unilateralism was still a problem at times, by and large Marshall Elliott, Donal Brown's successor, gradually stepped back to allow more space for others, including the increasingly strong NERC. Part of the reason for this was a surprise entrant into the mix: a new head of the UN Mission.

When Bintou Keita, a UNICEF veteran originally from Guinea, first arrived in March, Peter and I arranged to meet her on a Sunday morning, as we were both flying to Brussels for an Ebola conference that afternoon along with the President and some of the cabinet. We sat down over coffee at the Radisson, and I ran through a series of suggestions on how I thought UNMEER's role could complement what others were doing. For instance, up until that point, the key international responders had usually been interacting separately with the Sierra Leonean leadership, offering differing, occasionally even conflicting advice. I hoped Bintou could pull them together to form a unified position.

I liked Bintou immediately as she was frank and pragmatic. But I wasn't optimistic she would be able to have a significant impact on the response, particularly given that UNMEER's influence had been relatively marginal up to that point. However, in one of the clearest examples of how a single personality can have a significant impact, Bintou not only fulfilled my requests on coordination, but quickly became the moral compass of the response, winning the respect of the NERC as well as international actors.

Bintou was deliberative and jovial at the same time, with a gentle way of commanding respect that reminded me of my father. It had always amazed me how my nieces and nephews would suddenly shift from loud mischief to Zen-like calm within a short time of being in a room with him. And so it was with Bintou. She instantly commanded the respect of the UK, the NERC and the rest of the response community.

In one particular incident at an NERC meeting, a UK military official gave a presentation full of military language, like "attacking" the "enemy" of Ebola and maintaining a "battle rhythm" going after "escapees" from quarantine. Bintou sat quietly, writing down every military reference. She then took the official aside and showed him her notepad. She didn't have to say anything – he got the message and, after that, changed his tone. I was impressed, particularly with the discreet way she dealt with the situation, making sure nobody lost face. Supported by the then overall head of UNMEER, who had competently led the UN response in Liberia, Bintou showed us what the UN can be in its best incarnation.

I also had some experiences with the UN in its worst incarnation. One UN agency in particular infuriated me. They jumped to implement any idea that came up in the response that they thought they could mobilise funds for, even if it was a terrible idea. I had started raising the issue of this organisation's performance at the international level and when they sent a senior international manager over to Freetown to help with their Ebola response, I saw another opportunity. I sat down with this visitor to tell him just that, but only got as far as, "I need to talk to you about your country office . . . " before he responded: "You know what I'd like to do? I'd like to take our country office and throw it in the sea."

That conversation ended up being much easier than I'd thought it would be. I had quite a bit of experience in these kinds of difficult conversations about agencies' performance. The problem was, you didn't know in advance how the criticism would be received, as it depended on how open the person you were speaking to was, and on their relationship with the people you were complaining about. Frustrated though I was, it was also important for Irish Aid's reputation that I didn't come across as casting aspersions unjustifiably. So I had prepared notes on examples of what we felt the agency had done wrong, where and when. After that comment though, I was able to swiftly fold these notes up and put them back in my handbag. It was reassuring to see that UN agencies can identify poor performance and act firmly on it. That manager ended up helping to bring real changes, including much improved leadership, to the agency in-country.

So overall, both the national and international responses got stronger in 2015. But, as Mike had warned us, getting to zero wouldn't be straightforward. I got very excited when we got to two cases per week in early May, only to see another spike in the northern districts and Freetown, bringing us back up to fifteen cases in the first week of June. I remember sitting at my desk and getting the news about the fifteen cases. I just felt a wave of exhaustion come over me and I put my head in my hands. The most difficult part of it was that we were starting to see so many really worrying secondary impacts come to the fore, such as massive unemployment and the severely compromised health system. I was feeling impatient that we should all turn the attention we spent on Ebola to these issues, but if we did that too soon, we could see a spike and be back to square one.

OLIVER

Resilient zero

We realised quickly that survivors were going to be key to getting to a 'resilient' zero, which meant not just getting to zero but staying there. As our scientific understanding of Ebola had improved during the outbreak, we'd learnt more about how the virus could hide away from a survivor's immune system for months after they had been 'cured', in sites such as their eyeballs, in a woman's breastmilk and in a man's semen. This led to concern that survivors could still infect others through medical treatment, nursing of infants or unprotected sex. Various off-the-wall ideas were floated about how to tackle this, with furious MSF colleagues explaining one such scheme at a meeting with the UK: "We've heard that local leaders in Kailahun want to round up all our male survivors and lock them up in internment camps – this is unacceptable, it's outrageous!" Once again I worried that people could make these kinds of rash decisions when driven by fear. The truth is that nobody was quite sure how to handle this new challenge, although a lot of lessons were taken from HIV control programmes.

In practice, ETUs took a less punitive approach that focused on promoting safe sex and providing condoms to patients when they were discharged. Survivors commonly experienced ongoing medical problems after their recovery, such as eye problems and joint pain. I saw this first-hand with colleagues at the hospital who had survived their infections, including one lab technician whose vision was now so poor he could no longer take blood from patients and had to be transferred to an administrative role. Plans were put in place to provide free clinics for survivors.

In addition, with thousands of survivors potentially still harbouring low levels of the virus, it was clear the infection control measures introduced by the response would have to be maintained for months, even years, if we were to arrive at a resilient zero. Infection prevention and control across health facilities became a central part of the strategy and in January, King's volunteered to take this on at four of the government hospitals in Freetown. The CDC were spearheading this effort and offered a significant amount of funding through the US Office of Foreign Disaster Assistance. However, we soon encountered a challenge with this US grant as it explicitly banned us from building any permanent structures.

We found ourselves with plenty of money for improving infection control in hospital wards that often had no sinks or running water, only to be that we weren't allowed to buy new taps! Instead, we were told to buy temporary buckets, which could quickly break and end up costing us more in the long run. The reason behind this was that the US funding was designated for short-term emergency work, not long-term rehabilitation. Be that as it may, such lack of flexibility was crazy in situations where we would need improvements to be long-lasting in order to maintain zero cases of Ebola. I was incredulous and was keen to push back with the donor against these rules, but friends at the big international NGOs with past experiences like this convinced me not to waste my breath. Fortunately, DFID agreed to make up the gaps in US funding. It was a great example of donors coordinating and using common sense. The US funding would pay for our staff and the consumables (like soap), whilst the DFID funding would cover construction and repair.

Fixing the infrastructure was the easy part, however. The hard part was changing the behaviour of health workers, many of whom had spent decades doing things a different way. It wasn't uncommon to walk onto a ward and see nurses eating a snack while still wearing their medical gloves. On one memorable occasion earlier in the response, I was standing at the entrance to the unit at Connaught when I saw some terribly unsafe practice from a new burial team that had arrived to collect a corpse (who, amongst other things, sprayed me head to toe in chlorine as they walked past, ruining my clothes and leaving me spluttering). I marched up to their supervisor, who I knew well and who happened to be the lead trainer for infection control in Freetown at that time, to vent my outrage and give him a whole shopping list of complaints. "Ah Oliver, what on earth happened to your shirt?" he began, before apologising profusely and saying, "Wait one moment, let me get my pen, I want to make sure I write it all down so I don't forget." I then watched as he removed his industrial rubber gloves by putting his finger in his mouth so that he could pull them off with his teeth. I'm rarely left speechless, but this was one such occasion.

Getting doctors to wash their hands between every patient on their ward round, convincing nurses to dispose of dirty needles in a special 'sharps' bin, ensuring cleaners properly decontaminated wards with chlorinated water, getting everyone to protect themselves with rubber gloves and boots rather than working with their bare hands while wearing flip flops – it was going to be tough to change long-ingrained habits.

These might seem like basic changes, but infection control is an enormous struggle even in well-resourced countries. It's worth remembering what happened the only time an undiagnosed Ebola patient has ever been seen in the Emergency Department of a Western hospital – when Thomas Duncan walked into Texas Health Presbyterian in September 2014 inadequate infection control practices led to Ebola spreading from that single patient to two American nurses. Yet we were expecting Sierra Leonean health workers to do better than this, with far less training and fewer resources.

We recruited a team of international nurses to implement the project, supported by a wonderful engineer from California to help with the infrastructure improvements, but after a couple of months they had only been able to make limited progress.

It didn't help that many hospital staff felt betrayed that they had still not received all the hazard pay they were owed. Whilst the Ebola payment system had improved significantly, albeit slowly, after the establishment of the NERC, many of the earlier commitments had still not been honoured. What's more, some of the volunteer nurses had not been put on the government payroll as promised, including the few surviving volunteer nurses in Kenema who had been specifically highlighted by President Koroma in his announcement on 1 July 2014.[17] This contributed to low morale amongst many health workers and a wariness about engaging in the response.

Thus, when there was a flare-up in cases in June, we decided to be a bit more innovative in our approach, and set up a competition. The Ministry had appointed a new infection control nurse at every government hospital. We had a particularly determined and effective nurse at Connaught who, paired with an international nurse from King's, carried out an inspection and gave each ward a score. At lunchtime, the hospital staff came together in the grassy central courtyard, where the Deputy Matron announced the results. Wards that achieved a high enough score would be rewarded with bags of rice to be shared out amongst their staff. This may not seem an exciting prize to a foreigner, but it was enormously valued in Sierra Leone, where a plate of food isn't considered to be a meal until it includes rice. The results were left on display, meaning successful wards could be congratulated and failing wards would be publicly shamed.

That first week the results were really disappointing, with just two of the fifteen wards getting an acceptable score. The staff from the wards that failed were furious, and shouts of "Unfair, unfair, you cheated us!" and "What about us, where is our rice?" rang out across the courtyard.

When we reconvened a week later, however, the hospital had been transformed. All but two of the wards received a prize, including the Emergency Department, which was most at risk. Staff were routinely washing their hands. Soap and gloves were widely available. Waste had been separated into the right bins. The Deputy Matron stood at the centre of her cheering ward nurses and gave a powerful speech about working and learning together in the nation's fight against Ebola. After all we'd been through, seeing the whole hospital unite as one left me with tears in my eyes. Together we had started to achieve real change. Although standards started to dip again a few weeks later, when the prizes were stopped, they remained considerably higher than they had been before.

Building a centre of excellence

With the ETUs open, and the numbers of new infections dropping, many people in the government wanted to close the hospital isolation units, believing this would remove Ebola from the hospitals and help make them 'safe' again. This was backed by public pressure, as some patients complained they were afraid to go to the hospital in case they were exposed.

Although Marta and I agreed it was much better for Ebola patients to be treated in an ETU, and were directing any new

cases to ETUs immediately, we were desperate to keep the isolation units open. "The unit isn't bringing Ebola into the hospital,"
I said to colleagues from the Ministry, "it's the one thing that is
keeping Ebola out." Without these units, staff and patients would
be at risk if there was nowhere to isolate a suspected case. I was
exasperated that we were still caught up in these debates and felt
like the lessons from the start of the outbreak were already being
forgotten.

We were eventually successful when the NERC and WHO
swung behind the plan to keep the units open. DFID offered to
fund an upgrade of our existing isolation units, which aside from
now being too big, were often temporary structures made of tarpaulin and plywood. In their place, we proposed smaller but permanent screening and isolation. These refurbished units would
help hospitals reopen fully for normal patients during the tail end
of the outbreak, as well as having the potential to be reactivated
for any future emergency. Given the cramped, awkward layouts
of the urban hospitals, there was no one-size-fits-all design and
we had to work creatively with local staff in order to squeeze them
in.

Our focus at King's was on Connaught, where a decision was
made to be more ambitious. Since it was the national referral and
teaching hospital, it would be a natural place for suspected cases
to be referred to in small future outbreaks, be that of Ebola or
another disease like cholera or Lassa fever, as well as an ideal
training site for doctors and nurses.

Re-energised by this project, we soon got to work on a purpose-
built unit, called the Centre of Excellence for Infectious Diseases.
Engineers from the British military volunteered their help and we
worked with hospital staff to design our dream isolation unit. Now,
finally, we had the time and resources to do it properly, and were
able to include individual rooms for patients, windows in each

door so that people could view inside, and drains in the tiled floors. There was also a viewing area where relatives could safely speak with patients or view the bodies of those who had passed on. I was particularly pleased with the intercom and CCTV system that allowed us to communicate between the office and the red zone, keeping an eye on the wellbeing of patients from outside.

Construction started in May and the biggest challenge was installing the incinerator for medical waste at the back of the unit. DFID had arranged for a huge crane to come and hoist it over the Connaught building, but getting the crane into the hospital complex was a challenge.

I was in my office when I overheard they had decided to remove a ceremonial arch between two of the buildings in order to fit the crane through the middle. My eyes practically sprang out of their sockets, as the only ceremonial arch at Connaught was the gateway to the Old King's Yard, under which, roughly two hundred years previously, freed slaves had walked as they arrived in Freetown to settle in liberty. Sprinting through the hospital, I arrived just in time to save one of the country's most important historical monuments, which was under consideration by UNESCO as a site of Outstanding Universal Value. In the end, we found an alternative route.

For me, the Centre of Excellence remains one of our proudest achievements in Sierra Leone, and physical evidence that permanent legacies could be established even in the midst of a humanitarian crisis.

'Guinea pigs'

The reduced number of cases also provided an opportunity to finally do some research. The world had known very little about Ebola prior to this outbreak and many of us had been keen to do studies since it began. Most facilities had been too overwhelmed to engage, however, and many critical questions remained unanswered. What was the best way to identify a suspected case? How could we improve a patient's chance of survival? How effective were the new vaccines, treatments and diagnostic tests that had surfaced during the outbreak?

With the situation improving, we finally had time to think about these things, although we now had barely enough Ebola patients for any studies. The King's team were able to undertake several pieces of research, the most significant of which was to test out, under field conditions, a rapid diagnostic test for Ebola that had been invented by the UK military. Given all the challenges we'd had with labs during the response, we knew that this test could be a game-changer. The rapid test proved to be highly effective, but to my immense frustration the UK government refused to then make it available for use in the response, for reasons I never got to the bottom of. This left me feeling that our patients, who had volunteered to be part of the study, had been exploited and I was angry at my naïveté in allowing it to happen.

Dozens of other studies were undertaken in 2015 to address some of the key questions, perhaps the most ambitious being the trial of a potential Ebola vaccine. From early on in the response, there had been much excitement about the potential for a vaccine, although I remember being pretty sceptical myself. This was because, although there were three candidate vaccines, all of them were in the early stages of development and we didn't know if they would be safe or effective in humans and clinical trials usually take years. But after a huge global effort involving pharmaceutical companies, academics, ministries, WHO and donors, this was shrunk down to just a few months under some of the most challenging field conditions you can imagine. The Canadian vaccine proved safe and highly effective after a trial involving 12,000 people in Guinea, and from the middle of 2015 it was used in Sierra Leone to bring the outbreak to a more rapid close.[18] It will likely be a game-changer for future Ebola outbreaks.

However, few basic studies were done on the simple things we could have done to increase survival. Huge amounts of energy and funding were put into researching novel treatments like ZMapp, drugs that were both expensive and untested. But we never did any basic studies to definitively show, for instance, how much benefit there was to providing IV fluids instead of oral rehydration. Another unanswered question was whether we should be giving patients anti-diarrhoeal drugs to reduce dehydration. This was another key lesson for me, because maybe if we had taken the time to do this research earlier on, we could have saved hundreds more lives.

SINEAD

Isatu Kamara

As cases inched towards zero in the north, I went on a visit to Port Loko to try to understand the situation of survivors there.

Usually, if a foreigner drives into a village in Sierra Leone, there is quite a bit of interest – children swarm around your car and curious adults come out of their houses to say hello. So, it was an eerie experience arriving without any such fanfare in the village of Rolath, where almost half of the village had died of Ebola. My colleagues and I parked beside a cluster of deserted houses. Eighteen members of the Kamara family had lived in these houses, and sixteen of them had died, leaving only Isatu Kamara and her grandmother.

I spoke to Isatu, a shy fourteen-year old. She had also been infected with Ebola and spent a month at the International Medical Corps treatment centre. She told me about the terrifying hallucinations she had experienced whilst suffering from the virus. Her father, siblings, aunts, uncles and cousins had all succumbed, and her mother had already died when she was very young. So, when she came home to Rolath, only her grandmother was still alive. Isatu tried to go back to school, but had struggled and now sat all day in the quiet village next to her grandmother, who made soap to try to support them.

As I stood talking to Isatu, I was overwhelmed by a feeling of helplessness as I tried to think of any words of comfort that would not just be trite. All I could think of was that Isatu was about the same age as my eldest nephew in Ireland whose main preoccupations were basketball and video games.

There are over 4,000 known survivors of Ebola in Sierra Leone, and there are likely others who survived in the early phase of the epidemic, but were not recorded in all the chaos. Isatu was among the 'lucky' group in 2015 who were able to go to an ETU and get a bed right away. She was given good treatment, including psychosocial support. As a survivor, she was entitled to basic care for some of the physical problems many survivors have, but not much else. Leaving aside the very real challenges of health care, getting an education and making a living, how do you ever get over the loss of sixteen of your seventeen closest relatives?

I spoke to one of the IMC staff about Isatu's situation. A warm woman in her mid-forties and a former teacher, she was an Ebola survivor herself, and had lost her sister and her twenty-four-year-old daughter to Ebola. So she could understand the horror and grief Isatu had been through better than most, but even she had no idea how to help her.

Meeting with Isatu showed me the depressing reality for survivors in Sierra Leone. For a while they would be the focus of attention and promises would be made about supporting them. But, as in other disasters, these promises would rarely be kept.

As well as powerless, I also felt huge guilt as I drove away from Rolath. People like me would have the luxury of moving on to work on other things. Ebola would just be a memory for us and the subject of stories that we would tell our friends and family back home. But for many thousands of Sierra Leoneans like Isatu, Ebola would never be over.

The wider impact

While the situation was most acute for survivors and people who had lost relatives, the entire country had suffered due to the Ebola crisis. A group of our partners held meetings with more than 1,000 children around Sierra Leone and asked them how Ebola had affected them.[19] The statements the children made cut to the core of the wider impact of Ebola in terms of missed education and health care, job and income losses, and increased child labour:

> "I can no longer remember what I have previously learnt in school."

> "The only nurse in this village abandoned us during the Ebola outbreak and she comes to the village once or twice a month. We the children have suffered the most. We don't have a place to go when we are sick."

> "Before the Ebola I never sold anything because I was going to school – now I am a trader."

> "Sometimes I cry silently because my father has no money to care for me and my family . . . I am troubled because my dad has lost his job because of Ebola."

The statistics bore out these individual experiences of children. A study came out that showed that 2,819 more people died of tuberculosis, AIDS and malaria alone than would have been expected during the crisis.[20] It was a shocking figure, particularly when you compared it with the 3,956 deaths from Ebola.

The future of the health sector didn't look bright. Given so many health workers in the country had died of Ebola, it was estimated that, each year, an additional 1,845 pregnant women in Sierra Leone would not have access to medical care and would die in childbirth as a result.

For many Sierra Leoneans, the most difficult aspect of Ebola was the closure of schools. A total of 1.8 million school-going children were affected by the nine-month closure.[21] In a country where most children already have to drop out of school before they complete it, largely due to the pressures of poverty, many children who had an enforced break during Ebola might never go back.

The State of Emergency had included restrictions on movement, which had led to job or income losses for many people. For this and other reasons, an estimated 180,000 people had lost their jobs.[22]

These were some of the more tangible impacts, but there were myriad others.

For most of 2015, as Ebola numbers waxed and waned, my Irish Aid colleagues and I worked on the response in parallel with the process of helping the country to recover from these second-ary impacts. We expanded our nutrition programme. We helped farmers get back to work by providing seeds for the next season. We provided cash grants to vulnerable households to allow them to get by until they could start earning again from farming and trading. But the task just felt overwhelming at times, particularly because this was one of the poorest countries in the world before the epidemic had started.

'Business as usual?'

Because of the enormity of the recovery task, in February I convened a meeting of donors to talk about what a nationwide recovery programme could look like. I began the meeting by saying, "Throughout the Ebola crisis we have all said that we can't go back to 'business as usual' after Ebola. And this is our chance. What does 'not business as usual' look like in practice? And how do we get there?"

I recognised poor governance had been a key part of why the Ebola situation in Sierra Leone had been so catastrophic. The Ebola audit was a case in point – on 13 February, the Auditor-General of Sierra Leone released a report saying that 30% of Ebola funds from May to October 2014, around $14 million, were not adequately accounted for if at all.[23,24] It wasn't a great surprise. Every year the Auditor-General released damning findings in her annual report, but there was rarely much follow-up. For instance, by 2015, just 26 out of the 76 recommendations she had made between 2010 and 2012 had been implemented.[25]

However, it was not just the government that had improvements to make. We donors were also at fault, with the crisis having shone a critical light on some of our investments in the health sector. Going forward, how could we work with government to design a recovery programme that promoted better governance on their side and higher quality, longer-term investments from our side?

Unfortunately, despite my attempts to pull donors together for the recovery process to focus on how things had gone wrong pre-Ebola and how we should work jointly on a better approach, the UK started working unilaterally with the government, setting up a new recovery unit at State House and hiring international consultants to work with various stakeholders to draft a recovery plan that they would fund. This was presented to the rest of us as more or less a 'fait accompli' in a hastily arranged meeting in April at the Radisson. The plan had four sections: health, education, social protection and private sector development. I saw

nothing wrong with those as broad priorities, but as the Pow-
erPoints on each section were presented, I got more and more
annoyed. Some of the specific content of these plans was alarming
but even worse than that was how the planning had been done.

The main problem was that many key people had been left
out of the planning process, which was not surprising given the
consultants had literally just flown into the country and had no
idea who was who. What's more, most of the DFID people who
were managing this process were also fairly new in-country.

This had obvious implications for the content of the plan. So, for
example, in one sector we worked in, the proposed plan included
a programme that all donors in the sector had refused to fund for
years because we saw it as a vote-winning strategy for a particular
Minister, rather than being of any significant benefit to the population. Every year the Minister would put it in his plans, and every
year donors would not fund it. But the consultants didn't know
any of this and simply included what the Minister said he wanted,
word for word. All of a sudden, this pariah programme was part of
the official Ebola recovery plan. I was horrified.

I sent a stream of WhatsApp messages to Paula from my seat:
"You're not going to be believe this. UNICEF weren't consulted
on the social protection plan. They can't believe it either, since
they are leading on supporting the government on social protection!" "Oh my God, the agriculture component Paula! I have no
words."

When we were asked if we had any questions at the end, I knew
it was wiser if I didn't say much in this public forum given how I
actually felt at that moment. I restrained myself, but all this went
out the window when I called Peter from the car:

> Peter, this is just unacceptable. We agreed we were going to do
> this as a group. Remember that meeting? We talked about not
> going back to 'business as usual'. And then this? No mention of

governance whatsoever in the plan! But some of what did make
it in . . . Look, I get that we need to get a move on and not spend
ages in long planning processes, but you need to have the right
people in the room to come up with a proper plan that looks at
what happened pre-Ebola in these areas. The history of Sierra
Leone didn't start in 2014!

Another potential problem with the recovery programme was
that it repeated the NERC experience of helping the government
create a separate unit to manage recovery, rather than housing it
within the appropriate ministries of health, education, trade and
agriculture. Though I agreed that creating the NERC had been
the right thing to do for Ebola, which was a highly time-sensitive
emergency, was it the right thing to do in the long term? Would
it not be better to strengthen existing Ministries by having them
lead the plans in their sectors? The Ministries certainly had limitations, but wasn't it a vicious cycle not to invest in them?

A couple of days later, we had a working dinner with DFID
and the other donors to discuss the issues. I laid out my views,
but also acknowledged that it wasn't all bad news. The UK were
prepared to invest massive resources, to the tune of £240 million
(over $370 million at the time), in the recovery process, at a time
when the government was extremely cash strapped.[26,27] I appreciated this, and it was certainly vastly more than we could put on
the table. But I also said:

Colleagues, we have been here before. Billions of dollars have
been spent in this country since the end of the war. And this is
where we are. Let's face it, money is not the number one problem
in Sierra Leone. We have got to learn and change how we do
things if we want to really have an impact.

Other donors expressed similar sentiments although admittedly, no one seemed to feel the issues as keenly as I did. I had
been in Sierra Leone for four years by then, I had a seen a lot of

poorly planned programmes and a lot of waste. To my relief, the DFID team agreed that there needed to be a significant change of approach and trying to help them to revamp the recovery plan became a major focus for me and my colleagues in the second quarter of 2015.

Hope in enterprise

Apart from helping with the overall planning process, we engaged in some new activities on recovery, one being private sector development. As the final activity in our private sector match-making initiative, Irish Aid sponsored a trade fair at the Radisson hotel which my pal Memuna organised once more. This time we wanted to give the message that the international community should make better long-term use of the domestic private sector, beyond the Ebola response. We hoped for twenty-five companies but, on the morning of the event, thanks to Memuna's formidable marketing skills, forty-five Sierra Leonean companies arrived to set up stands to promote their goods and services, on top of which about fifteen other Sierra Leonean companies also showed up in the hopes of squeezing in.

We crammed as many tables as we could into the hall, and got the late-subscribers to share stands. When the fair kicked off, there was a strong attendance from the international community and the government, and by the end the room was completely packed. I had a few moments of worrying about asphyxiation, but the mass of people actually ended up creating a real buzz. It was the place to be. People squeezed between stands, shouting to be heard as they promoted their companies. For me it was a real moment of hope for Sierra Leone. These people had the ideas and the energy. Given the opportunity, and a few less obstacles, they could transform the country in long-term ways beyond what any of us aid actors could ever do.

Getting pregnant girls back to school

Another recovery priority close to my heart was a programme to get pregnant girls back into the formal education system, as they had been banned from school during pregnancy, due to a perception in this highly religious country that they would set a bad example for other girls and spread immorality. As someone who had grown up in a deeply Catholic society, I had some understanding of these dynamics and had pregnant schoolmates either drop out or be encouraged to drop out (I was never sure which). It had troubled me as a teenager, but this time I hoped to be able to do something about it.

This was a particularly salient issue in Sierra Leone since nearly one in three girls got pregnant as teenagers even before Ebola, and teenage pregnancy was widely thought to have skyrocketed during the crisis.[28] Some said this was because schools had been closed and teenagers had been hanging around with nothing to do, while others pointed to increased vulnerability of Ebola orphans or girls in quarantine to sexual abuse. In the same survey of over 1000 children, it was found that:

> Sexual violence against girls was observed to have increased across all districts . . . In nearly all of the [focus group discussions] where this issue was raised, children could relay a case of rape against a girl in their community, including attacks on girls in quarantine households.[29]

When I went to Brussels in March for the Ebola recovery conference, I had a meeting with President Koroma and some of his cabinet, along with Minister Seán Sherlock, who had visited us in October. Since schools were going to reopen in April, we raised the fact that pregnant girls would be banned from attending. I thought it was a long shot with all the other needs around, but to my surprise President Koroma seemed quite concerned about it. He talked about how many pregnant girls, as young as eleven years old, he had encountered while travelling around the country doing social mobilisation on Ebola and how shocking he had found this. I offered our support on the issue, although I still wasn't very hopeful that it would be prioritised.

One Friday evening a few weeks later, I was out running up a hilly main road when I got a call from the President's office. "Ambassador, I am calling from State House. His Excellency the President is interested in discussing with the Irish Embassy your offer of support with respect to education for pregnant girls." I ducked into an internet café to get away from the traffic noise and tried to catch my breath so that I could sound somewhat professional in my tank top and shorts. "Excellent," I managed to get out. "What are the next steps?" They asked me to come in to meet the President the following Monday.

Still standing in the internet café, I called the heads of DFID, UNICEF and UNFPA in quick succession. As I expected they were ready to jump on this opportunity and we arranged to meet the next morning at Balmaya restaurant. We strategised and ultimately put together a plan on how we could support the government to provide education for these pregnant girls, should the Ministry of Education remove the ban on their attendance.

On the Monday I sat with President Koroma, just the two of us in his enormous, ornate office at State House. I had been in dozens of meetings with the President over the years but this was the first time I had ever met him alone – usually there was the Minister for Foreign Affairs or the Chief of Protocol, or at the very least a note-taker. I had proposed bringing my UK and UN colleagues along to the meeting, but his staff had said I should come alone. This was a very sensitive topic in Sierra Leone and there were deep divisions in public opinion. I had even had a cabinet Minister ask me: "But if you let these girls continue in school, how will they be punished?" But, to his credit, the President got it. The solution to teenage pregnancy wasn't depriving girls of their education, quite the opposite. That day, he and I agreed on the outlines of a plan, and later the UK, UN, my colleague Emma and I worked with the Ministry of Education on the details.

Two months later, registration opened for a new 'bridging programme' for pregnant girls. We expected about 3,000 girls would register – we got 14,500. These girls had a hunger and a determination to continue with their education and they turned up in their droves. In my five years in Sierra Leone, that programme is one of the things I'm proudest of.

OLIVER

Here we are again: recovery

The optimistic mantra as the outbreak drew to a close in 2015 was to 'build back better'. During the crisis, there had been lots of remorse expressed by the government and the international community about how the severity of the outbreak was due to the weakness of the pre-existing health system. Promises had duly been made to learn the lessons from these mistakes and invest more into strengthening the overall health system in the future.

I grew frustrated with the UK-funded recovery process as I found myself summoned, along with technical leads from the Ministry and other NGOs, to tedious planning meetings in gloomy Radisson hotel conference rooms. Over endless rounds of coffee and biscuits, management consultants harvested our off-the-cuff suggestions and rehashed old policies, converting them into flashy PowerPoint slides without much in the way of strategic thinking or analysis, and with very little buy-in from the wider health sector. If I found this process patronising and superficial,

I can only imagine what my colleagues around the table from the Sierra Leone government must have felt.

While some of the promises from donors were ultimately kept – there was a significant increase in donor funding for health and an increase in technical support to the Ministry – many were forgotten as the spotlight moved on from Sierra Leone towards the next global crisis.

Before the outbreak, King's had been a small outfit with a handful of volunteers on the ground. When the music stopped and the outbreak wound down, things largely returned to the way they had been before. Although we were a bit bigger and had a higher profile, we still struggled to get donor funding for our long-term plans to strengthen the health system, which ironically included continuing our work on infection prevention and maintaining the new infectious disease unit, where we wanted to train staff for future outbreaks.

Arrivals and departures

By early 2015, I was totally exhausted and a bit broken. The loss of so many patients and colleagues haunted me and left me with a feeling of profound sadness, but it was somehow easier to come to terms with than the memories of the obstruction and corruption I'd witnessed when trying to set up the command centre and open new units. All the politics and frustration had left me pretty cynical, a far cry from the hopeful optimist I had been when I arrived. I decided it was time to hand over the reins of the King's Sierra Leone Partnership to new leadership.

In August 2015, as I prepared to depart, I got to see a new generation of King's volunteers arrive to take up their posts. A psychiatrist to support the opening of the country's first outpatient mental health clinic. An emergency medicine team to help convert the run-down rooms of our former Ebola isolation unit into a revamped resuscitation room for critically ill emergency patients. And, the day after I left, Marta admitted the first patient to the new Centre of Excellence for Infectious Diseases. The shortage of donor funding was a challenge, but I knew we would continue to have a meaningful impact on the ground thanks to our strong relationships with national partners and our committed team of volunteers.

On my final day, a few of us gathered in the hospital manager's office to say our goodbyes. Sister Cecelia Kamara, the lead nurse at the Connaught isolation unit who had stood shoulder-to-shoulder with us through the darkest days of the response, invoked the memory of the brilliant young nurse Hajara Serry. The reminder was overwhelming, as if it had triggered a dam to burst inside of me, and when it was my turn to talk, I started to cry uncontrollably and couldn't get a word out. My newly arrived colleagues looked at my breakdown with evident confusion and concern but stayed quiet. Like soldiers returning from the front, those who had not experienced it could never fully comprehend what we had been through.

Many of the original King's crew, such as Marta, Andy and Dan, had elected to stay behind and work on the recovery, and on my last night I met them for a final drink on the beach. The mood was subdued, we all had so much to say but none of us were ready for that yet. I knew, though, that I'd be seeing them, and Connaught, again one day.

As I boarded the speedboat for the airport, whilst feeling proud of what we had accomplished, my thoughts were occupied with regrets, with the things I wished I'd done differently. How I should have gotten in the car and travelled to Kenema with Marta and the team in June when I had heard how bad things were there. How I ought to have realised sooner that even a small team can make a real difference. And how I shouldn't have taken no for an answer when DFID turned down our $12,500 funding request, but should have kicked down the doors of the donors and of contacts back at King's to get the money we needed. It wasn't all regrets, however, and I stood by my decisions to take risks, hold my nerve when times were tough and constantly push the team to do more.

I returned to London to a hero's welcome, but felt hollow inside, haunted by the lives we could have saved but didn't. More than that, though, I missed the team, the band of brothers that we had become, and the sense of purpose we had shared in extraordinary circumstances.

SINEAD

Day 42
The end of the outbreak in Liberia was declared on 3 September 2015. After the last case was discharged from an ETU in late September, Sierra Leone's '42-day Ebola-free' milestone was due to be reached on 7 November, after seventeen-and-a-half long months. The days leading up to this date were tense. The NERC boss, Palo, told me that he dreaded hearing his phone ring, lest it be that dreaded 'suspected case', and he found himself snapping "WHAT?" at everyone who called.

A group of us convened at the NERC to mark midnight on the 7 November with champagne, and I have never seen President Koroma look as happy as he did that night. Peter gave the toast on behalf of the international community which I felt was very fitting given that he had played a key role since the beginning of the crisis and given that, quite simply, we would not have been where we were without the UK. No matter what criticisms I and others had of some of the ways the UK operated during the response, there was absolutely no doubt in my mind that they had turned the response around and invested enormous resources which had been central to getting to zero. They fully deserved to raise the first glass that night.

It was a fun, relaxed occasion after a long hard fight. The best moment was when the NERC military officer who usually read out the daily status reports projected his usual PowerPoint presentation, deadpan and with dramatic pauses. In exactly the same tone and with the same words we had listened to so many times before in that room he announced: "Good evening colleagues. Today . . . the number of confirmed Ebola cases in the Republic of Sierra Leone is . . . zero. The number of suspected cases is . . . zero." We all laughed and cheered.

There was a good bit of silliness then as the champagne kicked in and mixed with the euphoria and exhaustion in the room. I got some great pictures of Palo standing next to a life-sized cardboard cut-out of himself. Another big cheer when the WHO and CDC bosses hugged, as the two organisations had a famous rivalry, albeit good natured at the time. Ordinarily, I might have sent a tweet, but I was torn because I also felt it was inappropriate to publicly 'celebrate' the end of an outbreak that had destroyed so many lives. However, as I mused over such sensitivities, I started getting text messages from the Embassy staff from their homes saying, "We can see you." Apparently, the whole event was being shown live on national TV!

The ceremony the next day had much more of the standard formality of such events, taking place in the cavernous conference centre of a Chinese-built hotel adorned in yellow silk garlands. Yellow had been declared the colour of 'a resilient zero', so we had all scrambled around in our wardrobes and in the local market the day before to find something yellow and suitably official at the same time – a tricky task. I ended up recycling a traditional Sierra Leonean outfit that I had had made for St Patrick's day the year before. In truth, it was more green than yellow, which Peter helpfully highlighted to people at every opportunity that day, but I felt I got away with it.

In a charged atmosphere of joy and grief, Anders Nordström, the new WHO representative, made the official declaration that it was over. A total of 3,955 Sierra Leoneans, including 221 health care workers, had lost their lives to the virus.[30] Survivors appropriately took centre-stage in the event with one ten-year-old survivor in a snazzy suit stealing the show with a rap song. The speech I remember most clearly was Bintou's. While she spoke on behalf of the UN and the international community, the fact that she is from Guinea gave her a special insight into how Sierra Leoneans were feeling that day. In her speech she talked about the suffering that people had gone through during Ebola that just couldn't be expressed in words. She then let out a long, mournful and beautiful wail. You could have heard a pin drop in the enormous conference hall. It said more than any speech could have.

I had imagined that day so many times. When my human resources department had called me at the peak of the crisis in 2014 to confirm whether I would be leaving in the summer of 2015 as planned, I hadn't been able to think about their question in any kind of systematic way. Rather than weighing up pros and cons of leaving or extending as you should do in those situations, all I could think was that Ebola might not be over by the summer of 2015. So, I just went with my gut reaction, "No. I'll stay."

Now Ebola was over, and it felt surreal as I went back and forth between different parties that day. Like a lot of people I spoke to, I couldn't quite get my head around it. At the various parties everybody congratulated each other, but I felt a bit false as I was thanking people. Much had been achieved, yes, but so much had been lost for so many.

I didn't share this with anybody, it would have sounded a bit nuts, but around that time, I spent a lot of time wishing that I could turn back the clock to the start of the outbreak. I knew exactly what I would do. In June, I would go to Kailahun. I wouldn't get so caught up this time about whose mandate it was or whether I was wasting people's time by poking my nose in. I would run into Yoti Zabulon at the Taskforce and he would say, "I need $286,000," and I would say, "No problem." In another scenario, I would rock up to the the DHMT office in Freetown when things were at their worst and volunteer there . . . or I would base myself in Kenema in July. Or in Port Loko in September . . .

The reality, of course, is that you can't have everything. Painful as it was not to have been able to do more and do it more directly, I had to take comfort in the fact that, had I quit my job to go and volunteer somewhere, I wouldn't have been able to lobby the powers-that-be about issues that I cared about in the response, that might otherwise have been neglected. I woudn't have been able to raise the voices of frontline workers at the international level or cajole people to coordinate better. I knew this role made sense for me given how well I knew the country and given the relationships that I had built up over the years. And most of all, I knew that I was exceptionally lucky to work with our team at the Embassy. We were able to fund needs in the response as they emerged and also influence how some larger donors spent their money. I was proud that we had the flexibility to do that. It didn't stop me feeling guilty sometimes, but, as Sierra Leoneans would say: '*A don try-o*', I had tried.

The last round

The NERC's mandate ended on 31 December 2015, when they handed over responsibility for any further Ebola flare-ups or outbreaks to the Ministry and the Office of National Security. Many people thought that a transition of Ebola responsibility back to the Ministry should have taken place much earlier, while others lacked confidence that the Ministry would be able to do the job. We would soon find out.

Ten weeks after the end of the Ebola outbreak, on 14 January 2016, I was chatting with Peter and the US Ambassador at a reception, when all three of our phones rang in quick succession. It was almost comical, except for the fact we knew it was unlikely to be good news. Sure enough, there was a new Ebola case in the northern district of Tonkolili.

A 22-year-old female student, Marie Jalloh, had died. A swab had been taken and tested positive. Ebola was back.

The case was hardly a surprise, given there were many survivors who could potentially transmit Ebola through unprotected sex for months after they were cured. It had already happened in Liberia. Even so, it was a shock and it felt like we could be back to square one. There were 150 contacts of the late Marie Jalloh spread over four districts.[31]

On the positive side, this new case showed how much progress had been made since Ebola was first detected over a year and a half previously. Voluntary quarantine was used for high-risk contacts, who were also given the new vaccination. The biggest positive was that the Ministry surprised many people, myself included, by dealing pretty well with the situation. In my recent conversations with Ministry officials, there still seemed to be a lot of bitterness about the NERC taking over the health crisis, which didn't inspire confidence in me that the Ministry had changed much since the early days of infighting. But I was happy to be proven wrong.

There was strong coordination in the response to the new outbreak. Though there were some gaps, the experienced responders were still around, making it possible to get over these issues without too many consequences.

One more person, Marie Jalloh's aunt, developed Ebola; and she was taken to 34 Military Hospital in Freetown for treatment, which was successful. This was the end of the transmission, but unfortunately not the end of the story. The big negative of this last round of Ebola in Sierra Leone was an extraordinary example of Ebola denialism at almost the highest level of government.

Ever since Marie Jalloh's case had been announced, there had been doubts in Tonkolili.[32] Many people in the population found this new outbreak very confusing after all the announcements of November, and, as a result, denial of Ebola reared its head once more. Bafflingly, the Vice-President of Sierra Leone and the Minister for Education then made speeches to a large crowd in Tonkolili denying that Marie Jalloh's aunt had had Ebola. The news reached us in Freetown within minutes via WhatsApp. I then got a text from one of the NGOs to say that their staff and UN colleagues working in Tonkolili felt worried for their safety, concerned that an angry population might accuse them of fabricating Ebola for personal profit now that 'the government' had said it wasn't true.

I was livid. The problems ran beyond the risks to the staff working on Ebola in Tonkolili, this denialism also had implications for the future: what if Ebola were to recur in Sierra Leone? Would rural populations be sceptical, given such high-level individuals had denied the existence of this disease in a woman who had tested positive? After all of our struggles over so many months to convince people that Ebola was real? The President later made references in his speeches to government officials keeping their "personal views to themselves", but the moment had passed and a shadow of ambiguity remained. The incident was a stark reminder to me that governance and community engagement were still huge challenges after all this time.

Departure

There was no fanfare on 17 March when Sierra Leone marked the end of its part in the 2013–2016 Ebola outbreak for the second and last time. Because it happened to be St. Patrick's Day, we were holding our annual reception at the Embassy, so we observed a moment's silence for the 3,956 Sierra Leoneans who had died.

I remained in Sierra Leone for another five months. Guinea declared the end of their outbreak, and therefore the entire epidemic, on 1 June. In August 2016, after five years of the best of times and the worst of times, I left Sierra Leone.

For months before my departure, my friends at Balmaya restaurant contended there was no way I would actually leave, despite visible proof such as flight tickets and a reccie visit by my successor. "*Dis na Salone uman now*," Aunty Joy would pronounce to her posse, cigarette in hand. *She is a Sierra Leonean woman now.*

She had a point. I couldn't quite believe I was leaving this country that meant so much to me, and to which I had given so much of myself.

My last few weeks were a whirlwind of farewell parties and giving stuff away. The latter was quite a task as most expatriates stay in Sierra Leone for much shorter periods than me, so my spare room had become a dumping ground for possessions my friends didn't have space for at the last minute. Fortunately, Sierra Leone is an exceptionally easy place to give things away and for my last few weeks, I had a parade of friends and acquaintances coming to my apartment and staggering home with plastic bags stuffed with books, bedsheets and body lotion.

Surprisingly, I made it through my farewell parties without crying. I think this was because I knew that Freetown was merely moving from being my first home to being my second home.

I lasted a whole six weeks before going back for my first visit.

TEN | Conclusion

The epidemic changed everything – and nothing.[1]

(MSF)

Ebola changed both of us, as it did so many others. At least 11,310 people tragically lost their lives to the disease. Many of West Africa's over 10,000 Ebola survivors are still suffering from its physical after-effects, not to mention the trauma and the stigmatisation.[2] A much larger group of people in the three impacted countries have suffered the loss of family and friends or from the numerous secondary impacts.

At least 815 health care workers contracted Ebola. This included 328 health care workers in Sierra Leone, at least 221 of whom died.[3,4] Doctors like Sheik Humarr Khan, Modupeh Cole and Martin Salia. Nurses like M'balu Fonnie, Alex Moigboi, and Nancy Yoko in Kenema and Hajara Serry at Connaught. And so many other support staff, such as cleaners like Abdulai Sesay. They stayed at their posts despite the risks.

Many of their deaths could have been avoided, and these patients and health workers were ultimately let down by the system, let down by all of us. We owe it to them to have a frank and honest debate about the mistakes we made, and to ensure the lessons from this epidemic are learnt for the future.

Meaningful reform is vital. As Tom Frieden of the CDC said, this Ebola epidemic served as a test of the world's capacity to deal with biological threats: "We, the world, failed that test."[5] What's more, there are many infectious diseases that are more contagious than Ebola, particularly airborne diseases like variants of the flu.

We can't avoid outbreaks, but there are ways to ensure the next one does not needlessly destroy so many lives. As epidemiologist Larry Brilliant, who helped WHO eradicate smallpox in the 1970s, has said: "Outbreaks are inevitable. Pandemics are optional."[6] But have we really been honest about what happened, and has Ebola changed the key national and global institutions that would prevent a disaster of this magnitude from happening again?

Looking back and moving forward

There has been an enormous amount of reflection about the 2013–16 Ebola epidemic. One 2017 review found more than forty published studies that agree on what actions need to be prioritised in the aftermath.[7] The reflection, though, has been very unbalanced. Most of it has focused on WHO and the international health emergency system, and there has been very little about national government responses, the work of foreign governments, or the range of different approaches taken by international NGOs. This is a gap that we hope we have helped address with this book.

We commend organisations like MSF who have not only done extensive and critical reviews of their Ebola work, but also made them public. They are in the minority. Without critical self-reflection, it is difficult to see how organisations will learn for the future.

Unfortunately, even when lessons from Ebola outbreaks have been documented, they have rarely been translated into action. A review of the literature on the West African Ebola crisis in 2017 concluded that: "It is perhaps surprising to note that many of the recommendations suggested by these four panels and other experts mirror the main conclusions . . . after the Kikwit outbreak over 20 years ago."[8]

So is it any different this time?

At the international level, there have been some positive steps. The UN Secretary-General announced new arrangements for WHO to inform the wider UN of less serious outbreaks early on, so they can get more actively involved before outbreaks escalate too far.[9] Complementing this, the group that brings together all the main humanitarian organisations globally (known as the Inter-Agency Standing Committee) have now specified what exactly should happen the next time there is an infectious disease crisis such as Ebola.[10] This includes the immediate deployment of qualified people and supplies and the automatic release of funding from the Central Emergencies Relief Fund. It is a far cry from what we experienced and is very welcome.

Meanwhile, the World Bank has launched a Pandemic Emergencies Fund that can quickly provide resources to developing countries facing outbreaks, to enable a more rapid response.[11] One of the projected advantages of this fund is that it creates an incentive for countries to report infectious disease outbreaks early, since going public often has damaging economic effects, as we saw in West Africa.

There has also been progress in instituting an external evaluation of individual nations' health systems and preparedness for crises, although this review is still voluntary rather than required.[12] In addition, there is a new alliance to finance and coordinate the development of new vaccines for infectious disease epidemics.[13] And the Global Health Security Agenda, initiated by the US government shortly before Ebola began, now has fifty countries on board. It aims to build country-level capacity to prevent infectious diseases. At the regional level, a new institution, the African

Centres for Disease Control and Prevention, has been created with the objective of helping African countries to "close dangerous gaps" in their public health systems.[14]

These are some of a number of modest reforms and new initiatives demonstrating that at least some lessons have been learnt, although it is too early to judge whether these international programmes will actually translate to improved capacity on the ground, or for how long they will be sustained. Too often, we have seen a lot of great planning at a global level but no clarity on how the initiatives will actually be implemented and resourced at the country level, how they will interface with existing programmes on the ground and how they will ensure adequate national and local capacities.

A long way to go

The most crucial question remains: have we fundamentally addressed the root causes of the crisis, including weaknesses in the accountability, transparency, and capacity of WHO and at the national level?

WHO has undertaken some reorganisation, including introducing a new Health Emergency Programme, governed by an independent committee with access to its own funding stream, and a roster of seventy-five emergency medical teams on stand-by for health emergencies. The WHO Sierra Leone office has also been strengthened.[15]

But despite the enormous furore over their failures on Ebola, WHO has not initiated any other significant institutional reforms.[16] In addition, member governments refused to increase their mandatory contributions to WHO when requested to in 2015, meaning that the organisation is still deeply constrained by a constant need to raise voluntary funds. Calls for a redefinition of WHO's mandate, a transparency policy or an organisation-wide accountability system remain, to date, unanswered. The WHO African Regional Office remains overburdened with outbreaks and emergencies.

In 2017, WHO was once again accused of failing to stand up to governments that were trying to downplay an infectious disease epidemic. The initial claim from the governments of Ethiopia and Sudan that the cause of their outbreaks of "acute watery diarrhoea" was not cholera often went unchallenged by WHO, even though samples taken abroad for testing tested positive for the disease.

In Sierra Leone, the Ministry and its international partners have made significant investments in strengthening disease surveillance, establishing a national public health institute and a national office for infection control. They have also passed significant legislation to reform medical training and hospital governance. In addition, there is much greater emphasis on formulating strong national health plans and ensuring donors and NGOs are aligned with these and held accountable by the Ministry.

However, the government still lacks the resources to provide quality basic health services across the country, and critically, a lack of accountability and inadequate salaries for staff continue to hamper efforts to achieve meaningful reform. Whilst there has been a modest increase in international donors investing in specific programmes, there has been no radical shift towards financing the strengthening of key government health institutions. As one person involved in these programmes put it, "It's really disappointing, there was such an opportunity to strengthen the health system, but it just fizzled."

So, while some lessons have been learnt and acted upon, far too many seem to have been missed, ignored or forgotten. This situation will only change with stronger leadership and a shift in attitude and political will in the government of Sierra Leone, in

WHO, and in donors and other key institutions. Until we see that shift, the root causes of the Ebola crisis will remain unaddressed. In the Afterword we go into more depth about these root causes and what we and others should do differently the next time.

Finally

Whatever institutional reforms do or don't take place, they will not be enough to avoid the kind of catastrophic loss of life and unnecessary suffering we saw in the 2013–16 Ebola epidemic unless the right kind of individuals are involved.

Readers of this book may one day find themselves in situations where they can influence the response to a crisis or influence a development programme. We hope this book has given some insight into what to avoid and what to promote.

Fundamentally, our response to crises like this one comes down to how much we care. Do we truly hold every human life to be of equal value?

Afterword: If we had to do it all again . . .

After Sinead left Sierra Leone she took a year off work to work full time on this book at Harvard. Meanwhile, Oliver took a job with an NGO in Johannesburg. We reconvened in June in a hot and humid Boston, in an office a floor above that of Dr Paul Farmer. Whiteboard markers in hand, cups of coffee at the ready, we started brainstorming what we each thought the most important lessons from the response were and what we would love to have known if we were to do it all again.

In the beginning it felt like we were pretty far apart, but as we challenged each other and drilled a bit deeper, we started to find the same key things coming up again and again. These came from our experiences as well as from our interviews and readings. By the end, there were five key things that stood out to us.

We hope each of these will resonate and be useful to anyone who someday finds themselves in an outbreak, or really any type of emergency. Some of you might think it's not likely you'll end up in a situation like this, but bear in mind, we would have said the same ourselves . . .

Community engagement
The number one lesson we need to take from the Ebola crisis is the importance of good community engagement from the very beginning of a response.

Only the communities of Sierra Leone were ever going to be able to bring the Ebola epidemic under control. Only they could avoid unsafe practices. It was irrelevant how many ETUs we built if people didn't come to them, or how strong the safe burial system was if people didn't report deaths. Without communities pulling in the same direction as the response, it would never be successful.

But far too often and for far too long, we failed to sufficiently respect or empathise with communities, instead relying on punitive approaches. In our views, and in the views of most people we interviewed, this was the biggest failure of the response.

Why did we fail? One basic reason is that we simply didn't prioritise this area enough. As one NGO colleague said: "Generally, social mobilisation would be twenty-ninth on the agenda at meetings." For most of the response in 2014, we talked about how important community engagement was, but our attention and resources were mostly on other things. As one WHO representative said: "I think we were so caught up in the magnitude of the outbreak that we were focusing on the technical elements, like beds, surveillance or coordination mechanisms, and only turned our attention to the 'population problem' later."

But beyond how much priority we gave the area of community engagement, there was also the issue of *how* we did it and how we could do better next time. Let's start with what *not* to do.

Punitive approaches backfired

Of the three countries most affected by Ebola, Sierra Leone had the strongest and most systematic use of quarantine, as well as other mechanisms such as by-laws, where people could face imprisonment for not cooperating with the response.

Out of these approaches, household quarantine was the most widespread and contentious. Whilst it was strongly criticised by many people, some, particularly senior members of the Sierra Leone and UK governments, felt that quarantine was appropriate and a few people we interviewed felt it could have been used even more.

Fundamentally, household quarantine, and the punitive culture in general, stemmed from the attitude that Sierra Leonean citizens could not be trusted to collaborate with the response. One senior Sierra Leonean government official noted:

> I was a fan of quarantine because people in Sierra Leone lie. If you do this in the UK or somewhere, you can ask people: "Did you visit that house?" And they would tell the truth. But in Sierra Leone they will say no but have visited it five times. We couldn't risk this with the high-risk cases.

A senior UK official said similarly: "Communities were lying, absconding, this was a big factor, you can't trust contact tracing, you had to be sensible and know you didn't know. That's why we expanded quarantine to 'not sure' contacts."

These proponents of quarantine raised some valid points. While everybody agreed that it was necessary to restrict people's movement in some way during the epidemic, and that contact tracing for much of the response was weak, we and most people we interviewed are critical of quarantine and feel that it made things worse.

For one thing, it was enormously expensive and took up a lot of time that could have been spent on other aspects of the response. One UK staff member at the DERC level said: "you had to deal with health, food, water and sanitation. You were doomed to failure."

Still, despite all the effort and resources invested in it, quarantine often didn't work, in part because the security forces guarding quarantined homes could sometimes be bribed. One senior

Sierra Leone government official said: "How vigilant were the police? Some enriched themselves, like checkpoints, they took bribes."

But the main problem was that quarantine created the incentive to hide or flee, rather than to cooperate with the response. Apart from the basic human instinct not to be locked up, people avoided or escaped from quarantine for very practical reasons: they needed food, water or other necessities that weren't being adequately provided, and they were often worried about losing their livelihoods.

People went to enormous lengths to avoid being quarantined, which had negative impacts on the response as a whole. As one report says: "The fear of being quarantined at times resulted in some villagers scurrying into nearby bushes at the sound of sirens of ambulances or the sight of contact tracers. This has militated against contact tracing exercises." A DERC staff member recalled: "People would dump bodies to avoid quarantine. The team would ask, 'Where is the body from?' And nobody would answer."

Liberia largely stopped quarantine after the disaster of West Point, and community engagement is widely viewed as a major success of the response there. Dr Tom Frieden, Director of the CDC during Ebola, commented: "The quarantine policy most likely prolonged the outbreak in Sierra Leone by at least six months."

While quarantine was never lifted, the NERC stepped up in 2015 and, with the support of NGOs, made tangible improvements to quarantine that recognised the very real hardship being faced by communities, and tried to ease the burden. Examples include healthcare being provided to quarantined households and provisions for other community members to tend their farms.

In future, we think punitive approaches like forced quarantine should be avoided. Instead, we should focus on good contact tracing, using voluntary quarantine for high-risk contacts if necessary.

Respect and compromise were critical for engaging with communities

Key to any process of community engagement is respect. This meant being willing to sit down, listen, and then have a conversation with communities to find compromises between our preferred biomedical strategies and what they felt they could actually do. It took us a long time to get to that. Much of the community engagement in the early months was one-way, telling people what to do rather than understanding the kinds of challenges they faced and what ideas they had for how to protect themselves. After all, it was their health, their lives; communities in Sierra Leone had a far greater stake in this response than responders did.

As time went on though, we got better at listening. For instance, DERCs in the north heard that fear of ambulances was a key reason people didn't want to go to ETUs and began an 'ambulance exhibition' to reduce this fear. As part of this, community leaders got inside ambulances to show people that they were safe.

We also got better at compromising. The original biomedical burials evolved to include religious leaders and family attendance, albeit from a safe distance. There were successful negotiations with one community over how to conduct the safe burial of a pregnant woman, even though the final compromise arrangement still went against the spiritual norm for her Kissy ethnic group.[1] This notion that traditions are often flexible, and that compromise is possible, is the central theme of a book on the Ebola response by long-time anthropologist on Sierra Leone, Paul Richards. In it, he makes the case that there was eventually a convergence, whereby villagers began to think and act like epidemiologists, and epidemiologists like villagers.[2]

Respect also meant supporting communities' own initiatives. Even before the major NERC/UK response kicked in from October 2014, many communities in Sierra Leone had begun to take matters into their own hands. We saw it in Kailahun where mosques and churches became hubs for Ebola awareness-raising. We saw it in Koinadugu, the district which went five months without a case, helped by vigorous community mobilisation. We saw it in the rural parts of the Freetown peninsula where ultimately fifty-six taskforces took responsibility for keeping Ebola out of their communities.

In late 2014 a group of NGOs came together to form the Social Mobilisation Action Consortium, and, with help from a group of anthropologists, worked nationwide to help communities create their own action plans to prevent or overcome Ebola. This kind of approach was very welcome, but we should have started it from day one.

In future we should treat community engagement in a response as everyone's responsibility, while also engaging skilled professionals, such as anthropologists, to provide support, and giving them a seat at decision-making tables. But we must never forget that community members are the principal experts on their own lives.[3]

Empathy was put aside when it came to making decisions

Enormous demands were made of the people of Sierra Leone during the crisis. For those not directly affected this ranged from school closures to the burials policy to the constant fear that they might be next.

For people that were infected, it was of course far worse: long journeys to seek treatment, isolated from their families, seeing at least half of the people around them die. An MSF nurse gave one example of the mental health impact on patients:

> Someone had to hold babies in the red-zone of the ETU because the staff only came so often, so usually babies were given to teenage girls to take care of. Most of the babies died. One teenage girl, she lost her hair, a long time later she still didn't have her period. She was grieving and traumatised.

Families of patients frequently didn't know what had happened to their loved ones – had they died? And if so, where were they buried?[4] Apart from the grief of losing family members and friends, many people, including children, were thrust into economic insecurity when breadwinners died and some were exploited, including sexually exploited. There was often enormous stigma towards those affected by Ebola. The whole situation was devastating.

Some of this hardship was simply a consequence of how overwhelmed the response was for so many months, but some of it could, and should, have been avoided. All too often, we in the response, Sierra Leoneans and internationals alike, didn't put ourselves in the shoes of the people who were being affected. We failed to exercise empathy and compassion. Sometimes we even blamed communities for their 'exotic traditional practices' or their 'resistance'.

What lay behind this was, in part, that we often thought we had to choose between stopping Ebola transmission and improving care, and between public health and the rights of individuals. But these were false dichotomies. And by buying into them, consciously or sub-consciously, we failed the people of Sierra Leone.

One example was our lack of provision for non-Ebola health care for most of the response, either for people who were suspected of Ebola or the population more broadly. As a senior UK official said: "the goal had to be R_0 and that meant not maternal death or malaria or whatever . . . there was no space for anything else." While the laser-sharp focus of the UK was often helpful, in this case it was counterproductive. Our collective failure in the response to systematically provide health care for patients if they tested negative for Ebola became a factor preventing people from going to get tested in the first place and damaged an already shaky trust in the response. According to one MSF review: "When [communities] cannot find care for a child with diarrheal disease, they question the sincerity of response teams that seem eager to help them with Ebola."

Another example was the sub-standard care provided to Ebola patients for much of the response. This was not always a matter of resources, sometimes we just didn't think. For instance, training health workers in 'no-touch care' prioritised staff safety without adequately reflecting on how this would make patients feel.

But our mindset was focused on preventing transmission. Although there were a few notable exceptions, such as Dr Paul Farmer, not many voices were lobbying to improve care or increase survival in the first six months of the epidemic.

It stood to reason, though, that if ETUs are seen as places where people go to die, why would you go there if you had symptoms? Why would you be willing to send your relatives there? Too often and for too long, we overlooked this while making our policy decisions, failing to see that improving care would help our goal of reducing transmission, rather than being a distraction.

All of this comes back to human rights. It's to be expected that an infectious disease outbreak may require some curtailment of individual rights. Wider public health has to be prioritised. But this doesn't justify neglecting the rights of individuals as much as we did. As one senior UN staffer said: "The world forgot that this virus is in people."

We frequently lacked the indignation that we should have felt about the horrendous conditions that so many people were experiencing. Consciously or not, many of us had modified our standards to 'fit' the setting of a poor country where it was 'to be expected' that people died unnecessarily all the time. We wouldn't admit it, perhaps not even to ourselves, but we didn't always prioritise every single Sierra Leonean life the way we would have if this outbreak had been affecting Irish people or British people or Americans. We saw this when internationals were infected with Ebola; when this happened, we pulled out all the stops and went to great lengths to ensure their survival, and rightly so. But we did not apply this concern evenly.

This is not to suggest that people weren't working tirelessly to stop Ebola; they certainly were. Many people were risking their lives day-in, day-out. But in the response as a whole, we were collectively guilty of dehumanising people as we focused on the 'greater good'.

We did see significant improvements in 2015, when the response became more compassionate. And of course, there were more resources than in the early months. An example was ETUs systematically providing discharge packs to survivors to assist them in rebuilding their lives and changing their infrastructure to enable family visits.

Next time, alongside preventing transmission in an outbreak response, care and dignity must be prioritised because they are important in their own right, but also because this focus is a necessary part of reducing transmission. More broadly, we hope empathy will be a guiding principle for the next response from the very beginning and built into decision-making processes. This is not something that can be outsourced. We should ask ourselves, at every turn, how would I feel, or what would I do, if I were in that situation? What if this was my child?

Leadership and coordination

The second issue that we spoke a lot about was leadership and coordination. We found leadership was central to why the response initially failed, as well as to why we eventually succeeded. Of course, leadership will be important in any crisis, but because Ebola was new to Sierra Leone and the situation escalated so quickly and dangerously, it was even more important. We saw many examples of strong leadership, from the community health officer in Newton to the President of the United States, from the NERC to the UK government.

Are we talking about leadership from individuals or organisations? Both. But we think these are two sides of the same coin. For individual leaders to make a difference, they needed to have access to the resources of an organisation, such as an NGO or a district council. Similarly, organisations could only exercise leadership if the people on their team did too – often, the organisations that really stepped up were driven to do so by one or two of their staff, who argued passionately for that from inside. But the organisation had to be willing to listen and respond to those messages, and not all were. It was also key that leaders were given space to exercise leadership, rather than being micro-managed from afar.

We found a set of reasons why strong leadership did (or didn't) emerge. What also became clear is that effective leadership had to be linked with good coordination with others, and so often we didn't get that right.

Weak governance exacerbated poor leadership

Responsibility for managing the crisis rested with the government of Sierra Leone and WHO. Both failed to step up in those critical early months when the outbreak could have been contained.

There are a number of reasons for this failure, including a lack of resources and capacity, but we think that a central issue is that these organisations, in different ways, have long-standing governance problems.

For Sierra Leone, the heart of the problem was an institutional culture across government in which officials and politicians were not held to account, and often acted for personal and political reasons rather than the national interest. While the President eventually got heavily involved in the response, the dysfunction in the Ministry was allowed to continue for far too long. Even after the President took direct responsibility and the NERC was established, there were frequently serious instances where government officials and politicians continued to impede the response, such as in Freetown, and seemingly were not brought to book. This was not merely an issue with the Ministry of Health. As one Sierra Leonean NGO interviewee said: "The key issue is accountability all the way down in the civil service. There is no control of staff, no discipline."

Lack of accountability is not a new issue in Sierra Leone. In Connaught Hospital pre-Ebola the catchphrase was "Let them fall by their own weight", even when a porter dangerously posed as a surgeon for many years. The roots of this go back at least to colonial times when officials set up parallel political authorities to the central government with expedient side deals. Such arrangements persist today, and between chiefs, secret society leaders, businessmen and others, parallel political authorities are alive and well in the country's governance system.

In this context, leadership in Sierra Leone is often centred, first and foremost, around not upsetting the finely balanced apple cart of one's position. Whether a person is the president, a minister, a district council chairman or a junior official, their patronage networks must be carefully managed. As a result, keeping their leadership position often depends in significant part on *not* directly holding people to account.[5]

In some ways we see this dynamic in every country. A central part of politics is negotiation and compromise with different interest groups. In Sierra Leone, however, the sheer extent of the lack of accountability had deeply detrimental impacts on the population at large, as we saw.

There is no quick fix for this, since there doesn't seem to be any incentive for those in power to reform at the moment. What is clear is that the answer is not Sierra Leone conforming to a pre-cooked model of 'good governance' from other countries. What will actually work is much harder to say, but better education for the population and more local investment to create jobs would help to increase opportunities for more people to demand greater accountability from authorities at different levels.[6]

The same issue of poor leadership manifested itself in WHO in the early months of the Ebola crisis at country, regional and global levels. At all these levels, WHO initially prioritised politics over raising the alarm bell and, like the Government, gave us the message that things were under control when they weren't. They not only failed to act themselves, they also failed to coordinate or share relevant information with others. As one of the glaring examples, WHO Kenema staff were "screaming" for months about the horrific situation and their need for support, but WHO leadership failed to take adequate action.

A key issue here was the clash between WHO's governance structure (which led it to prioritise its relationship with host governments, who are members of its governing body) and its public health mandate. This close relationship with governments also influenced who was appointed to the WHO regional and (indirectly) country offices and this staffing was a central part of the problem in the early months. Finally, the organisation lacked transparency, a key enabler of good governance. For WHO to perform better in the next health crisis, how it is governed and funded by member states needs to better line up with and serve its global health mandate. Within this, holding staff accountable is critical.

While the UK government was ultimately vital to the response, it was slow to recognise the seriousness of the outbreak at the beginning or to play a significant role at the national level until the situation had already spiralled out of control, which compounded the lack of strong leadership from WHO and the government of Sierra Leone.[7]

Strong leadership came with resolve, integrity and a willingness to take risks

On the positive side, there were some great examples of strong leadership from organisations, as well as individuals within them, which were critical in eventually turning the crisis around.

Resolve was central here; some individual leaders made difficult decisions and showed great commitment in implementing them with urgency. Even when the national and international response was still weak in mid-2014, local leaders and government officials stepped up in some parts of the country. One government official in Kenema talked about how they managed to defeat the epidemic in their district, with some support from international partners, before the significant resources kicked in: "We did it with our bare hands. I believe that Kenema was sorted before the NERC/DERC came along. What made us different is that the Kenema politicians were resolved – they said let's do it for ourselves, there was zeal available . . . they were very committed."

Another excellent example of resolve was the UK government. The UK were unquestionably the game-changer in terms of leadership in the Sierra Leone response as a whole. They were focused, disciplined and well-resourced. One NGO said, "They got stuck in, they understood, they took strategic leadership." A donor official said, "The UK military came in and with ruthless efficiency really moved things. They sat down and gave people a bunch of cash and got things done."

The willingness to take risks was also a key aspect of leadership in this crisis. This was because the risk of some types of work, such as clinical work, was high and also because the perception of risk of all kinds of work on Ebola was heightened by fear and compounded by hysterical media coverage. When panic took hold in August 2014, and many international organisations were under pressure to evacuate their staff, it was important for organisations to keep a cool head.

Too many humanitarian organisations obsessed about the risks of taking action, without showing enough concern about the risks of inaction. This was particularly the case with ETUs, when many organisations, including the UK military, were hesitant to run them due to concern about the risks. As a result, the outbreak spiralled further out of control.

There were many notable exceptions to this however, of organisations holding their nerve despite the risks, going beyond their comfort zone, and doing whatever it took to get the response off the ground. They played an essential role in defeating Ebola. Concern Worldwide took on the challenge of running two cemeteries in Freetown and managing burial teams, despite having no experience of doing anything like this before. As their country director Fiona McLysaght said when interviewed, this was one of the many activities Concern ended up doing that had initially seemed out of the question: "We would say, 'we would never do that.' But then we would change. We did it because we are a humanitarian organisation. It was incumbent on us."

Integrity was also key: good leaders were honest and led by example. This quality stood out in the first national institution to really step up in the crisis: the Sierra Leone armed forces. Notably, the military medical corps had a strong leader in

Dr Foday Sahr who was seen as honourable. One military doctor said: "[The army] did well due to leadership . . . Foday Sahr, he was leading from the front. Looking after Ebola patients himself. When he asked us, we saw a logic to do it."

Similarly, when the NERC was established, part of its success was that people within were seen as having integrity and working hard for the country. NERC's Yvonne Aki-Sawyerr, for example, showed enormous dedication and worked tirelessly to bring the outbreak to a close. One NERC senior manager said: "NERC brought leadership, people like Yvonne who understand work ethic."

Organisations, including donor organisations, should prioritise these characteristics in their recruitment and training of future leaders, and they should have systems for assessing risk that include the risk of inaction.

Coordination needed trust, the right skills and prioritisation

Coordination was vital in the response as we needed so many different organisations to work together and so many activities like surveillance, treatment and burials to work in a joined-up way rather than in siloes.

In the early days of the crisis, coordination was a disaster. The dysfunction and lack of capacity of the Ministry prevented it from coordinating effectively. Plans would be made in coordination meetings but wouldn't be implemented, and nobody would be held accountable for it. This led to a lack of trust in the Ministry as a coordinator. Later in the response, coordination improved considerably with the NERC and DERCs, which showed competence and therefore gained the trust of many in the response. Coordination on the international side also generally improved with time, although aspects remained problematic.

Why was coordination so poor? Well for starters, there was a lack of coordination skills. In its early phase, the NERC put way too much emphasis on military-style decision making, often at the expense of discussion and analysis with the public health experts and frontline NGOs. There are plenty of people in the international humanitarian sector with coordination skills, but for much of the response they were not brought on board. As one report put it: "The structures and processes for responding to humanitarian disasters that have been developed and refined since 2005 were not activated . . . It was all a bit of a mess."[8] When these people were recruited later in the response, such as from the Office for the Coordination of Humanitarian Affairs, we could see what we had been missing.

Rather than tapping into such coordination skills from the outset, the UN set up a new structure, UNMEER, to lead international coordination. We and many others feel that setting up UNMEER was a mistake. Establishing a new organisation in the middle of a crisis is never ideal, but within a bureaucratic organisation like the UN, the challenges are multiplied. UNMEER struggled to find its footing in Sierra Leone and, for a long time, was seen as "peripheral".[9] While UNMEER ultimately managed to do some useful things, such as mobilising funds at the international level, paying salaries of many NERC staff and providing vehicles for the response, there is a wide consensus, even among UN interviewees, that UNMEER never should have existed, that its costs were not outweighed by its usefulness. As one donor representative said, "UNMEER was dead on arrival."

Beyond skilled people though, the bigger problem with coordination was that organisations often didn't make coordination enough of a priority, sometimes because they wanted to maintain control and so preferred to act unilaterally. The UK was criticised for not coordinating well enough with other organisations such as the UN and the US, the Ministry and sometimes the NERC itself. The example of the NERC is perhaps the most striking because, on the one hand, the UK integrated closely with the NERC and provided it with significant support. On the other hand, it seems the UK was reluctant to back the NERC wholeheartedly. One report noted:

> The agenda was what [UK] want out of the NERC. The conversation was how the NERC was getting too big for its boots. The NERC leadership was getting more independent and they [the British] were complaining about a sense of not being in control.' Some [interviewees contended] that although they set it up and were closely involved in running it, the British at times undermined the NERC's authority.[10]

Whilst the UK engaged in a huge number of partnerships, and provided a platform for various organisations to engage, unilateralism sometimes kicked in, seemingly when they felt the need to retain control of an agenda, or when they disagreed with the decisions of others. In 2015, on the whole, we saw a more collaborative approach by the UK and this clearly helped. Based on our experiences, we think the response would have been strengthened if the UK had prioritised coordination and collaboration much more from the outset.

So, in future we need trusted coordinators with the right skills, and we need everyone involved in the response to prioritise collaboration.

Politics and accountability

Politics and accountability issues were major and constant challenges in the response.

Politics can, of course, be good or bad. Many positive things that happened in the response, such as the UK intervention, resulted from favourable political dynamics. What we mean here is 'politicking', activity which aims to gain political or personal advantage. In some cases, people were trying to make money, in other cases, they were trying to gain political advantage for themselves or their party, or to boost the profile of their organisation. Politicking and weak accountability manifested themselves from the local level to the international level, including the international aid sector.

Politics trumped substance

Many of the reports that have been written about the Ebola crisis talk about the need for stronger health systems in the three countries to prepare for, and respond to, future outbreaks. However, very few of these reports talk about the political dimensions of this endeavour. The implication here is that health systems strengthening, or indeed outbreak responses, are primarily technical challenges. They are not.

One of the exceptions, the excellent lessons learnt report by IRC, talks about this "erasing of politics" in the Ebola reports:

> This includes the politics of poor, post-conflict countries, but also the politics of the UN, NGOs and the international aid world. These failures set the stage for a small Ebola outbreak to evolve into a catastrophic epidemic. The failure to anticipate and adapt to political realities then hobbled the response effort.[11]

We could not agree more. Whether we are talking about emergency response or longer-term development, we ignore political issues at our peril.

National and local politicking had a very tangible and negative impact on the Ebola response in Sierra Leone at all levels. We experienced this with the toxic internal divisions within the Ministry at national level and in Freetown. One senior Ministry official noted: "We spent more time fighting ourselves than the disease."

But it was broader than the Ministry of Health alone. One senior Ministry official talked about how other government ministers saw Ebola as a "free for all." In his interview for this book, President Koroma acknowledged that "political leadership, on both sides of the political divide, was a problem. This all fuelled the epidemic."

Politics was a huge issue at the local level. No surprises here if we think about the way in which politics at this level has, since colonial times, been fraught with tensions between the formal and 'traditional' authorities, such as local government and chiefs. One report found:

> Political parties were jockeying for primacy at the district
> level and using the Ebola response to lever their own political
> ambitions, sources said. One interviewee said the amount of time
> that had to be spent on governance analysis and navigating the
> 'riotous political battlefield' meant that in one district, getting to
> zero Ebola cases took about two or three months longer than in
> other places.[12]

This issue of politicking is not a new problem in Sierra Leone and is closely linked back to the issue of the lack of internal accountability in the government system. The combination of the President's frequent tours of the country and the work of the NERC and DERCs in collaboration with the UK quieted the politicking to the extent that the epidemic could end. But there is no indication that this has created any kind of lasting shift.

Internationally, we also saw how politics in the Western world affected the response from the donors. It wasn't until Ebola made the headlines and started being perceived as a threat by the public in Europe and the US that governments in those countries started taking the outbreak more seriously. Many decisions that they went on to make, such as cancelling direct flights, were made with a domestic politics in mind.

The first step for organisations to deal with politicking is to realise that it's happening. This requires hiring staff with political savvy, who can then push for political problems to be dealt with promptly in a crisis situation. Where leaders are internationals rather than nationals, they need to receive a strong induction to the context and stay in post for longer, to reduce the challenge of high turnover. It is also important for international organisations to retain flexibility in their funding and programming in order to be able to manoeuvre around changing political dynamics, negative and positive.

Weak accountability and corruption was pervasive

Lack of accountability was a huge problem in the Ebola response. One report lists some examples of corruption as including: "bribes required to get papers signed to build treatment centres; vehicles going missing; illegal charges for vehicle passes to enter or leave quarantine zones; and rain gear and personal protective equipment turning up on the black market."[13]

One of the most serious manifestations of corruption was the hazard pay debacle, which saw vast amounts of money being expended, with many demoralised health workers on the frontline not receiving what they were due. One NERC official recounted:

> Hazard pay was a disaster. The Ministry gave 12,000 names to be paid; 50% were either ghost workers or somehow not in the system. There were strikes all the time from August to October. Some hospital managers would give lists where some people were their relatives in freshly bought uniforms and some people were left off, there was no limit to the corruption.

Corruption had very real and tangible effects. One doctor in Port Loko recalled: "60% of the water sachets for the ETU were stolen. The cups we used to use for oral rehydration salts would get stolen. Billions of dollars in the response and I wouldn't have a cup to give to a patient."

Like politicking, this was not a new issue. Sierra Leone has a long history of corruption, from colonial times, to the Siaka Stevens era, to the Transparency International top ranking for bribery in 2013. One senior Ministry official noted, "The peripheries give their kickbacks to the relevant officers at headquarters – 'return to sender'. Things were rotten before and became even worse under Ebola."

And, corruption, along with politicking, fuelled the population's lack of trust in government during the crisis. Early in the response, a common reason why people didn't believe in Ebola was the assumption that politicians and government just wanted to 'eat money'. After all, the cow grazes where it is tethered. The national audit on Ebola, which found that 30% of Ebola funds were not adequately accounted for, if at all, is said to have "battered" public trust.[14] One military doctor said: "When I started working in the isolation unit, my relatives said to me: You want to kill yourself for these corrupt politicians?"

But one point which is perhaps less recognised about corruption is that it did not just cause action, such as misappropriation or bribery. It also prevented action, which could be even worse.

Some donors hesitated or declined to give funds to the Ministry, because they assumed the money would be misappropriated. Or donors refused to fund certain projects, such as infrastructure or vehicle purchases contracted by the government, because they saw a lot of potential for kickbacks in those kinds of transactions. Donors often gave their funds to NGOs and UN agencies to manage instead – which could often cost more or result in missed opportunities to strengthen the government system. So, corruption had indirect as well as direct effects.

This could work both ways. Sometimes government officials would avoid doing certain things because the activity didn't bring opportunities for personal gain. During the height of the crisis, when one official received an offer from mobile phone companies to provide Ebola messaging to their customers across the country for free, he astonished everyone present at the meeting by turning it down, and was then overheard complaining to a colleague that "10% of free is nothing".

Another dimension of how corruption indirectly prevented action was when government officials avoided taking part in potentially useful activities because they were worried about getting blamed if one of their colleagues misused the resources. For instance, after the release of the national audit report in February 2015, there was paralysis in the NERC. Nobody wanted to sign for anything, lest something go wrong and they get blamed. So corruption manifests itself in different ways, and things are not always as they seem.

A final point here is context. Discussions about corruption tend to be polarising because some people talk about corruption as a binary and clear-cut issue, i.e. corruption is simply wrong. While we have sympathy with this view and are not apologists for corruption, we also believe that it is not productive to talk about corruption without considering issues of context. For instance, a nurse demanding a payment from a patient for ostensibly 'free health care' is clearly a huge problem. But if that nurse has not received her salary in three months, this is also a huge problem. As one NGO representative said: "The problem is that corruption ends conversations. Rather, it should begin them."

There are no quick fixes to corruption issues in Sierra Leone. Political will (often lacking) is key, as is ensuring decent salaries for government workers. International support on anti-corruption efforts may sometimes be useful, but the impact of this will be limited if there isn't the political will for change nationally.

Accountability problems plagued international organisations too

Paul Farmer has written extensively about the tendency of people in the aid system to over-focus on weak accountability in developing countries, rather than questioning the role of developed countries, either today or historically. This is both about weak accountability within their international aid systems and about how they often contribute to corruption in developing countries.[15]

We agree that there are very real faults within the international aid system. We have largely spoken about politicking as it relates to politicians, and poor accountability to mean misappropriation of resources involving government officials. However, we believe that when national or international organisations of any kind exploit their positions for personal or organisational gain or use aid resources inefficiently or ineffectively, they also need to be held to account.

We have talked about failings in WHO's accountability already. More broadly, some people we interviewed expressed disappointment that UN agencies in general were too concerned with their budgets and their profile. One NERC official said:

> There were huge failures by the UN, they basically wanted the budget for themselves, they brought junk cars from Sudan and then they wouldn't pay to fix vehicles. Then you would see all these people at the Radisson with their phones paid for and their vehicles and UNMEER staff would be questioning a $300 monthly salary for a Sierra Leonean.

UN agencies across the board, as well as some donors, embassies and NGOs, paid large amounts of hazard pay to their staff from the early days of the Ebola crisis. For instance, from September 2014 onwards, all international UN staff were paid $1,200 per month on top of often generous salaries. However, some of these international UN staff were not working on Ebola at all, and very few were exposed to any risk of Ebola while doing their job.[16] Meanwhile, frontline Sierra Leonean health workers, who were working with Ebola patients and risking exposure on a daily basis, received $400 per month. It is difficult to see the justification for that use of UN resources, given that there were no significant cost-of-living increases in Freetown at the time.

There were specific criticisms of UNICEF as 'dropping the ball' on social mobilisation, for which they were co-lead with the Ministry. One NGO interviewee said that they failed to provide "strategic leadership", another said they were trying to "boost their profile and abuse their position, to have something for their newsletter."

Some international NGOs used the Ebola crisis as a profile-raising opportunity by misleading people on their role in the response. There was the example of the NGO who reopened a closed clinic in a slum area of Freetown for just one day to facilitate the visit of a camera crew. Another major international humanitarian NGO used dramatic images of people wearing PPE to fundraise for their organisation even though they had refused to get directly involved in Ebola treatment.

The international community as a whole went along with, and sometimes actively promoted, the per diem culture before and during Ebola, despite how this undermines accountability within the Ministry.

Perhaps the most shocking example of corruption in an international organisation was the revelation that over $5 million of International Federation of the Red Cross's Ebola funds had been misappropriated in Sierra Leone, Guinea and Liberia:

An investigation by Red Cross auditors has revealed that in Liberia $2.7m disappeared in fraudulently overpriced supplies, or in salaries for non-existent aid workers. In Sierra Leone, Red Cross staff apparently colluded with local bank workers to skim off over $2m while in Guinea, where investigations are ongoing, around $1m disappeared in fake customs bills.[17]

This was not a one-off event. The fact that the amounts were so huge and the corruption so widespread points to a major accountability failing within the organisation that goes beyond merely systems and speaks to the internal culture.

To combat weak accountability within governments, international organisations first need to tackle their own accountability problems. This includes being more open about their budgets and expenditure so that they can be held to account. They should also think harder about how some actions, like paying per diems to officials, might be undermining accountability in others.

Working through government systems

During a humanitarian emergency, it is normally the UN agencies and international NGOs that capture the attention of the world. But in reality, national governments are often the backbone of a response. They usually have the infrastructure and manpower to rapidly reach across a whole country, as others rarely can. And it is governments that have the democratic legitimacy to make decisions on behalf of their people. This frequently makes working with governments by far the best option for external organisations.

There are, of course, exceptions to this. In warzones, the government may be part of the conflict, while in 'failed' states, the government may have very limited presence in some regions. But that was not the case with the Ebola outbreak in Sierra Leone, where much of the response was delivered by government workers, using government infrastructure, under the overall leadership of the country's President.

Of course, working with government was easier said than done. Whilst there was sometimes strong leadership from within government, this book is also littered with examples of how politics, weak accountability and lack of capacity in the government were major challenges in the response.

Even bearing this in mind, there were still plenty of opportunities for collaboration between government and international organisations. While some were seized, others were missed, which didn't just undermine the response but also meant we failed to use the enormous resources flowing in to the country to strengthen government systems for the long term.

Collaborating with government often enabled a faster response

From the start, there were noticeable differences in approach between organisations that instinctively wanted to work through government, such as WHO and King's, and those that insisted on operating more independently, such as MSF.

There were several reasons why some preferred the more collaborative approach. Some saw benefits to using existing government systems and facilities, since these were already in place and could be converted quickly for the Ebola response. Many thought government officials should be the ones to make the decisions, on the grounds that they understood the local context and were in a better position to engage with communities. And in the face of an escalating crisis, a number believed that their limited staff and resources could have more impact if they were embedded with government across a wide range of sites. Finally, some believed that looking to government for leadership was more legitimate and democratic than making decisions about the lives of Sierra Leoneans independently.

There were some powerful examples of this model in practice including the isolation units that were run by King's and Partners in Health in partnership with the Ministry in Freetown and Port Loko.

By working collaboratively, the Ministry and King's were able to quickly set up five safe isolation units in Freetown that collectively diagnosed nearly 1,200 Ebola patients, which was nearly 40% of all Ebola patients in the district.[18]

This was important because speed matters in an outbreak response. Mathematical modelling was used after the crisis to predict what would have happened if we'd opened the Ebola beds more quickly. The study estimates that had the additional beds come online a month earlier, thousands of Ebola cases would most likely have been averted.[19] Perhaps this would have been possible if more organisations had been more willing to work directly with government health facilities instead of building independent purpose-built ETUs.

That said, the more independent organisations did have reasons for their approach. Avoiding staff infections was a top priority, and many organisations were anxious that they wouldn't be able to maintain the highest safety standards if they weren't in absolute control. And there was no denying that there could be risks to embedding staff in government-run services if this wasn't well managed. There was also the danger of becoming embroiled or implicated in any local politics or corruption issues that government institutions were experiencing.

Perhaps the clearest manifestation of this was with the ETU at Kenema Government Hospital in July, which was supported by a small WHO team. Despite valiant efforts by the health workers on the ground, conditions at the ETU became appalling, and the situation was unaddressed for weeks by the Ministry, as well as by WHO officials in Freetown and Geneva. It was understandable that other international organisations did not want to find themselves caught in a similar situation.

So the lesson we learnt was that partnership with government can be done to great effect, while recognising that it can also go wrong. In the future, working through governments should be the default position of humanitarian organisations, unless there's a clear reason not to. The key to success is getting the fundamentals of the partnership right, making sure that everyone's role is clear and that each side has leadership that can navigate any tensions or disagreements that are likely to emerge in this kind of collaboration.

Opportunities were missed to use the response to build capacity for the future

As one international health specialist noted in an address to the US Senate, "Ebola has taught us what works best in an emergency is not an emergency system – it is an everyday system that is robust, resilient, and functioning before the crisis begins."[20] The best way to manage a health crisis, or even to avoid one entirely, is to have a strong health system that is quick to detect new threats and has the capacity to respond. But the Ebola epidemic showed that over a decade of investment in rebuilding Sierra Leone's health system since the end of the war had failed to address many of its fundamental weaknesses. The Ministry still lacked capacity, whilst many health facilities had only minimal levels of trained staff, infrastructure or supplies.

But the example of the Sierra Leone military shows that it didn't have to be this way. Since the civil war in 2002, the UK military and others had given significant support to building the capacity of the Sierra Leone military, primarily through the UK-led International Military Advisory Training Team. Just over ten years later, the Sierra Leone military was called on to assist with the

Ebola response and they were quickly able to demonstrate their leadership, commitment and professionalism. Obviously there are significant differences between a military and a health system, but there's still plenty we can take away from the comparison.

The comprehensive and long-term approach to strengthening the army contrasts with donor and NGO investment in health programmes, which has tended to cherry-pick particular aspects, such as HIV or data systems, through separate projects. This fragmented the health system. On top of that, many of the methods used to deliver projects, such as paying additional salary to government workers for selected vertical programmes, also contributed to the dysfunction of the wider health system. The combination of a fragmented health system with weak accountability, along with a lack of resources and a demotivated and inappropriately incentivised workforce, meant that the early Ebola response was built on very weak foundations.

The international response was a missed opportunity to address some of these mistakes and use the massive influx of resources to improve the health system. Over a billion dollars was spent on the Ebola response in Sierra Leone but this investment was rarely used to leave a lasting legacy, although strong examples of how this could have been done do exist.

One positive example is how the UK funded the construction of a permanent isolation unit at 34 Military and an infectious diseases centre at Connaught. The UK and the CDC also invested in resuscitation equipment at Connaught and fixed the oxygen factory as part of the Ebola vaccine trial. More broadly, many international epidemiologists, health workers and logisticians made a deliberate effort to work closely with Sierra Leonean colleagues and share their skills.

Too often, however, opportunities to leave a permanent legacy were missed because nobody even stopped to think about them.

The US Office of Foreign Disaster Assistance were particular culprits here by refusing to allow their funding to be used for any refurbishments, such as installing sinks and taps, as part of an infection control project. The Community Care Centres were constructed at great expense in villages across Sierra Leone, but many could not be incorporated into the health system afterwards. A clear opportunity to extend and refurbish existing health clinics was missed. In August 2016, less than a year after the end of the outbreak, the BBC's Global Health Correspondent Tulip Mazumdar described how "the jewel in the crown [of the] response was the 100-bed Kerry Town Ebola treatment centre . . . When I visited this time, it was derelict and decaying. A few stray dogs and a family of goats had taken up residence in what used to be functioning wards."[21]

Smarter investments wouldn't just have benefited the health system in a broad sense, they would also have helped us to prepare for future possible outbreaks. As the Ebola virus is likely to be endemic in bats and other animals in West Africa, it's probably only a matter of time before a human gets infected once again. When that happens, will the leadership, the management systems, the trained staff, the infrastructure and the supplies still be in place for the countries to quickly detect and end the outbreak before it spirals out of control?

Clearly, in the heat of a crisis, strengthening the health system and leaving a legacy should not be the overriding priority or become a distraction. The task at hand is to quickly bring the emergency to an end. But this was an emergency that went on for twenty-one months in Sierra Leone and involved extensive planning and massive investment. What we learnt is that there is not necessarily a trade-off between emergency response and health systems strengthening – these can often be aligned in a way that delivers both simultaneously. Getting that alignment right should be more of a priority. And if we want to be better prepared for the next crisis, we've got to do a better job of building strong health systems in the first place.

The impact of individuals

When Sierra Leone began its preparedness efforts, having learnt about the outbreak in Guinea, no organisation in the country was set up to respond to a major outbreak.

Into that vacuum, we saw individuals step forward and take up pivotal roles in the response, often from unlikely backgrounds or from organisations with seemingly unrelated mandates. They demonstrated that, in an emergency, just one individual can have enormous impact. As one researcher on the outbreak in Sierra Leone put it, "Regardless of the systems and management structures that were put in place, it seemed that at nearly every level, personalities and personal relationships appeared to be key to the functioning of the response."[22]

Many such individuals had important roles in the response and their effectiveness often came down to their character, their motivation and their appreciation of the local context.

Impactful individuals were pragmatic, flexible and collaborative

The individuals who were widely acknowledged to have played key roles often shared certain key character traits.

In the crisis, pragmatism was essential to ensuring that things got implemented quickly and effectively. In the early part of the response, many people were proffering impractical solutions from around conference tables. There were reams and reams of policies and plans, but the gap between these and the reality on the ground were often staggering. As one WHO specialist, who had been asked to write new infection control guidelines, pointed out after a visit to Connaught, "I'm not so sure Connaught Hospital needs new guidelines, so much as they need soap."

Having strong plans was obviously important, but some people stood out for following through on them, and for rolling up their sleeves and taking responsibility for getting problems sorted. Lt Col Andy Garrow from the UK military was widely respected for his dedication and for focusing on solutions at the Freetown DERC. Similarly, Laura Miller from IRC provided vital practical support to the response in Kenema in the early days.

Stepping up and contributing to the response also meant being flexible. There were dozens of examples of individuals agreeing to take on challenging new roles and doing a superb job despite being stretched to their limits. People like Reynold Senesi, the Ministry lab scientist who helped set up the 117 hotline and then went on to coordinate the Ebola vaccine study. Or Amar Kamboz, the British former West End theatre manager who coordinated beds and ambulances at the Freetown DERC. They saw where the need was and were willing and able to adapt their roles accordingly.

The epidemic and the response were both constantly evolving, and as a result, people were often called on to adapt to circumstances at a moment's notice. A great example of this came from Dr Mohamed Boie Jalloh of the Sierra Leone army who recounted to us the opening of the ETU at Hastings.

> At 10 p.m. on that Friday, I got a call to say that the next morning I should go to Hastings to work as a physician. The ETU was opening the next morning. We arrived and made a plan for how to deal with incoming patients and started training the nurses. For the first week, myself and my colleague, we could not go home. We slept in the store. There were plenty of beds there; we would just put one down.

Without pause or protest, Mohamed and his colleagues had thought on their feet and simply gotten on with the job at hand with setting up the new site, which went on to admit over one hundred patients by the end of its first week.

Collaboration was also essential in the response, as discussed above, and when this worked well, it was normally when key individuals listened before making plans and brought people together. OB Sisay brought together many different groups at the NERC to get the job done, while Roeland Monasch, the UNICEF representative, exemplified respectful and collaborative relations with government.

The factor that seemed to underpin these three characteristics was motivation. These three positive traits seemed to be expressed intuitively from people who were committed for the right reasons, in contrast to the agendas and politicking.

To the bemusement of her colleagues at King's, Dr Marta Lado would hardly let candidates get a word in edgewise during their Skype interviews to join the international team at Connaught. Instead, she would emphasise to them the realities of the demeaning work that these highly qualified and ambitious doctors and nurses would have to undertake, from mopping the floors to carrying corpses and taking out the trash. When she was quizzed about her approach, she said she didn't want anyone on her team who was motivated by the idea of doing 'glamorous' Ebola work to further their careers. She needed people who were willing to do whatever was needed to help the patients. If they still wanted to come after hearing her discouraging description of the job, then they were the right people for it.

These personal traits, and the right motivation, were more central to an individual's success than their formal skills or their qualifications. Remarkably, even though the response was extremely complex and involved specialised subjects such as infectious diseases and epidemiology, many of the individuals who had real impact in the early phase of the response had little or no training in these areas. Instead, they found a way to learn the fundamentals quickly and draw on expert advice when they needed it.

As it turned out, it was sometimes the people who were most qualified technically who were least useful during the height of the crisis, either because they lacked the ability to translate what they knew into a low-resource and very fluid and challenging context, or because they struggled with the management and relationship-building that was needed to get things done. We lost count of the number of 'experts' who were flown in to great fanfare, only to watch them flounder as they tried to impose their ideas, sometimes with great arrogance. This stood in real contrast to people like WHO's Daniel Kertesz or CDC's Tom Frieden who combined technical expertise with a pragmatic and collaborative approach.

Individuals were particularly important in the early part of the response, when they helped to pioneer solutions that brought order to the chaos that had developed. As the systems matured and became effective, individuals could then step back and allow processes to function, and it was important that they did so.

Our lesson here is that almost anyone can make a difference in a crisis situation if they are motivated by the right reasons and can be practical, flexible and collaborate well with others. These are things we should all keep in mind for ourselves, but also qualities we should look for in others as we recruit staff and build a team. We may also find there are extraordinary individuals who are already working on the ground in other roles, who might be able to make a major contribution even though their technical skills are in a different field.

Appreciating the importance of context was essential
The response was only effective when policies were translated to the local context. In the words of one MSF doctor we interviewed, "It's not 'we know what to do', it's how to adapt what we know to the specific situation."

Many of the people who had a significant impact on the response were therefore either Sierra Leonean or had been in the country for a number of years. They knew the geography and the realities of life in Sierra Leone, issues like the road network, unreliable power and water supplies and a monsoon-like rainy season. They appreciated how to get things done in a small country that often relied on informal systems of decision making. This is why Sierra Leonean Saffea Senessie was such an effective leader of IRC, as they valiantly filled gaps in the Kenema response in the early days and went on to take a very prominent role in the national response to the crisis.

But there were other individuals who started to have a significant impact quite soon after arriving in the country. Although they hadn't come with a deep understanding of the context, they realised how important it was and made a real effort to engage with it. They quickly worked out the people who could advise them on the local context, and knew to ask the right questions when making decisions. WHO staff Yoti Zabulon and Chris Lane, who worked in Kailahun and Kenema respectively, valued their local colleagues' knowledge, engaged with communities, and as a result quickly became effective.

The thing that undermined contextually relevant solutions the most was the frenetic turnover of staff at many organisations. This also caused real problems with building institutional memory. The CDC stands out as the worst culprit here, with the 28-day turnover of many of their staff, including their leaders, although this did change in the later part of the response. People in leadership, management and coordination roles needed to stay long enough to build relationships and a proper understanding of the situation.

In the early days, we longed for the experts to arrive and take over from us. But as time went on, we realised that the people already on the ground were always going to be critical to getting the crisis under control. The notion of a 'cavalry' was a mirage, because nobody would be able to save the day if they didn't understand the intricacies of the context.

The thing we learnt here is that you've got to really understand the context when making decisions, and adapt ideas rather than just focusing on technical solutions or copying ideas wholesale from elsewhere. So it's vital to make sure that people who understand the context are part of the team making the decisions – and also that they stick around for as long as possible. If you don't know the context already, you can still hit the ground running and become useful quickly by remembering to ask the right questions and knowing who to get advice from.

A note on the writing of the book

We have used a memoir style for much of the book, so that readers can put themselves in our shoes as we faced the challenges of the crisis. At the same time, throughout the book, we also incorporated the knowledge we gained from a considerable amount of secondary research, mostly undertaken by Sinead. She conducted eighty-five interviews of key players in the response, read several hundred documents and attended a number of conferences on related topics, with Oliver also engaging with some of this research. In sum, we interviewed three groups, which sometimes overlapped:

- The leadership of the response at national and international levels, including the President of Sierra Leone, the Coordinator of the National Ebola Response Centre, both Ministers of Health who held office during the Ebola period, the UN Secretary-General and his Special Representative on Ebola, the head of the UK response, the US Ambassador to the UN, and the Director of the US Centers for Disease Control and Prevention (CDC).
- Individuals who were peers of ours during the response, from the government, donors, nongovernmental organisations (NGOs) and UN, some of whom were also among the leadership and some of whom were more operational.
- Other individuals with whom we didn't work directly, including Ebola survivors, who helped us to better understand different aspects of the crisis.

While many interviews are not directly referenced in the book, they helped us enormously in deepening our understanding of the response and in sometimes showing us an alternate perspective that challenged what we thought we knew. Interviews were off-the-record, and any references from interviews included in the book were based on subsequent written permission.

Similarly, while this book does not directly quote from all of the books, academic articles, media reports and organisational reviews that we read, these were vitally important to our final understanding of many topics.

Sinead led on structuring and editing of the book, with significant input from Oliver, as well as valuable support on editing and research from Madeleine Joung, our intern, in the later stages.

Interviewees (alphabetical by organisation)

State House

1. Dr Monty Jones
2. President Ernest Bai Koroma

Republic of Sierra Leone Armed Forces

1. Dr Mohamed Boie Jalloh
2. General Foday Sahr

Ministry of Health and Sanitation

1. James Bangura
2. Dr Donald Bash-Taqi
3. Dr Abu Bakarr Fofanah
4. Issa French
5. Dr Amara Jambai
6. Miatta Kargbo
7. Dr Mohamed Vandy

National Ebola Response Centre (NERC)

1. Yvonne Aki-Sawyerr
2. Chukwu-Emeka Chikezie
3. Major (Rtd) Palo Conteh
4. Stephen Gaojia
5. OB Sisay

Ebola survivors and workers

1. Yusuf Koroma
2. Mohamed Nao
3. Gibrilla Sheriff

UN

1. Dr Bruce Aylward – WHO
2. His Excellency Ban Ki-moon – UN
3. Dr Nahid Bhadelia – WHO
4. Dr Kande-Bure O'Bai Kamara – WHO
5. Dr Martin Cormican – WHO
6. Peter Graaff – WHO/UNMEER
7. Annette Hearns – OCHA
8. Bintou Keita – UNMEER
9. Dr Daniel Kertesz – WHO
10. Dr Margaret Lamunu – WHO
11. Roeland Monasch – UNICEF
12. Matthew Morgan – WHO
13. Dr David Nabarro – UN
14. Jo Nickolls – UNMEER
15. Dr Anders Nordström – WHO
16. Dr Ian Norton – WHO
17. Dr Yaron Wollman – UNICEF
18. Dr Yoti Zabulon – WHO

Diplomats/Donors

1. Ato Brown – World Bank
2. Esmee de Jong – European Commission's Humanitarian Aid and Civil Protection department (ECHO)
3. Kathleen Fitzgibbon – US Embassy

4. Dr Tom Frieden – US CDC
5. Sara Hersey – US CDC
6. Ambassador John Hoover – US Embassy
7. Dr Philippe Maughan – ECHO
8. Paula Molloy – Irish Embassy
9. Dr Oliver Morgan – US CDC
10 Emma Mulhern – Irish Embassy
11. Ambassador Samantha Power – US Government
12. Sonia Walia – Office for US Foreign Disaster Assistance

UK

1. Kate Airey
2. Dr Donal Brown
3. Edward Davis
4. Dr Marshall Elliott
5. Lt Col Andy Garrow
6. Dr Chris Lane
7. Brigadier Steven McMahon
8. Prof Dilys Morgan
9. John Raine
10. Peter Rees-Gildea
11. High Commissioner Peter West
12. Prof Chris Whitty

NGOs

1. Clare Bader – Save the Children
2. Dr Jean-Clément Cabrol – MSF-Switzerland
3. Dr Corrado Cancedda – Partners in Health
4. Brice de la Vigne – MSF-Belgium
5. Dr Paul Farmer – Partners in Health

6. Hussein Ibrahim – International Medical Corps
7. Mohammad Jalloh Sr – Focus 1000
8. Mohammad Jalloh Jr – Focus 1000
9. Dr Joanne Liu – MSF
10. Else Kirk – Goal
11. Dr Marta Lado – King's Sierra Leone Partnership
12. Jon Lascher – Partners in Health
13. Steve McAndrew – International Federation of the Red Cross and Red Crescent Societies
14. Amanda McClelland – International Federation of the Red Cross and Red Crescent Societies
15. Fiona McLysaght – Concern Worldwide
16. Laura Miller – International Rescue Committee
17. Jochen Moninger – Welt Hunger Hilfe
18. Katherine Owen – Goal
19. Victoria Parkinson – Africa Governance Initiative
20. Will Pooley – King's Sierra Leone Partnership
21. Saffea Senessie – International Rescue Committee
22. Dr Amanda Tiffany – MSF-Switzerland
23. Dr Dan Youkee – King's Sierra Leone Partnership

Requested but unavailable for interview

1. Dr Margaret Chan WHO
2. Kate Foster DFID
3. Dr Jacob Mufunda WHO
4. Dr. Alie Wurie MOHS

Notes

PREFACE

1 Farrar and Piot (2014, p. 1545)
2 WHO Ebola Response Team (2014)
3 Meltzer et al. (2014)
4 Farrar and Piot (2014, p. 1545)
5 Kupferschmidt (2014)
6 Lee (2017)

ONE

1 Jalloh et al. (2013, p. 132)
2 Byaruhanga (2008)
3 Kargbo (2006, p. 24)
4 Richards (1996, p. 40-41)
5 Kargbo (2006, p. 29)
6 Richards (1996, p. 12)
7 Kargbo (2006, p. 15)
8 Jackson, 2004 (p. 63)
9 Keen (2005, p. 109)
10 Stockholm International Peace Research Institute (2016)
11 Kaifala (2017)
12 Kargbo (2006, p. 37)
13 Sierra Leone Truth and Reconciliation Commission (2004, vol. 3A ch. 1 p. 5)
14 *Ibid.* (p. 6)
15 Bundu (2001, p. xv)
16 Reno (1995, p. 28)
17 Harris (2014)
18 *Ibid.*

19 "While in Sierra Leone 'traditional' authorities retain considerable legitimacy, they have also undergone so much change through colonialism and post-colonialism, that 'traditional' is a problematic descriptor" (Harris 2017, Personal correspondence with author, 28 July).

20 United Nations Development Programme (2013b)

21 Ferme (2014)

22 Kron (2011)

23 Secret societies are gendered community groups in Sierra Leone and in other countries such as Liberia whose internal affairs are kept highly confidential within the group. While their cultural and spiritual roles are commonly emphasised, they are often central in local and national politics. Their precise functions vary with factors such as geography and ethnic group, but in Sierra Leone they tend to play significant roles in the spiritual life of communities (and thus in events such as funerals), in initiation ceremonies (including the conduct of female genital mutilation by female secret societies), and in health care.

24 United Nations Development Programme (2013a, p. 2)

25 United Nations Development Programme (n.d.)

26 United Nations Development Programme (2015, p. 6)

27 In fellow Commonwealth countries, ambassadors are known as "high commissioners". This applies to the UK in Sierra Leone.

28 Department for International Development (2012, p. 2)

29 In this book, "donors" refers to these official or governmental donors who had a presence in Sierra Leone. There are also very significant private donors, such as the Gates Foundation, but these did not have an in-country presence at this time and so, unless specified, are not being discussed here.

30 The World Bank (n.d.) *Data: Sierra Leone*

31 United Nations Development Programme (n.d.)

32 The World Bank (2012, p. 1)

33 For simplicity, we refer to the Ministry of Health & Sanitation as the "Ministry of Health" in the remainder of the book.

34 Kargbo (2017)

35 High-level Panel on the Global Response to Health Crises (2016, statistics from 2012)

36 Mankad et al. (2015)

37 Kargbo (2017)

38 Sierra Leone Ministry of Health and Sanitation (2016)

39 Mankad et al. (2015)

40 The World Bank (n.d.) *Data: United Kingdom*

41 Government of Sierra Leone (2013, p. 5)
42 Kieny et al. (2014, p. 850)

TWO

1 Fitzpatrick et al. (2015, p. 1752)
2 Agence France-Presse (2014)
3 PBS Frontline (2014)
4 High-level Panel on the Global Response to Health Crises (2016, p. 21)
5 World Health Organization (2014b)
6 Centers for Disease Control (n.d.)
7 Ibid.
8 Sack et al. (2014)
9 Médecins Sans Frontières (2014)
10 Médecins Sans Frontières (2015, p. 6)
11 Sack et al. (2014)
12 World Health Organization (2006)
13 Sack et al. (2014)
14 Nossiter (2014b)
15 Sack et al. (2014)
16 Gostin (2015)
17 World Health Organization (2006)
18 Gostin (2015)
19 Moon et al. (2015, p. 2216)
20 Mankad et al. (2015)
21 Nebehay and Lewis (2011)
22 Gostin and Friedman (2015, p. 1904)
23 Gostin and Friedman (2015, p. 1904)
24 High-level Panel on the Global Response to Health Crises (2016, p. 46)
25 Sack et al. (2014)
26 Funk et al. (2017, p. 6)
27 Reaves et al. (2014)
28 Sack et al. (2014)
29 Funk et al. (2017, p. 6)
30 *Ibid.*
31 Sack et al. (2014)
32 World Health Organization (2015b)
33 Sack et al. (2014)
34 The World Bank (n.d.) *Population living in slums*
35 Much of this section draws on Sack et al. (2014)

36 Médecins Sans Frontières (2015)
37 Allié et al. (2016)

THREE

1 Wauquier et al. (2015)
2 *Ibid.* (p. 4)
3 Fairhead (2014, p. 9)
4 Richards et al. (2014, p. 9)
5 Sack et al. (2014)
6 *Ibid.*
7 International Crisis Group (2015)
8 Niang (2015)
9 Sprecher et al. (2015)
10 Médecins Sans Frontières (2015, p. 7)
11 *Ibid.* (p. 6)
12 Wolz (2014, p. 1083)
13 Happily, Mamie Lebbie survived the virus.
14 Niang (2015)
15 Garrett (2014)
16 World Health Organization Global Task Force on Cholera Control (2013, p. 1)
17 It is worth noting that President Koroma did carry out some actions on Ebola. On 1 July, he recorded radio messages where, most significantly, he tried to address misconceptions about Ebola. He also engaged with the Ministry early on in negotiations with MSF on the opening of the Kailahun ETU.
18 Médecins sans Frontières (2014)
19 Centers for Disease Control (2016) and Glassman (2016)
20 Nardelli (2015)
21 Unless otherwise noted, all historical currency conversions in this book are calculated using Bloomberg Markets: Currencies, see Anon (n.d.) *Bloomberg Markets*.
22 Schieffelin et al. (2014, p. 14 in Supplementary Appendix)
23 World Health Organization (2014f)
24 Johnson et al. (2015, p. 8)
25 Sierra Leone Ministry of Health and Sanitation (2014b)
26 This was 8 billion Leones at the exchange rate 4300 Leones to US$1.
27 Nsenga (2015)

FOUR

1 Sierra Leone Ministry of Health and Sanitation (2014c)
2 Brett-Major (2016)
3 Senga et al. (2017)
4 Lane (2017), Personal correspondence with author, 6 August.
5 Chris worked for Public Health England at the time and had volunteered under the Global Outbreak Alert and Response Network (GOARN), a partnership of over 150 institutions based at WHO that mobilizes technical support from around the world to assist countries with outbreak response. GOARN ultimately sent 895 people to work on the Ebola response, including the doctors at the Kenema ETU. World Health Organization (n.d.) *Partners: Global outbreak alert*
6 This is also mentioned in Brett-Major (2016). Dr Fukuda did take some action to assist Kenema by lobbying for an increased security presence there to help the staff.
7 Associated Press (2015)
8 Fofana (2014)
9 Associated Press (2016)
10 Koroma (2014b)
11 O'Dempsey (2017, p. 175)
12 Brett-Major (2016, p. 86–87)
13 Pollack (2014)
14 Much of this section draws from a description of Dr Khan's treatment in an excellent chapter in the MSF book *Ebola: Politics of Fear* (2017, p. 175–186) written by the WHO Clinical Lead, Tim O'Dempsey.
15 World Health Organization (2015a)

FIVE

1 Sierra Leone Ministry of Health and Sanitation (2014a)
2 NestBuilders International (2016)
3 Campbell (2012); The World Bank (n.d.) *Data: Guinea*; (n.d.) *Data: Liberia*; (n.d.) *Data: Sierra Leone*
4 Koroma (2014a)
5 The WHO website description of the event makes no mention of the fact that the centre was closed when the President arrived (World Health Organization, 2014d). However, the State House website retained the original story we heard until they updated the site in August 2017.
6 CBS News and Associated Press (2014)

7 Freeman and Akkoc (2014)

8 Centers for Disease Control and Prevention (2016)

9 World Health Organization (2014b)

10 Sierra Leone Ministry of Health and Sanitation (2014b)

11 Beaubien (2014)

12 World Health Organization, 2014c

13 This quote is from p. 268 of Helene Cooper's book *Madame President: The Extraordinary Journey of Ellen Johnson Sirleaf* which is a key source for this section. The next quote is from p. 269–70.

14 UNICEF-Liberia (2014)

15 Roos (2014)

16 Cooper (2014, p. 270)

17 Johnson et al. (2015)

18 Médecins Sans Frontières (2015, p. 9)

19 Médecins Sans Fontières (2016)

SIX

1 Liu (2014)

2 Tavernise (2014)

3 Cooper (2014); Flynn (2014)

4 UNICEF-Sierra Leone (2014)

5 One international responder at the time, Daniel Cohen, coined this phrase in relation to the plight of health care workers but to me, it is also apt to describe the entire response at that time.

6 World Health Organization (n.d.) *Ebola Virus Disease Fact Sheet*

7 Kamara (2014)

8 Women made up 51% of Ebola cases in Sierra Leone (World Health Organization, 2016a) and were 51% of the population (Sierra Leone 2015 Population and Housing Census, 2016).

9 As I pointed out in my rebuttal at the time, this is not to suggest that there were no gendered impacts to Ebola. There were many, for example, while there are no firm statistics on this, it is widely thought that there was increased sexual violence during the Ebola period, for various reasons. But the data did not suggest that women were more likely to be infected or to die, which was the point being made.

10 Government of Sierra Leone Emergency Operations Centre (2014a)

11 Lu et al. (2016, p. 199)

12 http://www.cnn.com/2014/09/19/world/africa/sierra-leone-ebola-lock-down/ (Accessed 24 April 2017)

13 Cooper (2017, p. 274)

14 Cooper et al. (2014)

15 Department for International Development and Foreign and Commonwealth Office (2014a, 2014b)

16 United Nations Security Council (2014)

17 UNFPA (2014)

18 Government of Sierra Leone Emergency Operations Centre (2014a)

19 Al Jazeera (2014)

20 Marah (2014)

21 Meltzer et al. (2014)

SEVEN

1 World Health Organization (2014a, p. 3)

2 NestBuilders International (2016, p. 18)

3 Government of Sierra Leone Emergency Operations Centre (2014a)

4 UNICEF-Sierra Leone (2014, p. 1)

5 Nossiter (2014a)

6 Government of Sierra Leone Emergency Operations Centre (2014a)

7 Whitty et al. (2014, p. 193)

8 Sack et al. (2014)

9 Evans et al. (2016, p. 52)

10 The World Health Organization (2014e)

11 UNICEF-Sierra Leone (2014, p. 1)

12 Government of Sierra Leone Emergency Operations Centre (2014a)

13 Meltzer et al. (2014, p. 13)

14 Ross et al. (2017)

15 Kamradt-Scott et al. (2015, p. 20)

16 Fink (2015)

17 *J R Army Med Corps* (2016, p. 201)

18 World Health Organization (2014a)

19 UNICEF-Sierra Leone (2014)

20 World Health Organization (2015b)

EIGHT

1 Freeman (2014)

2 Connor (2014)

3 Bricknell et al. (2016)

4 Connor (2014)

5 Alexander (2012)

6 Anon (2015)

7 Moyer (2014)

8 National Ebola Response Centre (2014)

9 World Health Organization (2014h)

10 Nossiter (2014c)

11 Government of Sierra Leone Emergency Operations Centre (2014b, p. 2)

12 At the time, the WHO called these Ebola Care Units, but these were renamed Community Care Centres during the development process.

13 UNICEF (2016, p. 11) came to the same conclusion in their internal review, that their approach to CCCs led to poor referral with clinics and was a missed opportunity to strengthen primary health care.

14 Bricknell et al. (2016)

15 Department for International Development et al. (2014)

16 Bricknell et al. (2016)

17 *Ibid.*

NINE

1 World Health Organization (2014a)

2 World Health Organization (2014b)

3 Whitty et al. (2014, p. 193)

4 World Health Organization (2014b, p. 6)

5 DuBois et al. (2015, p. 18)

6 Pronyk et al. (2016, p. 730)

7 *Ibid.*

8 WHO Ebola Response Team (2014)

9 Whitty (2017)

10 National Ebola Response Centre (2015)

11 National Ebola Response Centre (2015)

12 Ross (2017, p. 6)

13 UNMEER et al. (2015)

14 O'Bai Kamara (2017), Personal correspondence with author, 1 August.

15 Lane (2017), Personal correspondence with author, 15 August.

16 NERC (2015)

17 This is apparently still the case at the time of writing.

18 Henao-Restrepo et al. (2015)

19 Risso-Gil and Finnegan (2015)

20 Brolin Ribacke et al. (2016, p. 10)

21 BBC (2015)

22 High-level Panel on the Global Response to Health Crises (2016, p. 26)
23 Fofana (2017)
24 Audit Service Sierra Leone (2014)
25 *Ibid.*, p. 1
26 Bloomberg Markets: Currencies (2015)
27 Duddridge and Foreign and Commonwealth Office (2016)
28 The Demographic and Health Surveys Program (2013)
29 Risso-Gil and Finnegan (2015, p. 19)
30 Hofman and Au (2017)
31 World Health Organization (2016b)
32 Kabba (2016)

TEN

1 Hofman and Au (2017, p. xix)
2 World Health Organization (2016c)
3 World Health Organization (2015a, p. 4)
4 Hofman and Au (2017, p. 186)
5 Sun et al. (2014)
6 Brilliant (2014)
7 Moon et al. (2017)
8 Coltart et al. (2017, p. 20)
9 Moon et al. (2017, p. 4)
10 Inter-Agency Standing Committee (2016). I am grateful to Joe Cook, Belinda Holdsworth and Bruce Aylward at OCHA for directing me to the relevant documents.
11 The World Bank (2017)
12 Alliance for Country Assessments for Global Health Security and IHR Implementation (accessed 2017)
13 Coalition for Epidemic Preparedness Innovations (accessed 2017)
14 Africa CDC (accessed 2017)
15 15 Moon et al. (2017)
16 Ibid.

AFTERWORD

1 Grant et al. (2014)
2 Richards (2016)
3 Part of the reason these skilled professionals are useful is that community engagement is rarely easy or straightforward. It is as complex as we are as people. Important questions range from who constitutes 'a

community', to who speaks for 'the community', to simply how best to engage in each different situation.

4 Bayntun and Zimble (2016, p. 24)

5 David Harris (2017, Personal correspondence with author, 18 December) makes the point that, "Arguably, there is some accountability, but in a patron-cliental or familial obligations sense. In many ways, this is what makes reform doubly hard and contributes to an explanation of why the system continues."

6 I am grateful to Paul Richards for his insights on this point.

7 One of our interviewees did, however, make the point that the lack of leadership from the Sierra Leone government and WHO in the early months made it difficult for the UK to accurately assess the situation or to act.

8 Kamradt-Scott et al. (2015, p. 9)

9 Kamradt-Scott et al. (2015, p. 9)

10 Ross et al. (2017, p. 29)

11 International Rescue Committee (2016, p. 2)

12 Ross et al. (2017, p. 35)

13 Ross et al. (2017, p. 36)

14 Spencer (2015, p. 11)

15 Farmer (2013)

16 Personal correspondence of author with UN international staff [3rd August 2017].

17 BBC (2017)

18 Johnson et al. (2016, p. 1)

19 Kucharski et al. (2015, p. 14367)

20 Panjabi (2016, p. 3)

21 Mazumdar (2016)

22 Ross et al. (2017, p. 40)

Bibliography

Africa CDC (n.d.) *Africa Centres for Disease Control and Prevention: Safeguarding Africa's health.* Available at: https://au.int/en/africacdc (Accessed 11 August 2017).

Agence France-Presse (2014) 'I would sit next to Ebola sufferer on Tube', says scientist who discovered deadly virus. *The Telegraph*, 31 July. Available at: http://www.telegraph.co.uk/news/worldnews/africaandindianocean/sierraleone/11002041/I-would-sit-next-to-Ebola-sufferer-on-Tube-says-scientist-who-discovered-deadly-virus.html.

Alexander, R. (2012) Which is the world's biggest employer? *BBC News*, 20 March. Available at: http://www.bbc.com/news/magazine-17429786 (Accessed 12 August 2017)

Alliance for Country Assessments for Global Health Security and IHR Implementation (n.d.) *JEE Alliance.* Available at: https://www.jeealliance.org/about/ (Accessed 12 August 2017).

Allié, M.-P. et al. (2016) *OCB Ebola review: Part 1: Medico-operational* (March). Stockholm: Stockholm Evaluation Unit. Available at: http://evaluation.msf.org/evaluation-report/ocb-ebola-review-2016 (Accessed 28 February 2018)

Anon (n.d.) *Bloomberg Markets: Currencies.* Available at: https://www.bloomberg.com/markets/currencies (Accessed 8 August 2017).

Anon (2015) *Report from UK-Med-recruited NHS health workers contracted to Emergency NGO.* Freetown. (Unpublished)

Associated Press (2015) Political considerations delayed WHO Ebola response, emails show. *CBS News*, 20 March. Available at: http://www.cbsnews.com/news/political-considerations-delayed-who-ebola-response-emails-show/ (Accessed 6 August 2017).

Associated Press (2016) Investigation: U.S. company bungled Ebola response. *CBS News*, 7 March. Available at: http://www.cbsnews.com/news/american-company-metabiota-problems-during-ebola-outbreak/ (Accessed 6 August 2017).

Audit Service Sierra Leone (2014) *Report on the audit of the management of the Ebola funds.* (October). Freetown: Audit Service Sierra Leone.

Available at: http://www.auditservice.gov.sl/report/assl-report-on-ebola-funds-management-may-oct-2014.pdf (Accessed 28 February 2018).

Bayntun, C. & Zimble, S. A. (2016) *Evaluation of the OCG response to the Ebola outbreak: Lessons learned from the Freetown Ebola Treatment Unit, Sierra Leone.* Vienna: MSF Vienna Evaluation Unit. Available at: http://cdn.evaluation.msf.org/sites/evaluation/files/attachments/sierra_leone_evaluation_of_the_ocg_response_to_the_ebola_outbreak_3_may_2016_final_1.pdf (Accessed 28 February 2018).

BBC (2015) Schools reopen in Sierra Leone as Ebola threat recedes. 14 April. Available at: http://www.bbc.com/news/world-africa-32299543 (Accessed 6 August 2017).

BBC (2017) Red Cross apologise for losing $5m of Ebola funds to fraud. 3 November. Available at: http://www.bbc.com/news/world-africa-41861552 (Accessed 6 August 2017).

Beaubien, J. (2014) Back on its feet, a Liberian hospital aims to keep Ebola out. *NPR*, 14 October. Available at: http://www.npr.org/sections/goatsa ndsoda/2014/10/14/355873770/back-on-its-feet-a-liberian-hospital-aims-to-keep-ebola-out (Accessed 6 August 2017).

Brett-Major, D. (2016) *A year of Ebola: A personal tale of the weirdness wrought by the world's largest Ebola virus disease epidemic.* Bethesda: Navigating Health Risks, LLC.

Bricknell, M. et al. (2016) Operation GRITROCK: The Defence Medical Services' story and emerging lessons from supporting the UK response to the Ebola crisis. *Journal of the Royal Army Medical Corps*, 162, 169–175.

Brilliant, L. (2014) Revenge of the superbugs: How can we outsmart killer microbes. Panel presentation at Milken Institute Global Conference. Los Angeles: April 2014. Available at: http://www.milkeninstitute. org/events/conferences/global-conference/2014/panel-detail/4879 (Accessed 28 February 2018)

Brolin Ribacke, K. J. et al. (2016) Effects of the West Africa Ebola virus disease on health-care utilization – a systematic review. *Frontiers in Public Health*, 4 (October). Available at: http://journal.frontiersin.org/article/10.3389/fpubh.2016.00222/full (Accessed 6 August 2017).

Bundu, A. (2001) *Democracy by force? A study of international military intervention in the conflict in Sierra Leone from 1991–2000.* USA: Universal Publishers.

Byaruhanga, F. K. (2008) The Athens of West Africa: A history of international education at Fourah Bay College, Freetown, Sierra Leone. *African Studies Review*, 51 (1), 195–196. Available at: https://muse.jhu. edu/article/242490 (Accessed 6 August 2017).

Campbell, J. (2012) This is Africa's new biggest city: Lagos, Nigeria, population 21 million. *The Atlantic*. Available at: https://www.theatlantic.

com/international/archive/2012/07/this-is-africas-new-biggest-city-lagos-nigeria-population-21-million/259611/ (Accessed 12 August 2017).

CBS News & Associated Press (2014) *U.S. Peace Corps volunteers exposed to Ebola.* 30 July. Available at: http://www.cbsnews.com/news/peace-corps-volunteers-in-liberia-isolated-for-ebola-exposure/ (Accessed 6 August 2017).

Centers for Disease Control (n.d.) *Outbreaks chronology: Ebola virus disease.* Available at: https://www.cdc.gov/vhf/ebola/outbreaks/history/chronology.html (Accessed 26 February 2018).

Centers for Disease Control (2016) *Cost of the Ebola epidemic.* Available at: http://www.cdc.gov/vhf/ebola/pdf/cost-response.pdf (Accessed 6 August 2017).

Centers for Disease Control and Prevention (2016) *2014 Ebola outbreak in West Africa – Case counts.* Available at: https://www.cdc.gov/vhf/ebola/outbreaks/2014-west-africa/case-counts.html (Accessed 12 August 2017).

Coalition for Epidemic Preparedness Innovations (n.d.) *CEPI: New vaccines for a safer world.* Available at: http://cepi.net/ (Accessed 12 August 2017).

Coltart, C. E. M. et al. (2017) *The Ebola outbreak , 2013–2016 : Old lessons for new epidemics.* Available at: http://rstb.royalsocietypublishing.org/content/372/1721/20160297 (Accessed 28 February 2018).

Connor, S. (2014) Sierra Leone criticises Save the Children's running of Ebola centre. *The Independent,* 9 December. Available at: http://www.independent.co.uk/news/world/africa/sierra-leone-criticises-save-the-childrens-running-of-ebola-centre-9913438.html (Accessed 6 August 2017).

Cooper, H. (2014) Liberian president pleads with Obama for assistance in combating Ebola. *The New York Times,* 12 September. Available at: https://www.nytimes.com/2014/09/13/world/africa/liberian-president-pleads-with-obama-for-assistance-in-combating-ebola.html (Accessed 6 August 2017).

Cooper, H. (2017) *Madame President: The extraordinary journey of Ellen Johnson Sirleaf.* New York: Simon and Schuster.

Cooper, H. et al. (2014) U.S. to commit up to 3,000 troops to fight Ebola in Africa. *The New York Times,* 15 September. Available at: https://www.nytimes.com/2014/09/16/world/africa/obama-to-announce-expanded-effort-against-ebola.html (Accessed 6 August 2017).

Department for International Development (2012) *Operational Plan 2011-2015. DFID Sierra Leone.* Freetown: UK Department for International Development. Available at: https://www.gov.uk/government/uploads/system/uploads/attachment_data/file/67408/sierra-leone-2011.pdf (Accessed 28 February 2018).

Department for International Development et al. (2014) *First British Ebola treatment facility opens in Sierra Leone.* 5 November. Available at:

https://www.gov.uk/government/news/first-british-ebola-treatment-facility-opens-in-sierra-leone (Accessed 6 August 2017).

Department for International Development & Foreign and Commonwealth Office (2014a) *The UK is leading the international drive against Ebola in Sierra Leone*. 23 September. Available at: https://www.gov.uk/government/news/the-uk-is-leading-the-international-drive-against-ebola-in-sierra-leone (Accessed 6 August 2017).

Department for International Development & Foreign and Commonwealth Office (2014b) *UK to increase support to Sierra Leone to combat Ebola*. 17 September. Available at: https://www.gov.uk/government/news/uk-to-increase-support-to-sierra-leone-to-combat-ebola--2 (Accessed 6 August 2017).

DuBois, M. et al. (2015) *The Ebola response in West Africa: Exposing the politics and culture of international aid*. Available at: https://www.odi.org/publications/9956-ebola-response-west-africa-exposing-politics-culture-international-aid (Accessed 6 August 2017).

Duddridge, J. and Foreign & Commonwealth Office (2016) *Minister for Africa speech at UK-Sierra Leone Trade and Investment Forum*. Available at: https://www.gov.uk/government/speeches/minister-for-africa-speech-at-uk-sierra-leone-trade-and-investment-forum (Accessed 14 August 2017).

Evans, N. G. et al. (eds) (2016) *Ebola's message: Public health and medicine in the twenty-first century*. Cambridge: Massachusetts Institute of Technology Press.

Grant C. et al. (2014) *Ebola – local beliefs and behaviour change*. London: Health & Education Advice & Resource Team. Available at: http://www.heart-resources.org/wp-content/uploads/2014/11/Final-Ebola-Helpdesk-Report.pdf (Accessed 28 February 2017).

Fairhead, J. (2014) *The significance of death, funerals, and the after-life in Ebola-hit Sierra Leone, Guinea and Liberia: Anthropological insights into infection and social resistance*. (October). Available at: http://www.heart-resources.org/wp-content/uploads/2014/10/FairheadEbolaFunerals8Oct.pdf (Accessed 6 August 2017).

Farmer, P. (2013) Rethinking foreign aid: Five ways to improve development assistance. *Foreign Affairs*, 12 December. Available at: https://www.foreignaffairs.com/articles/2013-12-12/rethinking-foreign-aid (Accessed 6 August 2017).

Farrar, J. and Piot, P. (2014) Editorial: The Ebola emergency – immediate action, ongoing strategy. *New England Journal of Medicine*, 371, 1545–1546. Available at: http://www.nejm.org/doi/full/10.1056/NEJMe1411471 (Accessed 28 February 2018).

Ferme, M. (2014) Hospital diaries: Experiences with public health in Sierra Leone. *Cultural Anthropology*. Available at: https://culanth.org/

fieldsights/591-hospital-diaries-experiences-with-public-health-in-sierra-leone (Accessed 6 August 2017).

Fink, S. (2015) Pattern of safety lapses where group worked to battle Ebola outbreak. *The New York Times*, 12 April. Available at: https://www.nytimes.com/2015/04/13/world/africa/pattern-of-safety-lapses-where-group-worked-to-battle-ebola-outbreak.html?_r=1 (Accessed 6 August 2017).

Fitzpatrick, G. et al. (2015) The contribution of Ebola viral load at admission and other patient characteristics to mortality in a Médecins Sans Frontières Ebola Case Management Centre, Kailahun, Sierra Leone, June–October 2014. *The Journal of Infectious Diseases*, 212 (11), 1752–1758.

Flynn, D. (2014) Liberian president appeals to Obama for U.S. help to beat Ebola. *Reuters*, 13 September. Available at: http://www.reuters.com/article/health-ebola-usa-idUSL5N0RE12I20140913 (Accessed 6 August 2017).

Fofana, U. (2014) Ebola center in Sierra Leone under guard after protest march. *Reuters*, 26 July. Available at: http://www.reuters.com/article/us-health-ebola-africa-idUSKBN0FV0NL20140726 (Accessed 6 August 2017).

Fofana, U. (2017) Where are Sierra Leone's missing Ebola millions? *BBC Africa*, 23 January. Available at: http://www.bbc.com/news/world-africa-38718196 (Accessed 6 August 2017).

Foreign and Commonwealth Office (2015) *FCO press release: Honours for the best of Britain overseas*. Available at: https://www.gov.uk/government/uploads/system/uploads/attachment_data/file/434651/Birthday_Honours_2015_FCO_press_release.pdf (Accessed 6 August 2017).

Freeman, C. (2014) British Ebola clinic opens for patients in Sierra Leone. *The Telegraph*, 5 November. Available at: http://www.telegraph.co.uk/news/worldnews/ebola/11212080/British-Ebola-clinic-opens-for-patients-in-Sierra-Leone.html (Accessed 6 August 2017).

Freeman, C. and Akkoc, R. (2014) Ebola outbreak: BA suspends flights to Sierra Leone and Liberia over virus. *The Telegraph*, 5 August. Available at: http://www.telegraph.co.uk/news/aviation/11013996/Ebola-outbreak-BA-suspends-flights-to-Sierra-Leone-and-Liberia-over-virus.html (Accessed 12 August 2017).

Funk, S. et al. (2017) The impact of control strategies and behavioural changes on the elimination of Ebola from Lofa County, Liberia. *Philosophical Transactions of the Royal Society B*, 372 (1721). Available at: https://www.ncbi.nlm.nih.gov/pubmed/28396473 (Accessed 28 February 2018).

Garrett, L. (2014) Sierra Leone's Ebola epidemic is spiraling out of control. *Foreign Policy*, 10 December. Available at: http://foreignpolicy.

com/2014/12/10/sierra-leones-ebola-epidemic-is-spiraling-out-of-control/ (Accessed 6 August 2017).

Glassman, A. (2016) After Ebola. *Finance & Development*, 53(2), 25. Available at: http://www.imf.org/external/pubs/ft/fandd/2016/06/pdf/glassman.pdf (Accessed 28 February 2018).

Gostin, L. O. (2015) World Health Organization reform: Lessons learned from the Ebola epidemic. *Hastings Center Report*, 45 (2), 6–7. Available at: http://onlinelibrary.wiley.com/doi/10.1002/hast.424/abstract;jsessio nid=DDF6EC95CAD973DF0DDD12D765D43B58.f03t02 (Accessed 28 February 2018).

Gostin, L. O. and Friedman, E. A. (2015) A retrospective and prospective analysis of the West African Ebola virus disease epidemic: Robust national health systems at the Foundation and an empowered WHO at the apex. *The Lancet*, 385 (9980), 1902–1909. Available at: http://www.thelancet.com/journals/lancet/article/PIIS0140-6736(15)60644-4/abstract (Accessed 28 February 2018).

Government of Sierra Leone (2013) *Connaught Hospital Taskforce Report*. Freetown: Government of Sierra Leone.

Government of Sierra Leone Emergency Operations Centre (2014a) *Ebola Outbreak Updates 8, 14, 24 and 25 September, 1-7 and 16 October 2014*. Freetown: Government of Sierra Leone.

Government of Sierra Leone Emergency Operations Centre (2014b) *Sierra Leone Emergency Management Program Standard Operating Procedure for Interim Home Protection and Care*. Freetown: Government of Sierra Leone.

Harris, D. (2014) *Sierra Leone: A political history*. New York: Oxford University Press.

Henao-Restrepo, A. M. et al. (2015) Efficacy and effectiveness of an rVSV-vectored vaccine expressing Ebola surface glycoprotein: Interim results from the Guinea ring vaccination cluster-randomised trial. *The Lancet*, 386 (9996), 857–866. Available at: http://www.thelancet.com/journals/lancet/article/PIIS0140-6736(15)61117-5/abstract (Accessed 28 February 2018).

High-level Panel on the Global Response to Health Crises (2016) *Protecting humanity from future health crises* (January). Available at: http://www.un.org/News/dh/infocus/HLP/2016-02-05_Final_Report_Global_Response_to_Health_Crises.pdf (Accessed 6 August 2017).

Hofman, M. and Au, S. (eds) (2017) *The politics of fear: Médecins sans Frontières and the West African Ebola epidemic*. New York: Oxford University Press.

Inter-Agency Standing Committee (2016) *Reference Document: Level 3 (l3) Activation procedures for infectious disease events*. Available at: https://interagencystandingcommittee.org/principals/documents-public/final-iasc-system-wide-level-3-l3-activation-procedures-infectious (Accessed 6 August 2017).

International Crisis Group (2015) The politics behind the Ebola crisis. *Crisis Group Africa Report*. Issue 232. Brussels: International Crisis Group. Available at: https://www.crisisgroup.org/africa/west-africa/politics-behind-ebola-crisis (Accessed 28 February 2018).

International Rescue Committee (2016) *The Ebola Lessons Reader: What's being said, what's missing and why it matters*. New York: International Rescue Committee. Available at: https://www.rescue.org/report/ebola-lessons-reader-whats-being-said-whats-missing-and-why-it-matters (Accessed 28 February 2017).

Jackson, M. (2004) *In Sierra Leone*. Durham, NC: Duke University Press.

Jalloh, A. B. et al. (2013) The geology, mineral resources of Sierra Leone and how the resources can be used to develop the nation. *Procedia Earth and Planetary Science*, 6, 131–138. Available at: http://linkinghub.elsevier.com/retrieve/pii/S1878522013000192 (Accessed 16 July 2017).

al Jazeera (2014) *Sierra Leone quarantines over one million*. 25 September. Available at: http://www.aljazeera.com/news/africa/2014/09/sierra-leone-quarantines-over-one-million-ebola-201492591852825986.html (Accessed 15 August 2017).

Johnson, G. et al. (2015) *Evaluating the impact of safe and dignified burials for stopping Ebola transmission in West Africa. Summary findings from the anthropological study in Sierra Leone*. Geneva: International Federation of the Red Cross and Red Crescent Societies.

Johnson, O. et al. (2016) Ebola holding units at government hospitals in Sierra Leone: Evidence for a flexible and effective model for safe isolation, early treatment initiation, hospital safety and health system functioning. *BMJ Global Health*. Available at: http://kslp.org.uk/students/research-projects/ (Accessed 6 August 2017).

Kabba, M. (2016) Sierra Leone news: Tonkolili Ebola saga . . . 9 released, 37 more to go with no positive case. *Awoko*, 2 February. Available at: http://awoko.org/2016/02/02/sierra-leone-news-tonkolili-ebola-saga-9-released-37-more-to-go-with-no-positive-caseby-mohamed-kabba/ (Accessed 6 August 2017).

Kaifala, J. (2017) *Free slaves, Freetown, and the Sierra Leonean civil war*. New York: Palgrave Macmillan.

Kamara, J. (2014) We can no longer ignore Ebola's wider impact – particularly on women. *The Guardian*, 14 October. Available at: https://www.theguardian.com/global-development/poverty-matters/2014/oct/14/ebola-women-sierra-leone (Accessed 6 August 2017).

Kamradt-Scott, A. et al. (2015) *Saving lives: The civil-military response to the 2014 Ebola outbreak in West Africa*. Sydney: University of Sydney.

Kargbo, M. S. (2006) *British foreign policy and the conflict in Sierra Leone, 1991–2001*. Bern: Peter Lang.

Kargbo, S. (2017) Too many health clinics hurt developing countries. *Project Syndicate*. Available at: https://www.project-syndicate.org/ commentary/health-clinics-hurting-poor-countries-by-samuel-kargbo-2017-05 (Accessed 6 August 2017).

Keen, D. (2005) *Conflict and collusion in Sierra Leone*. New York: Palgrave Macmillan.

Kieny, M. et al. (2014) *Health-system resilience: Reflections on the Ebola crisis in western Africa*. Geneva: Bulletin of the World Health Organization. Available at: http://www.who.int/bulletin/volumes/92/12/14-149278/en/ (Accessed 28 February 2018).

Koroma, E. B. (2014a) *Address to the nation on the Ebola outbreak by His Excellency the President Dr. Ernest Bai Koroma, July 30, 2014*. Freetown: Government of Sierra Leone. Available at: http://www.parliament.gov. sl/portals/0/2014%20document/ebola/outbreak%20address%20by%20 the%20president%2030%20july%202014.pdf (Accessed 28 February 2018).

Koroma, E. B. (2014b) *President Koroma's address to the nation on the Ebola disease*. Available at: http://www.sierra-leone.org/Speeches/ koroma-070114.html (Accessed 8 August 2017).

Kron, J. (2011) Somalia: Sierra Leone to send troops. *The New York Times*, 3 November. Available at: http://www.nytimes.com/2011/11/04/world/ africa/somalia-sierra-leone-to-send-troops.html (Accessed 6 August 2017).

Kucharski, A. J. et al. (2015) Measuring the impact of Ebola control measures in Sierra Leone. *Proceedings of the National Academy of Sciences*, 112(46), 14366–14371. Available at: http://www.pnas.org/content/112/46/14366 (Accessed 28 February 2018).

Kupferschmidt, K. (2014) WHO, CDC publish grim new Ebola projections. *Science*, 23 September. Available at: http://www.sciencemag.org/ news/2014/09/who-cdc-publish-grim-new-ebola-projections (Accessed 6 August 2017).

Lee, B. (2017). Bill Gates warns of epidemic that could kill over 30 million people. *Forbes*, 19 February. Available at: https://www.forbes.com/sites/ brucelee/2017/02/19/bill-gates-warns-of-epidemic-that-will-kill-over-30-million-people/ (Accessed 15 August 2017).

Liu, J. (2014) United Nations Special Briefing on Ebola. *Médecins sans Frontières*, 2 September. Available at: http://www.doctorswithoutborders. org/news-stories/speechopen-letter/united-nations-special-briefing-ebola (Accessed 13 August 2017).

J R Army Med Corps. (2016) Chinese military medical teams in the Ebola outbreak of Sierra Leone. *Journal of the Royal Army Medical Corps*, 162, 198–20Mankad, M. et al. (2015) *A wake-up call: Lessons from Ebola for the world's health systems*. Available at: http://www.savethechildren.org.uk/ sites/default/files/images/A-Wake-Up-Call.pdf (Accessed 6 August 2017).

Marah, K. (2014) Remarks at the high-level ministerial side event on peace and capable institutions as stand-alone goals in the post-2015 development agenda. *Awoko*, 1 October. Available at: http://awoko. org/2014/10/01/sierra-leone-news-remarks-by-dr-kaifala-marah/ (Accessed 15 August 2017).

Mazumdar, T. (2016) Is Sierra Leone ready for the next epidemic? *BBC News*, 8 August. Available at: http://www.bbc.com/news/world-africa-37007088 (Accessed 6 August 2017).

Médecins sans Frontières (2014a) *Ebola in West Africa: Epidemic requires massive deployment of resources*. Brussels: Médecins sans Frontières. Available at: http://www.msf.org/en/article/ebola-west-africa-epidemic-requires-massive-deployment-resources (Accessed 28 February 2018).

Médecins Sans Frontières (2014b) *Guinea: Mobilisation against an unprecedented Ebola epidemic*, 31 March. Available at: http://www.msf.org/en/article/guinea-mobilisation-against-unprecedented-ebola-epidemic (Accessed 6 August 2017).

Médecins Sans Frontières (2015) *Pushed to the limit and beyond*. Available at: http://www.msf.org.uk/sites/uk/files/ebola_-_pushed_to_the_limit_and_beyond.pdf.

Médecins Sans Frontières (2016) *OCB Ebola review: Summary report*. Stockholm: Stockholm Evaluation Unit. Available at: http://evaluation.msf.org/evaluation-report/ocb-ebola-review-2016 (Accessed 28 February 2018)

Meltzer, M. I. et al. (2014) Estimating the future number of cases in the Ebola epidemic – Liberia and Sierra Leone, 2014–2015. *Morbidity and Mortality Weekly Report (MMWR)*, 63(3), 1–14. Available at: https://www.cdc.gov/mmwr/preview/mmwrhtml/su6303a1.htm?s_cid=su6303a1_w (Accessed 6 August 2017).

Moon, S. et al. (2015) Will Ebola change the game? Ten essential reforms before the next pandemic. The report of the Harvard-LSHTM Independent Panel on the Global Response to Ebola. *The Lancet*, 386(10009), 2204–2221. Available at: http://dx.doi.org/10.*1016*/S0140-6736(15)00946-0 (Accessed 6 August 2017).

Moon, S. et al. (2017) *Post-Ebola reforms: Ample analysis, inadequate action*. 2801–8. Available at: http://dx.doi.org/doi:10.1136/bmj.j280.

Moyer, J. W. (2014) Ebola victim Thomas Eric Duncan's family has settled with Dallas hospital. *The Washington Post*, 12 November. Available at: https://www.washingtonpost.com/news/morning-mix/wp/2014/11/12/family-of-ebola-victim-thomas-eric-duncan-has-settled-with-dallas-hospital/?utm_term=.47c0672df229 (Accessed 6 August 2017).

Nardelli, A. (2015) How the UK civil service has changed in 10 charts. *The Guardian*, 19 November. Available at: https://www.theguardian.com/politics/2015/nov/19/how-the-uk-civil-service-has-changed-in-10-charts (Accessed 6 August 2017).

National Ebola Response Centre (2014) *Ebola Outbreak Updates, 24 November 2014*. Freetown: National Ebola Response Centre.

National Ebola Response Centre (2015) *Ebola outbreak updates, 1 and 7 February and 1 and 7 March 2015*. Freetown: National Ebola Response Centre.

Nebehay, S. and Lewis, B. (2011) WHO slashes budget, jobs in new era of austerity. *Reuters*, 19 May. Available at: https://www.reuters.com/article/us-who/who-slashes-budget-jobs-in-new-era-of-austerity-idUSTRE74I5I320110519 (Accessed 28 February 2018).

NERC (2015) *Annex to NERC Official Guidance, Western Area DERC Stay-at-Home Campaign 26 March, Version 3.0*. Freetown: National Ebola Response Centre.

NestBuilders International (2016) *Lessons learned: National and local responses to the Ebola outbreak in Sierra Leone: Research report and case studies of Koinadugu, Kono and Port Loko districts*. Freetown: Nestbuilders International.

Niang, C. I. (2015) *Ebola diaries: Lessons in listening*. Available at: http://www.who.int/features/2015/ebola-diaries-niang/en/ (Accessed 3 August 2017).

Nossiter, A. (2014a) A hospital from hell, in a city swamped by Ebola. *The New York Times*, 1 October. Available at: https://www.nytimes.com/2014/10/02/world/africa/ebola-spreading-in-west-africa.html?_r=0 (Accessed 6 August 2017).

Nossiter, A. (2014b) Ebola now preoccupies once-skeptical leader in Guinea. *The New York Times*, 30 November. Available at: https://www.nytimes.com/2014/12/01/world/africa/ebola-now-preoccupies-once-skeptical-leader-in-guinea.html (Accessed 6 August 2017).

Nossiter, A. (2014c) Officials admit a 'defeat' by Ebola in Sierra Leone. *The New York Times*, 10 October. Available at: https://www.nytimes.com/2014/10/11/world/africa/officials-admit-a-defeat-by-ebola-in-sierra-leone.html?_r=0 (Accessed 6 August 2017).

Nsenga, N. (2015) *Ebola diaries: Crossing the border, Ebola enters Sierra Leone*. Available at: http://www.who.int/features/2015/ebola-diaries-nsenga/en/ (Accessed 15 August 2017).

O'Dempsey, T. (2017) Failing Dr Khan, in *The Politics of Fear: Médecins sans Frontières and the West African Ebola Epidemic*. Oxford: Oxford University Press, pp. 175–186.

Panjabi, R. (2016) *Testimony of Dr. Raj Panjabi on behalf of Last Mile Health before the Senate Foreign Relations Subcommittee on Africa and Global Health Policy*. Available at: https://www.foreign.senate.gov/imo/media/doc/040716_Panjabi_Testimony.pdf (Accessed 28 February 2018).

PBS Frontline (2014) Ebola's patient zero, the child at the epidemic's start. *Frontline*. Available at: http://www.pbs.org/wgbh/frontline/article/

exclusive-video-where-the-ebola-outbreak-began/ (Accessed 2 August 2017).

Pollack, A. (2014) Opting against Ebola drug for ill African doctor. *The New York Times*, 12 August. Available at: https://www.nytimes.com/2014/08/13/world/africa/ebola.html (Accessed 6 August 2017).

Pronyk, P. et al. (2016) The effect of community-based prevention and care on Ebola transmission in Sierra Leone. *American Journal of Public Health*, 106(4), 727–732. Available at: https://www.ncbi.nlm.nih.gov/pmc/articles/PMC4816080/ (Accessed 28 February 2018).

Reaves, E. et al. (2014) Control of Ebola virus disease – Firestone District, Liberia, 2014. *Morbidity and mortality weekly report*, 63, 959–965. Available at: http://www.cdc.gov/mmwr/pdf/wk/mm6342.pdf (Accessed 6 August 2017).

Reno, W. (1995) *Corruption and state politics in Sierra Leone*. New York: Cambridge University Press.

Richards, P. (1996) *Fighting for the rainforest: War, youth and resources in Sierra Leone*. Suffolk: James Currey.

Richards, P. (2016) *Ebola: How a people's science helped end an epidemic*. London: Zed Books.

Richards, P. et al. (2014) Social pathways for Ebola virus disease in rural Sierra Leone, and some implications for containment. *PLOS Neglected Tropical Diseases*. Available at: http://journals.plos.org/plosntds/article?id=10.1371/journal.pntd.0003567 (Accessed 28 February 2018).

Risso-Gil, I. & Finnegan, L. (2015) *Children's Ebola Recovery Assessment Report (CERA): Sierra Leone*. Available at: http://www.savethechildren.org/atf/cf/%7B9def2ebe-10ae-432c-9bd0-df91d2eba74a%7D/EBOLA_REPORT_CHILDRENS_RECOVERY_ASSESSMENT_SIERRA_LEONE.PDF (Accessed 28 February 2018).

Roos, R. (2014) As Ebola outbreak grows, WHO notes case-count difficulties. *Center for Infectious Disease Research and Policy*, 22 August. Available at: http://www.cidrap.umn.edu/news-perspective/2014/08/ebola-outbreak-grows-who-notes-case-count-difficulties (Accessed 6 August 2017).

Ross, E. (2017) Command and control of Sierra Leone's Ebola outbreak response: Evolution of the response architecture. *Philosophical Transactions of the Royal Society B*. 372 (1721) Available at: http://rstb.royalsocietypublishing.org/content/372/1721/20160306.long (Accessed 28 February 2018).

Ross, E. et al. (2017) *Sierra Leone's response to the Ebola outbreak: Management strategies and key responder experiences*. London: Chatham House. Available at: https://www.chathamhouse.org/publication/sierra-leones-response-ebola-outbreak-management-strategies-key-responder (Accessed 28 February 2018).

Sack, K. et al. (2014) How Ebola roared back. *The New York Times*, 29 December. Available at: http://www.nytimes.com/2014/12/30/health/how-ebola-roared-back.html (Accessed 6 August 2017).

Schieffelin, J. S. et al. (2014) Clinical illness and outcomes in patients with Ebola in Sierra Leone. *New England Journal of Medicine*, 371(22), 2092–2100. Available at: http://www.nejm.org/doi/full/10.1056/NEJMoa1411680 (Accessed 28 February 2018).

Senga, M. et al. (2017) Contact tracing performance during the Ebola virus disease outbreak in Kenema district , Sierra Leone. *Philosophical Transactions of the Royal Society B.*, 372 (1721). Available at: http://rstb.royalsocietypublishing.org/content/372/1721/20160300.long (Accessed 28 February 2018).

Sierra Leone 2015 Population and Housing Census (2016) *Provisional Results*. Available at: https://www.statistics.sl/wp-content/uploads/2016/06/2015-Census-Provisional-Result.pdf (Accessed 6 August 2017).

Sierra Leone Ministry of Health and Sanitation (2014a) *Ebola Outbreak Update, 25 July 2014*. Freetown: Ministry of Health and Sanitation.

Sierra Leone Ministry of Health and Sanitation (2014b) *Ebola Update June 26, 2014*. Freetown: Ministry of Health and Sanitation.

Sierra Leone Ministry of Health and Sanitation (2014c) *Ebola Updates: 26 June, 4 and 11 and 25 July, 1 August*. Freetown: Ministry of Health and Sanitation.

Sierra Leone Ministry of Health and Sanitation (2016) *Human Resources for Health Strategy 2017–2021*. Freetown: Ministry of Health and Sanitation. Available at: http://www.afro.who.int/sites/default/files/2017-05/hrhstrategy2017.pdf (Accessed 28 February 2018).

Sierra Leone Truth and Reconciliation Commission (2004) *Witness to Truth*. Freetown: Sierra Leone Truth and Reconciliation Commission. Available at: http://www.sierraleonetrc.org/ (Accessed 28 February 2018).

Spencer, S. N. (2015) Invisible enemy: Translating Ebola prevention and control measures in Sierra Leone. Working papers of the priority programme 1448 of the German Research Foundation. Leipzig and Halle: DFG. Available at: https://lostresearchgroup.org/wpcontent/uploads/2017/05/SPP1448_WP13_Spencer_upd.pdf (Accessed 28 February 2018).

Sprecher, A. G. et al. (2015) Personal protective equipment for Filovirus epidemics: A call for better evidence. *The Journal of Infectious Diseases*, 212(S2), S98–S100.

Stockholm International Peace Research Institute (2016) *UN arms embargo on Liberia*. Available at: https://www.sipri.org/databases/embargoes/un_arms_embargoes/liberia (Accessed 2 August 2017).

Sun, L. et al. (2014) Out of control: How the world's health organizations failed to stop the Ebola disaster. *The Washington Post*, 4 October. Available at: http://www.washingtonpost.com/sf/national/2014/10/04/how-ebola-sped-out-of-control/?utm_term=.81279661b8e5 (Accessed 6 August 2017).

Tavernise, S. (2014) Head of World Bank makes Ebola his mission. *The New York Times*, 13 October. Available at: https://www.nytimes.com/2014/10/14/science/a-bank-chief-makes-ebola-his-mission.html (Accessed 6 August 2017).

The Demographic and Health Surveys Program (2013) *Sierra Leone: Standard demographic and health survey, 2013*. Available at: http://dhsprogram.com/what-we-do/survey/survey-display-450.cfm (Accessed 9 August 2017).

The World Bank (n.d.) *Data: Guinea* [online]. Available at: http://data.worldbank.org/country/guinea (Accessed 12 August 2017).

The World Bank (n.d.) *Data: Liberia* [online]. Available at: http://data.worldbank.org/country/liberia?view=chart (Accessed 12 August 2017).

The World Bank (n.d.) *Data: Sierra Leone* [online]. Available at: http://data.worldbank.org/country/sierra-leone (Accessed 2 August 2017).

The World Bank (n.d.) *Data: United Kingdom, physicians (per 1,000 people)* [online]. Available at: http://data.worldbank.org/indicator/SH.MED.PHYS.ZS?locations=GB (Accessed 26 February 2018)

The World Bank (n.d.) *Population living in slums* [online]. Available at: http://data.worldbank.org/indicator/EN.POP.SLUM.UR.ZS?locations=SL (Accessed 2 August 2017).

The World Bank (2012) *Project appraisal document on a proposed (loan/credit) in the amount of SDR 11 million (US $17 million equivalent) to the Republic of Sierra Leone for a pay and performance project*. Washington DC: The World Bank. Available at: http://documents.worldbank.org/curated/en/893711468336621509/text/674470PAD0P1280Official0Use0Only090.txt (Accessed 28 February 2018).

The World Bank (2017) *Pandemic emergency financing facility: Frequently asked questions*. Available at: http://www.worldbank.org/en/topic/pandemics/brief/pandemic-emergency-facility-frequently-asked-questions (Accessed 12 August 2017).

UNFPA (2014) *Double Ebola threat for pregnant women*. 27 October. Available at: http://pacific.unfpa.org/en/news/double-ebola-threat-pregnant-women?page=5%2C2 (Accessed 28 February 2018).

UNICEF (2016). *Ebola Community Care Centers: Lessons learned from UNICEF's 2014-2015 Experience in Sierra Leone*. Available at: https://www.unicef.org/health/files/CCCReport_FINAL_July2016.pdf (Accessed 15 August 2017).

UNICEF-Liberia (2014) *Ebola Virus Disease: SitRep #47, 15 August 2014*.

Available at: https://www.unicef.org/appeals/files/UNICEF_Liberia_ Ebola_Viral_Disease_SitRep47_15_August_2014.pdf (Accessed 6 August 2017).

UNICEF-Sierra Leone (2014) *Ebola Virus Disease weekly update 7 September, 15 and 29 October 2014*. Freetown: UNICEF.

United Nations Development Programme (n.d.) *About Sierra Leone*. Available at: http://www.sl.undp.org/content/sierraleone/en/home/ countryinfo.html (Accessed 2 August 2017).

United Nations Development Programme (2013a) *Explanatory note on 2013 HDR composite indices*. Available at: http://hdr.undp.org/sites/default/ files/Country-Profiles/SLE.pdf.

United Nations Development Programme (2013b) *Human Development Reports*. Available at: http://hdr.undp.org/en/content/ under-five-mortality-rate-1000-live-births.

United Nations Development Programme (2015) *Briefing note for countries on the 2015 Human Development Report: Sierra Leone*. New York: UNDP, p. 6. Available at: http://www.sl.undp.org/content/dam/ sierraleone/docs/HDRs/Sierra%20Leone%20Explanatory%20Note. pdf?download. (Accessed 26 February 2018).

United Nations Security Council (2014) *With spread of Ebola outpacing response, Security Council adopts Resolution 2177 (2014) urging immediate action, end to isolation of affected states*. 18 September. Available at: https://www.un.org/press/en/2014/sc11566.doc.htm (Accessed 6 August 2017).

UNMEER et al. (2015). *Sierra Leone: Ebola, situation report no. 22, 30 March – 12 April*. Freetown: UNMEER. Available at: https://reliefweb. int/report/sierra-leone/sierra-leone-ebola-emergency-situation-report- no-22-30-march-12-april (Accessed 28 February 2018).

Wauquier, N. et al. (2015) Understanding the emergence of Ebola Virus Disease in Sierra Leone: Stalking the virus in the threatening wake of emergence. *PLOS*. Available at: http://currents.plos.org/outbreaks/ article/understanding-the-emergence-of-ebola-virus-disease-in-sierra- leone-stalking-the-virus-in-the-threatening-wake-of-emergence/.

Whitty, C. J. et al. (2014) Infectious Disease: Tough choices to reduce Ebola transmission. *Nature*, 515 (7526), 192–194. Available at: http://www.nature.com/news/infectious-disease-tough-choices-to-reduce- ebola-transmission-1.16298.

Whitty, C. J. M. (2017) The contribution of biological, mathematical, clinical, engineering and social sciences to combatting the West African Ebola epidemic. *Philosophical Transactions of the Royal Society B*. 372 (1721). Available at: https://www.ncbi.nlm.nih.gov/pubmed/28396466 (Accessed 28 February 2018).

WHO Ebola Response Team (2014) Ebola Virus Disease in West Africa

– the first 9 months of the epidemic and forward projections. *The New England Journal of Medicine*, 371 (16), 1481–1495. Available at: http://www.nejm.org/doi/full/10.1056/NEJMoa1411100 (Accessed 28 February 2018).

Wolz, A. (2014) Face to face with Ebola – an emergency care center in Sierra Leone. *Perspective*. 371(12), 1081–1083. Available at: http://www.nejm.org/doi/full/10.1056/NEJMp1410179 (Accessed 28 February 2018).

World Health Organization (n.d.) *Ebola virus disease fact sheet*. Available at: http://www.who.int/mediacentre/factsheets/fs103/en/ (Accessed 3 August 2017).

World Health Organization (n.d.) *Partners: Global Outbreak Alert and Response Network (GOARN)*. Available at: http://www.who.int/csr/disease/ebola/partners/en/ (Accessed 8 August 2017).

World Health Organization (2006) *Constitution of the World Health Organization, forty-fifth edition*. Available at: http://www.who.int/governance/eb/who_constitution_en.pdf (Accessed 6 August 2017).

World Health Organization (2014a) *Ebola response roadmap situation report, 1 and 8 October and 31 December 2014*. Available at: http://apps.who.int/iris/bitstream/10665/136020/1/roadmapsitrep_8Oct2014_eng.pdf (Accessed 6 August 2017).

World Health Organization (2014b) *Ebola virus disease in Guinea*. Available at: http://www.who.int/csr/don/2014_03_23_ebola/en/ (Accessed 2 August 2017).

World Health Organization (2014c) *Ebola virus disease in Sierra Leone situation report 13 August 2014*. Freetown: WHO.

World Health Organization (2014d) *President Koroma visits the Emergency Operational Centre at the WHO complex*. Available at: http://www.afro.who.int/news/president-koroma-visits-emergency-operational-centre-who-complex (Accessed 12 August 2017).

World Health Organization (2014e) *Sierra Leone: A traditional healer and a funeral*. Available at: http://www.who.int/csr/disease/ebola/ebola-6-months/sierra-leone/en/ (Accessed 14 August 2017).

World Health Organization (2014f) *Sierra Leone: How Kailahun district kicked Ebola out*. Available at: http://www.who.int/features/2014/kailahun-beats-ebola/en/ (Accessed 9 August 2017).

World Health Organization (2014g) *Statement on the 1st meeting of the IHR Emergency Committee on the 2014 Ebola outbreak in West Africa*. Available at: http://www.who.int/mediacentre/news/statements/2014/ebola-20140808/en/ (Accessed 12 August 2017).

World Health Organization (2014h) *Weekly Partner Brief, 25 November, 2 and 16 December 2014*. Available at: http://www.who.int/csr/disease/ebola/situation-reports/archive/en/ (Accessed 28 February 2018).

World Health Organization (2015a) *Health worker Ebola infections in*

Guinea, Liberia and Sierra Leone – a preliminary report. Geneva: World Health Organization. Available at: http://www.who.int/hrh/documents/21may2015_web_final.pdf (Accessed 28 February 2018).

World Health Organization (2015b) *Liberia: A country – and its capital – are overwhelmed with Ebola cases,* January. Available at: http://www.who.int/csr/disease/ebola/one-year-report/liberia/en/ (Accessed 6 August 2017).

World Health Organization (2015c) *The Ebola outbreak in Liberia is over,* 9 May. Available at: http://www.who.int/mediacentre/news/statements/2015/liberia-ends-ebola/en/ (Accessed 15 August 2017).

World Health Organization (2016a) *Ebola data and statistics: Situation summary by sex and age group.* Available at: http://apps.who.int/gho/data/view.ebola-sitrep.ebola-summary-latest-age-sex (Accessed 3 August 2017).

World Health Organization (2016b) *Ebola situation report 3rd February 2016.* Available at: http://apps.who.int/ebola/current-situation/ebola-situation-report-3-february-2016 (Accessed 28 February 2018).

World Health Organization (2016c) *Interim Guidance: Clinical care for survivors of Ebola virus disease.* Available at: http://apps.who.int/iris/bitstream/10665/204235/1/WHO_EVD_OHE_PED_16.1_eng.pdf?ua=1 (Accessed 6 August 2017).

World Health Organization Global Task Force on Cholera Control (2013) *Cholera Country Profile: Sierra Leone.* Available at: http://www.who.int/cholera/countries/SierraLeoneCountryProfile2013.pdf (Accessed 28 February 2018).

Further reading

The list below consists of documents we read and that influenced us, despite them not being directly referenced in the text.

Ansumana, R. et al. (2014) Ebola in Freetown area, Sierra Leone – A case study of 581 patients. *The New England Journal of Medicine*, 372(6), 587–588. Available at: http://www.nejm.org/doi/full/10.1056/NEJMc1413685 (Accessed 28 February 2018).

Baize, S. et al. (2014) Emergence of Zaire Ebola virus disease in Guinea. *The New England Journal of Medicine*, 371(15), 1418–1425. Available at: http://www.nejm.org/doi/full/10.1056/NEJMoa1404505 (Accessed 28 February 2018).

Bausch, D. G. (2015) The year that Ebola virus took over West Africa: Missed opportunities for prevention. *The American Journal of Tropical Medicine and Hygiene*, 92(2), 229–232. Available at: https://www.ncbi.nlm.nih.gov/pmc/articles/PMC4347318/ (Accessed 28 February 2018).

Cheng, M. et al. (2015) AP Investigation: Bungling by UN agency hurt Ebola response. *Associated Press*, 21 September. Available at: https://apnews.com/3ba4599fdd754cd28b93a31b7345ca8b/ap-investigation-bungling-un-agency-hurt-ebola-response (Accessed 6 August 2017).

Coltart, C. E. M. et al. (2017) The 2013–2016 Ebola epidemic: Multidisciplinary success conceals a missed opportunity. *Philosophical Transactions of the Royal Society B.*, 372. (1721). Available at: https://www.ncbi.nlm.nih.gov/pmc/articles/PMC5394632/ (Accessed 28 February 2018).

Cormican, M. (n.d.) *Infection justice: Infectious disease control and human rights*. Unpublished paper.

Cormican, M. (2015) Concerns about cohorting of patients with suspected Ebola. *BMJ*, 350. Available at: http://www.bmj.com/content/350/bmj.h564.long (Accessed 28 February 2018).

D'Harcourt, E. (2015) Three myths about Ebola: The stories the west tells itself. *Foreign Affairs*, 8 January. Available at: http://www.foreignaffairs.com/articles/142762/emmanuel-dharcourt/three-myths-about-ebola (Accessed 6 August 2017).

Dhillon, R. S. & Kelly, J. D. (2015) Community trust and the Ebola endgame. *The New England Journal of Medicine*, 373(9), 787–789. Available at: http://www.nejm.org/doi/full/10.1056/NEJMp1508413 (Accesssed 28 February 2018).

Fink, S. (2015) Tracing the Ebola outbreak, scientists hunt a silent epidemic. *The New York Times*, 5 May. Available at: https://www.nytimes.com/2015/05/06/health/frontline-tracing-the-ebola-outbreak.html.

GOAL Sierra Leone (2014) *Support to Quarantined Homes*. Dublin: GOAL. Available at: https://www.humanitarianresponse.info/en/operations/sierra-leone/document/ebola-response-lessons-learned-series-support-quarantined-homes (Accesssed 28 February 2018).

Harris, J. (2015) Infections in the Sierra Leone healthcare workforce: Combined data from VHF, passive reporting, and active case-finding. Presentation at the NERC, Freetown, 6 January.

House of Commons International Development Committee (2016) *Ebola: Responses to a public health emergency*. London: House of Commons. Available at: https://www.parliament.uk/business/committees/committees-a-z/commons-select/international-development-committee/inquiries/parliament-2015/follow-up-to-the-responses-to-the-ebola-crisis/ (Accesssed 28 February 2018).

Kentikelenis, A. et al. (2014) The International Monetary Fund and the Ebola outbreak. *The Lancet Global Health*, 3(2), e69–e70. Available at: http://dx.doi.org/10.1016/S2214-109X(14)70377-8 (Accessed 6 August 2017).

Kutalek, R. et al. (2015) Ebola interventions: Listen to communities. *The Lancet Global Health*, 3(3). Available at: http://www.thelancet.com/pdfs/journals/langlo/PIIS2214-109X(15)70010-0.pdf (Accessed 28 February 2018).

Lokuge, K. et al. (2016) Successful control of Ebola virus disease: Analysis of service based data from rural Sierra Leone. *PLoS Neglected Tropical Diseases*, 10 (3). Available at: https://www.ncbi.nlm.nih.gov/pubmed/26959413 (Accessed 28 February 2018). .

Maxmen, A. (2015) Frontline health workers were sidelined in $3.3bn fight against Ebola. *Newsweek*, 19 May. Available at: http://pulitzercenter.org/reporting/sierra-leone-frontline-health-workers-were-sidelined-33bn-fight-against-ebola (Accessed 6 August 2017).

National Academy of Medicine (2016) *The neglected dimension of global security: A framework to counter infectious disease crises*. Washington DC: National Academies Press. Available at: https://www.ncbi.nlm.nih.gov/books/NBK368394/ (Accessed 28 February 2018).

Olu, O. O. et al. (2016) Incident management systems are essential for effective coordination of large disease outbreaks: Perspectives from the coordination of the Ebola outbreak response in Sierra Leone. *Frontiers in Public Health*, 4, 254. Available at: https://www.ncbi.nlm.nih.gov/pmc/articles/PMC5117105/ (Accessed 28 February 2018).

Piot, P. et al. (2017) Preface: The 2013 – 2016 West African Ebola epidemic: Data, decision-making and disease control. *Philosophical Transactions of the Royal Society B.*, 372 (1721). Available at: https://www.ncbi.nlm.nih.gov/pubmed/28396482 (Accessed 28 February 2018).

Sharma, A. et al. (2014) Evidence for a decrease in transmission of Ebola virus – Lofa County, Liberia. *Morbidity and Mortality Weekly Report*, 63 (46), 1067–1071.

de Waal, A. (2014) Militarizing global health. *Boston Review*. Available at: http://bostonreview.net/world/alex-de-waal-militarizing-global-health-ebola (Accessed 6 August 2017).

Wilkinson, A. et al. (2017) Engaging 'communities': Anthropological insights from the West African Ebola epidemic. *Philosophical Transactions of the Royal Society B.*, 372 (1721). Available at: https://www.ncbi.nlm.nih.gov/pmc/articles/PMC5394643/ (Accessed 28 February 2018).

Index

ZED

Zed is a platform for marginalised voices across the globe.

It is the world's largest publishing collective and a world leading example of alternative, non-hierarchical business practice.

It has no CEO, no MD and no bosses and is owned and managed by its workers who are all on equal pay.

It makes its content available in as many languages as possible.

It publishes content critical of oppressive power structures and regimes.

It publishes content that changes its readers' thinking.

It publishes content that other publishers won't and that the establishment finds threatening.

It has been subject to repeated acts of censorship by states and corporations.

It fights all forms of censorship.

It is financially and ideologically independent of any party, corporation, state or individual.

Its books are shared all over the world.

www.zedbooks.net
@ZedBooks